Nelson's
INSTRUCTIONS
FOR
PEDIATRIC PATIENTS

Nelson's
INSTRUCTIONS
FOR
PEDIATRIC PATIENTS

ALBERT J. POMERANZ, MD
Professor, Department of Pediatrics
Medical College of Wisconsin
Children's Hospital of Wisconsin
Milwaukee, Wisconsin

TIMOTHY O'BRIEN
Writer and Editor
Specializing in the Health Sciences
Chicago, Illinois

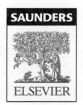

SAUNDERS

ELSEVIER

SAUNDERS
ELSEVIER

1600 John F. Kennedy Blvd.
Ste 1800
Philadelphia, PA 19103–2899

NELSON'S INSTRUCTIONS FOR PEDIATRIC PATIENTS   ISBN: 978-1-4160-0296-3

Notice

Library of Congress Cataloging-in-Publication Data

Pomeranz, Albert J.
  Nelson's instructions for pediatric patients / Albert J. Pomeranz, Timothy O'Brien.
    p. cm.
  ISBN-13: 978-1-4160-0296-3
    1. Pediatrics.   2. Patient education.   I. O'Brien, Timothy.   II.Title.
RJ26.3.P66 2007
616.8—dc22   2006050642

Publishing Director: Judith Fletcher
Developmental Editor: Melissa Dudlick
Project Manager: Mary B. Stermel
Design Direction: Steve Stave
Marketing Manager: Todd Liebel
Multimedia Manager: Paul Coker

Printed in the United States of America

Last digit is the print number: 9   8   7   6   5   4   3   2   1

To Emily and Kate and to our children's children
                                        —A.P.

To Lisa and Maggie
                    —T.O'B.

Preface

Nelson's Instructions for Pediatric Patients was written for physicians and other health care providers as a tool to help parents understand the most common medical problems and psychosocial issues that their children may face. Depending on the issues discussed, we have included instructions on caring for the child and on when to contact a provider for specific signs or symptoms.

We have spent considerable time and effort to ensure a broad view of physicians' approaches to and treatment for the conditions discussed. The information presented is the most up-to-date available, based on an extensive review of the research and literature.

For many conditions, we have provided trustworthy resources for additional information that parents can access via the Internet or telephone. Although Internet addresses and phone numbers were accurate at press time, some of this information may change.

We think we have succeeded in producing a text that covers a host of issues affecting the health of children, and presents the information in a way that will be very easy for parents to read and understand. Most important, we hope this work adds to the health and well-being of all children and their families.

Albert J. Pomeranz
Timothy O'Brien

x ■ Contents

Lead Poisoning **141**

Nosebleeds **143**

Poisoning **145**

Seizures Without Fever (Nonfebrile Seizures) **147**

Skin Wounds (Lacerations, Punctures, and Abrasions) **149**

Section X ■ Endocrine Disorders **151**

Breast Enlargement in Boys (Gynecomastia) **153**

Breast Enlargement in Infants (Premature Thelarche) **155**

Diabetes Mellitus, Type 1 **157**

Diabetes Mellitus, Type 2 **160**

Puberty: Normal, Early, and Late Development **162**

Short Stature (Below Normal Height) **164**

Thyroid Disorders (Hypothyroidism, Hyperthyroidism) **166**

Section XI ■ The Eye **169**

Blocked Tear Duct **171**

Conjunctivitis (Pinkeye) **172**

Corneal Abrasions **173**

Glaucoma **175**

Strabismus **177**

Stye (Hordeolum) **179**

Section XII ■ Gastrointestinal **181**

Anal Fissure **183**

Celiac Disease (Sprue) **185**

Colic **187**

Constipation **189**

Gastroesophageal Reflux Disease **191**

Hirschsprung's Disease **193**

Inflammatory Bowel Disease **195**

Inguinal Hernia **197**

Intestinal Obstruction **199**

Irritable Bowel Syndrome **201**

Pancreatitis **203**

Peptic Ulcer Disease **205**

Pyloric Stenosis **207**

Section XIII ■ Genetics **209**

Down Syndrome (Trisomy 21) **211**

Fragile X Syndrome **213**

Genetic Counseling **215**

Klinefelter's Syndrome **217**

Marfan's Syndrome **219**

Turner's Syndrome **221**

Section XIV ■ Genitalia **223**

Epididymitis **225**

Foreskin Problems **227**

Hydrocele **229**

Hypospadias **231**

Testicular Torsion **233**

Undescended Testicles **235**

Varicocele **237**

Section XV ■ The Heart **239**

Arrhythmias and Palpitations **241**

Heart Murmurs (Innocent Murmurs) **243**

High Blood Pressure (Hypertension) **244**

Kawasaki Disease **246**

Rheumatic Fever and Rheumatic Heart Disease **248**

Section XVI ■ Infections **251**

Acute Diarrhea (Gastroenteritis) **253**

Bacterial Vaginosis **255**

Bronchiolitis **256**

Cat-Scratch Disease **258**

Chickenpox (Varicella) **260**

Chronic Diarrhea **262**

Cold Sores (Herpes Simplex) **264**

Colds **266**

Croup **268**

Fifth Disease **270**

Food Poisoning **272**

German Measles (Rubella) **274**

Hand-Foot-and-Mouth Disease and Related Infections **275**

Hepatitis (Hepatitis A, B, or C Virus) **277**

HIV/AIDS **279**

Impetigo **281**

Influenza **282**

Laryngitis **284**

Lyme Disease **285**

Measles (Rubeola) **287**

Meningitis—Viral and Bacterial **289**

Mononucleosis (Infectious Mononucleosis) **291**

Mumps **293**

Pertussis (Whooping Cough) **294**

Contents

Section I ▪ Health Maintenance and Preventive Health Issues 1

Adoption 3
Child Passenger Safety 5
Childproofing Your Home 7
Day-Care Guide 9
Discipline—The Basics 11
Fever Management 13
Habits: Thumb Sucking, Nail Biting, Etc. 14
Immunizations (Vaccinations) 16
Sleep Problems and Bedtime Issues 18
Smoking: Risks and How to Quit 20
Talking to Your Teen about Sex 22
Toilet Training 25

Section II ▪ Allergy 27

Anaphylaxis 29
Asthma 31
Bee Stings and Other Insect Stings 33
Food Allergies 35
Hay Fever (Allergic Rhinitis) 37
Hives 39

Section III ▪ Behavior—Psychology 41

Adjustment Disorder 43
Anxiety 45
Attention Deficit–Hyperactivity Disorder (ADHD) 47
Bipolar Disorder 49
Bullying 51
Conduct Disorder 53
Depression 55
Divorce 57
Drugs and Alcohol: Use and Abuse 59
Eating Disorders 61
Nightmares and Night Terrors 63
Obsessive-Compulsive Disorder 65
Panic Attacks and Panic Disorder 67
Phobias 69
Suicide 71
Temper Tantrums 73

Section IV ▪ Blood Disorders 75

Blood Clots (Thrombotic Disorders) 77
Enlarged Lymph Nodes 79
Iron-Deficiency Anemia 80
Sickle Cell Disease and Sickle Cell Trait 82

Section V ▪ Cancer 85

Hodgkin's Disease 87
Leukemia 89

Section VI ▪ Dental 91

Dental Trauma 93
Preventive Antibiotics for Children with Heart Disease 94
Tooth Decay and Dental Care 96

Section VII ▪ Development 99

Autism 101
Fetal Alcohol Syndrome 103
Learning Disabilities 105
Stuttering 107

Section VIII ▪ The Ear 109

Earwax Problems 111
Middle Ear Infection (Acute Otitis Media) 112
Otitis Media with Effusion 114
Outer Ear Infection (Swimmer's Ear) 116

Section IX ▪ Emergency 119

Acute Appendicitis 121
Animal and Human Bites 123
Carbon Monoxide Poisoning 125
Dehydration 127
Fainting (Syncope) 129
Febrile Seizures (Seizure with Fever) 131
Foreign Bodies (Swallowed Objects) 133
Frostbite 135
Head Trauma (Minor) 137
Heat-Related Illnesses 139

Pinworm Infection **296**

Pneumonia **297**

Rabies **299**

Sexually Transmitted Diseases (STDs) **301**

Shingles (Herpes Zoster) **303**

Sinusitis **304**

Skin Abscesses **306**

Skin Infection (Cellulitis) **307**

Sore Throat **309**

Strep Throat and Scarlet Fever **311**

Tetanus (Lockjaw) **313**

Transient Synovitis of the Hip **315**

Tuberculosis **316**

Vulvovaginitis (Infection of the Vagina) **318**

West Nile Virus Infection **320**

Yeast Infections (*Candida* Vaginitis) **322**

Section XVII ■ Kidney and Urinary Tract **325**

Bed-Wetting (Nocturnal Enuresis) **327**

Glomerulonephritis **329**

Hemolytic-Uremic Syndrome **331**

Henoch-Schönlein Purpura **333**

Kidney Stones (Urolithiasis) **335**

Posterior Urethral Valves **337**

Urinary Tract Infections **339**

Vesicoureteral Reflux **341**

Section XVIII ■ Musculoskeletal—Orthopedic **343**

Bowlegs and Knock-Knees **345**

Flatfoot (Pes Planus) **346**

Fractures **347**

Ganglion Cyst **349**

Growing Pains **350**

Legg-Calvé-Perthes Disease **351**

Nursemaid's Elbow (Pulled Elbow) **353**

Osgood-Schlatter Disease **354**

Patellofemoral Pain Syndrome **355**

Scoliosis **356**

Slipped Capital Femoral Epiphysis (SCFE) **358**

Sprains and Strains **360**

Tendinitis and Tennis Elbow **362**

Torticollis **363**

Section XIX ■ Nervous System **365**

Bell's Palsy **367**

Cerebral Palsy **368**

Guillain-Barré Syndrome **370**

Headaches (Tension and Migraine Types) **372**

Hydrocephalus **374**

Muscular Dystrophy **376**

Tics and Tourette's Syndrome **378**

Section XX ■ Newborn **381**

Ambiguous Genitalia and Intersex Conditions **383**

Apnea of the Newborn (Interrupted Breathing) **385**

Baby's First Weeks—Newborn Care **387**

Circumcision **389**

Cleft Lip and Cleft Palate **391**

Clubfoot (Talipes Equinovarus) **393**

Collarbone Fractures in Newborns **395**

Common Newborn Rashes **396**

Congenital Diaphragmatic Hernia **397**

Cradle Cap (Seborrheic Dermatitis of Newborns) **399**

Developmental Dysplasia of the Hip **400**

Diaper Rash **402**

Feeding Your Newborn: Breast Feeding and Bottle Feeding **404**

Group B Streptococcal Infection **406**

Human Immunodeficiency Virus and Your Newborn **408**

Infants of Diabetic Mothers **410**

Jaundice of the Newborn **412**

Meconium-Stained Amniotic Fluid **413**

Myelomeningocele **415**

Natal and Neonatal Teeth **417**

Newborn Screening **418**

Prematurity and Low Birth Weight **420**

Respiratory Distress Syndrome in Newborns (Hyaline Membrane Disease) **422**

Sacral Dimple (Pilonidal Dimple) **424**

Spitting Up (Gastroesophageal Reflux) **425**

Swollen Scalp (Caput Succedaneum and Cephalohematoma) **427**

Thrush **429**

Umbilical Cord Care **430**

Section XXI ■ Nutrition **433**

Healthy Diet **435**

High Cholesterol **437**

Obesity **439**

Section XXII ■ Respiratory 441

Cystic Fibrosis 443
Laryngomalacia 446
Obstructive Sleep Apnea 448
Peritonsillar and Retropharyngeal Abscesses 450
Sudden Infant Death Syndrome 452
Vocal Cord Nodules (Screamer's Nodes) 454

Section XXIII ■ Skin and Nails 457

Acne 459
Athlete's Foot (Tinea Pedis) 461
Eczema 462
Fungal Infections of the Nails (Onychomycosis, Tinea Unguium) 464
Head Lice (Pediculosis Capitis) 465

Heat Rash (Milaria Rubra) 467
Ingrown Toenails 468
Jock Itch (Tinea Cruris) 469
Minor Burns 470
Pityriasis Rosea 472
Poison Ivy 473
Psoriasis 475
Ringworm (Tinea Corporis) 477
Ringworm of the Scalp (Tinea Capitis) 478
Scabies 480
Sunburn 482
Tinea Versicolor 484
Warts 485

Index of Topics 487

Section I ▪ Health Maintenance and Preventive Health Issues

Adoption

Most adopted children thrive in their new family. Your pediatrician can offer helpful advice if your family is considering adoption or has adopted a child. It is important that you talk to your child about being adopted as soon as he or she is old enough to understand. Children adopted from other countries and from foster care may have special health needs.

What is adoption?

Adoption is the process of providing a new family for a child whose birth family cannot or will not care for the child. Adoption is not only a legal process, but also a social and emotional process. For the most part, adopted children share the same bonds with their parents as birth children do.

Most adopted children and families adjust well and lead healthy, productive lives. It is normal for adopted children to wonder about their birth family—open communication is important. Children should be told they are adopted as soon as they are old enough to understand—usually in the toddler years.

In the United States, a growing number of children are being adopted from other countries or from foster care. These children may have special health and developmental needs and should be screened for health problems soon after adoption. Your pediatrician's office can answer questions and provide useful information if you are considering adoption or are raising an adopted child.

Some important facts on adoption

- Adoption is common. There are approximately 1 million adopted children in the United States—2% to 4% of American children are adopted.

- Today, an increased number of adoptions take place through public agencies or international adoptions. In the past, most adoptions either went through private adoption agencies or were family adoptions (children adopted by relatives or stepparents).

- More older children are being adopted, as opposed to newborns. Brothers and sisters may be adopted together. Many families are adopting children with special medical, developmental, or educational needs.

- The Internet has had a major impact on the adoption process, including putting families in touch with adoption resources and children who need families. The Internet has been especially important in driving the trend toward increased international adoption. Unfortunately, it has also led to an increase in unethical practices related to adoption.

Do adopted children have any special medical concerns?

The pediatrician's office can play an important role in assessing the health of your adopted child. Most adopted children are perfectly healthy, both physically and developmentally. Their medical care is no different from that of other children.

Depending on the birth mother's health and the circumstances of her pregnancy, some adopted children may have preexisting medical or developmental issues. This is especially likely for children adopted from foster care or from other countries. (Of course, many families knowingly adopt children with special medical needs.)

Your child should have a thorough medical evaluation as soon as he or she joins your family. Some parents who have identified a child they hope to adopt will have a doctor look over the child's medical records before adoption. This helps prepare for any special medical needs the child may have. Important information includes possible alcohol or drug abuse by the mother during pregnancy, diabetes during pregnancy, any complications during delivery, and, if available, family history of genetic (inherited) disorders. Information on the biological father's medical history may be helpful as well.

Children adopted from other countries—especially from developing countries—may need to be screened for certain health problems, including hepatitis B and C, tuberculosis, parasites, and syphilis. They may also need repeated or new vaccinations.

How do adopted children and their new families adjust to each other?

In general, families and adopted children adjust well. Older children, children adopted from foster care, and other special cases may need more time to adjust. Responsible adoption agencies will usually assess your family's ability to handle the child and help integrate him or her into your family before finalizing the adoption.

What should I tell my child about being adopted?

The truth! Children should be told they are adopted as soon as they are old enough to understand.

- If the child is of a different race than the parents, the child will notice this difference at a young age—in fact, you may want to start talking about adoption sometime after age 2 or 3. Otherwise, discussions about being adopted should take place sometime after age 5 or 6. Certainly by the teen years, children should know the truth about their adoption.

- The information should be repeated, at a level your child can understand as he or she grows and develops. It is completely normal for adopted children to wonder about their birth parents, about why they were placed for adoption, and other questions regarding their history. They may even imagine that their birth parents "gave them up" because of something they did wrong.

- Parents should be aware of their own feelings related to being adoptive parents. For example, it is normal for toddlers to "push away" from their parents, as a sign of becoming more independent. Adoptive parents shouldn't interpret this as rejection any more than birth parents would.

- Other issues will come up as your child grows and develops. It's sometimes hard to tell how much these problems are related to being adopted, rather than just the normal stress and strain of growing up. Adoption issues may be a focus of attention during adolescence, especially as teens "try on" new identities. Some of these identities may resemble your child's birth parents—or how he or she imagines them to be.

By the teen years, your child should know the whole story about his or her adoption. Be truthful, even if the truth is difficult to tell and hear. Some children have had traumatic experiences before they were adopted, especially if they were adopted at an older age. In these situations, counseling may be helpful for your child and family.

Are there any special issues related to cross-cultural adoptions?

Especially with the rise in international adoptions, many families have adopted children of other racial or ethnic backgrounds. The racial difference may be obvious, even to young children.

Many parents of international adoptees look for ways of letting their child remain in touch with his or her racial/ethnic identity—for example, through language, cultural and religious activities.

Parents may hear some insensitive comments regarding the racial differences. As they get older, the children may be the targets of racial prejudice. Be prepared to discuss these issues with your child, including strategies for handling rude or racist comments.

Adoptions by gay or same-sex couples are increasingly common and accepted. Studies suggest that these children have no more social or emotional problems than other children.

When should I call your office?

Call our office if:

- You are considering adopting a child and have questions about mental or physical health issues.

- You have just brought your adopted child home. An initial medical examination and screening is especially important for children adopted from foster care or from other countries.

- You need advice on helping your family and child adjust to their new situation. Talking to a mental health professional or counselor may be helpful.

- You have questions about your child's health and development (whether he or she is adopted or not!).

Where can I get more information about adoption?

Our office may be able to put you in touch with adoption resources and support in the community.

The U.S. Department of Health and Human Services provides a wealth of adoption-related information and resources. Online at *www.childwelfare.gov/adoption*.

Child Passenger Safety

> Motor vehicle injuries are the leading cause of serious and fatal injuries in all age groups, including children. Precautions are needed to keep your child as safe as possible when riding in a car. Infants should ride in a backward-facing car seat until they are at least 1 year old and weigh 20 pounds. Until age 4, your child should ride in a forward-facing car seat or toddler seat. The back seat is the safest place to ride for all children. Seatbelts should always be worn.

How can I keep my child safe in the car?

The most important thing you can do to reduce your child's risk of serious injury and death is to provide proper child seat restraints. Using recommended car seats, booster seats, and seatbelts greatly reduces your child's risk of being injured or killed in an accident.

Recommendations are based on your child's age, height, and weight. You must have an appropriate, backward-facing car seat before you drive your newborn home from the hospital. *All child car seats belong in the back seat, never the front seat!*

After outgrowing car seats, your child should ride in a booster seat until he or she is tall enough to wear lap and shoulder belts. Seatbelts greatly reduce the risk of serious injury or death for adults as well as children. The driver and all passengers should "buckle up" every time they ride in their vehicle.

What kind of car seat do I need for my infant?

Infants who are less than 1 year old and weigh less than 20 pounds (9 kilograms) should ride in a backward-facing car seat. Some models are "infant-only" seats; these are smaller and more portable, among other advantages. Others are "convertible" seats, which you may be able to continue using until your baby is bigger.

Infant and child car seats must always be placed in the back seat, never in the front seat! If you're in an accident and the car's air bags deploy, they can cause serious or even fatal injuries to the baby if he or she is in the front seat. The back seat is the safest place for all children.

- Follow the manufacturer's instructions carefully to be sure that you are installing the car seat properly. It can be a little difficult to figure out at first! Many local police departments offer safety checks to be sure car seats are correctly placed.

- Make sure the seatbelts are securely fastened to hold the car seat in place. Make sure your baby is buckled into the seat. Remember to check and adjust the straps as your baby grows.

Infants older than 1 year and who weigh more than 20 pounds can ride in a forward-facing car seat. Convertible infant seats can be turned to face forward, or you can obtain a special toddler seat. It's best to keep your baby "rear-facing" as long as he or she fits in the car seat.

- Again, make sure to follow the manufacturer's instructions for installation. With convertible seats, make sure you use the proper "forward-facing" slots.

Your baby or toddler must be properly secured in his or her car seat every time you drive. While driving, don't turn around to attend to your child. If necessary, pull off the road and park the car in a safe place before checking on your infant.

What kind of safety equipment do I need for my older child?

In general, children should ride in a car seat as long as possible before moving to a *booster seat*—usually when they reach about 40 pounds (18 kilograms). The maximum height and weight may be listed by the manufacturer. "Shield" booster seats are not recommended because of safety concerns.

The booster seat raises your child up a few inches, allowing the lap and shoulder belts to fit properly around his or her body. The lap belt should lie across your child's thighs and the shoulder belt across the chest.

When can my child use a regular seatbelt?

In general, children no longer need a booster seat when they are about 8 years old and 4 feet, 9 inches (145 centimeters) tall. However, your child should stay in the booster seat until the seatbelts (lap and shoulder belt) fit correctly. Your child should be able to sit back with his or her legs over the seat. Make sure the shoulder belt is not over your child's neck.

Children who are under 13 years old and less than 4 feet, 9 inches tall should ride in the back seat. In general, the back seat is the safest place to ride (for adults as well as children). Also, in a crash, front seat air bags may cause injury to child passengers (and small adults).

When should I call your office?

Talk to the doctor if you have any questions about child passenger safety. We may be able to put you in touch with helpful community resources (for example, safety checks, low-income assistance).

Where can I get more information?

- The National Highway Traffic Safety Administration has a list of locations providing free child safety seat inspections. On the Internet at *www.seatcheck.org*, or call 1-866-SEATCHECK (1-866-732-8243).

- The American Academy of Pediatrics offers a Car Seat Guide on the Internet at *www.aap.org/family/carseatguide. htm*.

Childproofing Your Home

After the first few months, injuries are the leading cause of death in infants and children. Many serious injuries happen at home. Some simple steps can greatly reduce the risk of injuries to your baby or toddler, including poisoning, burns, falls, and drowning. The most important step is to make sure your infant or toddler is appropriately supervised at all times.

What is childproofing?

Babies and toddlers are naturally curious. They love to explore their world, especially as they become able to crawl and climb. It's important to be aware of the possible hazards in your home and to remove or eliminate as many of these dangers as you can. Childproofing means going through each room, removing dangerous objects, and taking the simple steps needed to reduce the risk of injury.

How can I childproof my home?

- *Prevent poisoning.* All medicines, household cleaners, chemicals, laundry products, and other poisonous substances should be placed out of reach. Place these items up high, preferably where children can't even see them.
  - Buy medicines in child-resistant packages. Avoid putting medicines or poisons into other containers that are not child-resistant or could be confused for something to eat or drink. Use safety latches or locks for further protection.
- *Put safety latches or locks on cabinets and drawers.* Simple, inexpensive devices can keep babies and toddlers from opening cabinets and drawers. Safety latches are designed to be easily opened by adults but not by babies and tots. Put latches on cabinets in the bathroom, kitchen, basement, garage—any room your child can get into.
- *Prevent fire and burns.* Make sure smoke detectors are installed in your home. Check batteries regularly.
  - Keep hot objects out of reach, for example, pots and pans on the stovetop. Don't leave the stove burners on. Don't use cooking utensils, curling irons, or other appliances with long electrical cords; children can pull these items down.
  - Use approved flame-retardant children's sleepwear.
- *Cover electrical outlets.* Simple devices are available to prevent children from putting their fingers or small objects into electrical outlets.
- *Keep toys and other small objects out of reach.* For babies and toddlers under age 3, remove all objects small enough to be swallowed (for example, small toys, coins, watch batteries).
- *Install safety gates.* Install safety gates to keep your child from entering unsafe areas, especially staircases.
- *Avoid walkers.* They don't improve walking skills but do increase the risk of injuries by letting toddlers get into places they shouldn't (for example, near stairways and hot stoves).
- *Prevent bath hazards.* Many serious injuries to babies and toddlers occur at bath time. Prevent burns by making sure the bath water is not too hot. If possible, set the temperature of your water heater to around 120°F (49°C). Another option is to install antiscald devices on your sink and bath. Always test water temperature before placing your baby in the bath.
  - *Never leave your baby or toddler alone in the bath, even for a minute!* Drowning can occur in the time it takes to answer a phone call. Cordless phones are a good option for homes with infants or young children.
  - Swimming pools are another drowning hazard. Just like in the bath, don't leave your child alone in or near a pool. For home pools, lock doors to make sure your child can't enter the pool area alone.
- *Secure windows and doors.* Simple devices are available to keep windows from opening wide enough to allow children to fall out. Other types of window guards or safety nets may be installed as well. Young children may be strangled by the cords on window blinds. Cut the cords or install special safety devices. Lock doors or install doorknob covers to keep your child from getting into unsafe areas.
- *Keep your child safe in the car.* Use a car seat or booster seat appropriate for your child's age. Talk to your doctor if you have any questions about child passenger safety.
  - Never leave your child alone in the car. On warm days, the inside of a car can become dangerously hot within minutes.

Are there any other steps I can take?

- Recheck your home every few months to make sure it is safe. This is especially important as your child reaches new milestones, for example, crawling or climbing.
- When your child is old enough to understand, teach him or her about safety precautions.
- As your child grows, emphasize important safety messages about playing with matches, watching out for cars, and so forth.

Where can I get more information?

The U.S. Consumer Product Safety Commission provides information on product safety, including recalls of defective products on the Internet at *www.cpsc.gov* or *www.recalls.gov*.

Day-Care Guide

There are a lot of factors to think about when choosing a day-care provider for your child. There are several options for day care, each with advantages and disadvantages. For most families, the decision depends on factors such as cost, distance from home, and safety. This chapter reviews some of the important questions to ask when evaluating day-care options.

What is day care?

Many families rely on day care to look after their children during the day or after school so that they can work. Children of all ages may spend at least part of their day in child care. Day care may be provided in several settings, such as private homes or child-care centers. Most larger child-care centers are licensed by the states.

Choosing a day-care center is a big decision. Some important questions to ask include how many children are cared for in the center, how many caregivers are present, what the caregivers' experience is, and whether the day-care provider is accredited. Standards and guidelines vary by state.

Once you have chosen a day-care provider, it's important to pay attention to how your child is doing there and to stay involved with your child's caregivers. The best type of day care for your child may change as he or she grows.

What types of day-care options are there?

Although local options vary, day-care settings fall into some general categories:

- *Family-home day care.* Many caregivers provide day-care services in their homes. It's important to make sure there are enough adults to care for the number of children present. If toddlers are present, there needs to be more supervision. Make sure that the home has been "childproofed."

- *Day-care centers.* Other facilities provide care for larger numbers of children. Some day-care centers are private businesses, independent or part of a chain. Others are sponsored by the government, a church or a religious organization, or an employer. Each state has its own licensing regulations.

- *In-home day care.* Some families hire a nanny or regular babysitter to watch children in their own home. This is usually the most expensive option.

Other types of day-care situations include:

- "Drop-in" facilities, which generally provide only occasional care.

- Various types of facilities that provide after-school care.

- Other types of facilities for children with medical problems or other special needs.

How do I choose a day-care provider?

Start early. Day care can be hard to find in some communities, and high-quality day care may be even harder to find. Some important questions to ask are:

- *How many children are present?* Especially for babies and toddlers, smaller groups of children are better. Larger groups may increase the risk of catching infections and other diseases.

- *How many caregivers are present?* Recommended numbers of staff members per child often vary according to the children's age:

  - Birth to 12 months: At least one staff member for every three infants.

  - Ages 13 to 30 months: At least one staff member for every four children.

  - Ages 31 to 35 months: At least one staff member for every five children.

  - Age 3 years: At least one staff member for every seven children.

  - Ages 4 to 5 years: At least one staff member for every eight children.

  - Ages 6 to 8 years: At least one staff member for every ten children.

  - Ages 9 to 12 years: At least one staff member for every twelve children.

- *Are the caregivers qualified?* Do they have experience and/or training in the care and education of children?

- *Is the facility licensed,* if required by state regulations? Is it accredited by national organizations, such as the National Association for the Education of Young Children (NAEYC) or the National Association for Family Child Care (NAFCC)?

- *What is the facility like?* Make visits to the centers. Does the facility look safe, clean, and well-maintained? How are the children behaving? Do the setting and activities look appropriate and inviting for your children? Ask the caregiver to give you the names of other parents as references.

- *How is your child doing?* After your child starts day care, pay attention to how your child seems to be doing. Does he or she seem well cared for at pickup time? Have there been any types of changes in his or her behavior since starting day care? Especially if it's your child's first

9

experience with day care, he or she may be a little anxious at first. Normally, children get used to the change within a few days.

Stay involved with your child's day-care center or provider. Talk to and meet with caregivers on a regular basis. Ask questions and voice any concerns you may have.

When should I call your office?

Call our office if you have questions or concerns about day care or need advice about choosing a day-care provider.

Where can I get more information?

A good place to start is the National Resource Center for Health and Safety in Child Care and Early Education. Visit its new "Healthy Kids, Healthy Care" website at *www.healthykids.us*, or call 1-800-598-KIDS (1-800-598-5437). The website offers lots of useful information, including a parents' guide, state licensing regulations, and more.

Discipline—The Basics

Effective discipline is based on a positive, supportive relationship between parents and children. Strategies based on praising and rewarding desired behaviors and removing privileges are generally better than strategies based on punishment. For young children, "time-outs" are a useful strategy. Most pediatricians don't recommend spanking because other approaches seem to work better.

How should I discipline my children?

There's no "right" way to discipline children; every family must find an approach that works for them. However, some key concepts can help you develop an effective approach to teaching children proper behavior.

The approach to discipline should be consistent for all children in your family, with limits set and enforced for all. Both parents, as well as other care providers, should be consistent in disciplining children.

It's important to consider your child's developmental level in setting expectations and responding to behavior problems. For example, it would be normal for a one-year-old to play with the family stereo, possibly causing damage. An appropriate response would be to distract the child and put the stereo out of reach.

The family atmosphere should be a safe, loving, and supportive one for your child. It is also very important for parents to be good role models. Show the kind of behavior you would like your child to follow—children learn from their parents!

What are the principles of discipline?

"Positive reinforcement" means praising and rewarding desired behaviors. This is more effective than "negative reinforcement"—yelling or punishment for undesired behaviors.

When punishment is necessary, "time-outs" are a good tool to use with young children. By age 5, children are old enough to understand the consequences of their behavior. Strategies based on removing privileges are recommended for this age group.

- *Time-outs.* For toddlers and preschoolers, the idea behind time-outs is to remove the child from playtime or other desired activities as a direct consequence of undesired behavior.

  - Tell your child you are giving him or her a time-out. During the time-out, your child must sit by himself or herself away from play or other activities.

  - Especially for toddlers, the time-out should happen immediately after the undesired behavior. Two-year-olds can't make the connection between misbehaving earlier in the day and the time-out they are getting later.

  - Time-outs shouldn't last too long: 1 minute per year of age is a good guideline. Stay calm and don't argue or bargain with your child.

  - Time-outs only work when they are used consistently. If you are just starting to use time-outs, at first your toddler may respond by having a tantrum. *When tantrums happen, ignore them if possible, and remove the child from the situation if necessary.* Don't give in to tantrums, or you will reinforce that behavior. Your child will learn that he will get what he wants eventually. Parents who stick with it usually find time-outs effective in reducing undesired behaviors.

- *Removing privileges.* After age 4 or 5, children are old enough to understand why they are being disciplined.

  - Taking away some privilege or activity that your child really wants provides consequences for misbehavior. For younger children, this may mean taking away TV or video game privileges. Older children may be "grounded" (not allowed to go out with friends). Teens may have their driving privileges taken away.

  - Be clear, direct, and consistent each time the undesired behavior occurs. Be calm when discussing the misbehavior with your child. If you can't stay calm, it may be best to discuss the problem later.

What discipline strategies are less effective?

- *Negative verbal statements.* If used infrequently, negative verbal statements can be helpful in pointing out misbehavior. However, if used often, negative comments and criticisms become less effective; they can actually be a way of giving the child attention. Negative statements should refer to the behavior ("What you did was wrong because..."), not the child's character ("You're a bad boy.").

- *Spanking.* Although spanking is not necessarily bad, most pediatricians think other strategies are more effective. Parents who were spanked while growing up are more likely to spank their own children.

  - Spanking is defined as hitting a child with an open hand on the buttocks, arm, or leg without causing physical harm. Even when used correctly, spanking is not as effective as the other methods discussed.

  - Any other type of physical punishment is *not* spanking. This includes hitting a child in anger; hitting hard; hitting with a fist or object; kicking; hitting hard enough to leave a mark; or pulling hair, jerking arms, or shaking a child. All of these types of hitting could injure a child. They also show him or her that aggressive, angry behavior is an OK way to solve problems.

If you ever feel so angry that you might hurt a child, remove yourself from the situation. Leave the room and try to calm down, or call your spouse or a friend.

When should I call your office?

Call our office if:

- The methods of discipline you are using do not seem to be working.

- You are getting very frustrated with your child and feel like you might harm him or her.

Fever Management

Many different illnesses can cause a fever. The most common causes of fevers in children are minor infections, such as a cold or sore throat. Most fevers less than 102°F (39°C) do not need any treatment. Fever-reducing medicines may help your child feel better.

Never give aspirin for fever in young children. Call your doctor's office if your child has a fever lasting longer than 2 or 3 days, or if he or she is acting very ill, has a temperature of 104°F (40°C) or higher, or has a fever and is less than 2 to 3 months old.

What are fevers?

Fever is a higher than normal body temperature. Average body temperature is about 98.6° Fahrenheit (F) or 37.0° Celsius (C). Most doctors define a fever as a temperature of 100.4°F or 38.0°C when taken rectally. Many different illnesses can cause fevers. The most common cause is some type of infection—usually with a virus or bacteria. Fever may help your child's body fight the infection.

In a child over ages 2 to 3 months who isn't acting very ill, fevers up to 102°F (39°C) are usually nothing to worry about, especially if accompanied by other symptoms of a cold or other minor illness. It's usually not necessary to give medicines to lower the fever, unless you think it will make your child feel better. Use only acetaminophen (for example, Tylenol) or ibuprofen (for example, Advil).

- *Never give aspirin for fever in young children.* This can increase the chances of developing a serious illness called Reye's syndrome.

Fevers sometimes cause seizures (involuntary movements). These "febrile seizures" are usually not serious, but you should call our office if they occur.

When should fevers be checked by the doctor?

Call our office or see a doctor if any of the following occurs:

- Fever in a child who is acting very ill: not easily soothed, crying a lot, very tired or sleepy—more than expected than for just "being sick."
- Fever lasting 3 or more days.
- Very high temperature: 104°F (40°C) or higher.
- Fever in an infant less than 2 to 3 months old.
- Fever developing later in an illness; for example, your child has a cold for 4 or 5 days and then gets a fever.
- Seizures related to a fever.

Which fevers should be treated with medications?

Treatment with fever-reducing drugs does not affect how long your child will be sick. However, lowering your child's temperature may help to make him or her feel better. You may give fever-reducing drugs in certain situations:

- If your child is uncomfortable or in pain. Fevers higher than 102°F (39°C) often make children uncomfortable, so it's reasonable to give drugs to bring the fever down.
- If your child is at risk of becoming dehydrated (not drinking enough liquids or losing fluids through vomiting or diarrhea). Fevers cause increased loss of water from the body (through evaporation).
- Children with certain diseases, such as heart disease or febrile seizures, may benefit from treatment to control fever.

What medications should I use?

If giving medications to lower your child's fever, use acetaminophen or ibuprofen. Both drugs can help reduce fever and make your child feel better. They are available in liquid, chewable, or pill form.

- Ibuprofen may be somewhat more effective and last longer than acetaminophen, but both work.
- Some doctors recommend alternating between doses of acetaminophen and ibuprofen or using them together for difficult-to-control fevers. However, it's not clear how much better this approach works.
- Acetaminophen can be used every 4 to 6 hours, at the dose recommended on the label (based on your child's weight). Ibuprofen can be given no more frequently than every 6 hours.
- Both acetaminophen and ibuprofen are relatively safe drugs:
  - Ibuprofen is more likely to cause inflammation of the stomach (gastritis) and abdominal pain. Rarely, it can affect the kidney.
  - Large overdoses of acetaminophen can cause liver damage, sometimes serious. Large overdoses of ibuprofen have less serious consequences.

Occasionally, lukewarm sponge baths can be helpful if your child's fever is hard to control, but these usually aren't necessary. There is never a reason to use rubbing alcohol to bring the fever down.

If the fever is still present after 2 to 3 days of treatment, see the doctor.

Habits: Thumb Sucking, Nail Biting, Etc.

Most habits are behaviors your child has developed as a way of dealing with stress. Some habits can have harmful effects; for example, thumb sucking can lead to problems with your child's teeth. Generally, the best thing to do about habits is ignore them. Rather than criticizing your child's habit, praise him or her for substituting other behaviors.

What are childhood habits?

Parents are often concerned about their children's habits, such as thumb sucking, nail biting, hair pulling, and others. Children sometimes seem to develop habits as a way of dealing with stress. At other times, they learn habits by imitating adults.

Most childhood habits are harmless. Some habits can cause physical harm, for example, possible dental problems caused by thumb sucking or tooth grinding. Other habits can be socially embarrassing or annoying. In general, it's best not to pay too much attention to your child's habit or to nag him or her about it. Children generally outgrow habits or learn to control them, especially in social situations.

Less often, habits such as head banging or hair pulling can cause pain or injury to children. These habits may develop in children who have been abused or neglected or in children with mental retardation or other forms of developmental delay. Habits are different from tics, which are repeated, involuntary movements such as facial twisting or eye blinking. Any habit that is causing physical harm or interfering with your child's life in any way should be evaluated by a doctor.

What do they look like?

Many kinds of habits may develop.

- Thumb sucking is normal in infants and toddlers but may cause problems with tooth development in some children if it is prolonged.

- Tooth grinding, especially at night (bruxism). This may cause some dental problems.

- Rocking: children may rock back and forth, often when put to bed or alone.

- Head banging—sometimes hard enough to raise fears of the child's injury to himself or herself.

- Nail biting.

- Hair twirling.

- Hair pulling—sometimes severe enough to leave bald spots (trichotillomania).

How are childhood habits managed?

General issues. Usually, no treatment is necessary. Most childhood habits go away on their own, generally within a few weeks or months.

- Try not to pay too much attention to your child's habit. Calling attention to or commenting on habits may actually reinforce them.

- Praise substitute behaviors. Give your child alternatives to the habit. For example, if you see your child biting her nails, say, "Let's take out the crayons and color." Don't comment on the nail biting at all.

- Try to reduce stress in your child's life, especially if there is any stressful situation that may be contributing to the habit.

Thumb sucking and tooth grinding. If they are severe and persistent, these habits can cause dental problems. In some children, special methods may be needed to stop them.

- Thumb sucking is normal in infants and toddlers. However, if the habit continues, it may interfere with the way your child's teeth come in. The best way to deal with thumb sucking is to praise your child when he or she isn't sucking his or her thumb or is keeping busy with other activities (like coloring or playing).

- In the past, putting bitter substances on the fingers was recommended as a way of "breaking the habit" of thumb sucking. It's not clear how well this works, so it's usually not recommended at first. If all else fails and the habit needs to be stopped, the doctor may suggest trying this approach.

- Tooth grinding may be related to anxiety. It may help to work with your child to find other ways of reducing anxiety. If the habit continues, we may recommend evaluation by a dentist.

If habits persist or are causing other problems. If habits are causing any physical harm or social embarrassment, or are interfering with your child's life in other ways, the doctor may suggest a visit to a child psychologist or other mental health professional.

When should I call your office?

Call our office if:

- Your child has a habit you are concerned about, which doesn't improve or go away within a few months.

- Your child has habits that could cause him or her physical harm (for example, head banging) or are severe (for example, hair pulling that leaves bald patches).

- Your child is having social problems, problems at school or at home, or other issues that you think might be contributing to or resulting from the habit.

Immunizations (Vaccinations)

Because of modern immunizations, many once serious childhood diseases are now rare. Vaccines are carefully tested and monitored to be sure they are safe. Several new vaccines have been introduced in the past few years. It is very important to make sure your child receives all recommended immunizations.

What are immunizations?

Immunizations (also called vaccinations) are recommended to help prevent infection with disease-causing germs. Vaccines are made up of either a part of a germ (such as viruses or bacteria) but not the complete germ that's capable of causing disease, or of a *live* germ that has been changed so that it can't cause serious infection. Immunizations cause the body to produce antibodies, which then protect the person from catching specific diseases.

Immunizations are given by injection (a shot), orally (by mouth), or through the nose (intranasal). Recommended immunizations are given in a series, starting soon after your baby is born. Some diseases can be particularly serious in infants and toddlers, so it is important to get immunizations at the appropriate time.

Most vaccines are given in a repeated series to make sure they are effective. The recommended schedule of immunizations requires up to 16 to 20 shots by age 2 years. If your child has missed any immunizations at the usual age, they can usually be given later. New combination vaccines are being developed that will reduce the number of shots needed.

What are all these immunizations for?

Immunization recommendations are updated frequently. The following list presents the routine immunizations recommended for *nearly all* children as of 2006. It also provides some information on the diseases prevented by immunizations.

- *Hepatitis B.* Infection of the liver caused by a virus, which can lead to chronic liver disease. The hepatitis B virus is spread mainly through contaminated blood or sexual contact; a pregnant woman who is infected may pass the virus to her baby.

  - The first dose of hepatitis B vaccine is given soon after birth. Two more doses are given between 1 and 18 months.

- *Diphtheria, tetanus, pertussis (DTP).* These diseases are caused by bacteria. Diphtheria results in severe infections of the tonsils and throat, causing difficulty breathing. It can also damage the heart. Tetanus results in severe muscle spasms, caused by a toxin produced by the bacteria (usually found in soil). Pertussis (whooping cough) is an infection of the airways and lungs that is especially severe in infants.

  - Four doses of DTP vaccine are given in the first 18 months, another dose between 4 and 6 years, and another dose at 11 to 12 years. Regular "booster shots" against diphtheria and tetanus (Td) are recommended every 10 years.

- *Haemophilus influenzae type B (Hib).* Bacteria that can cause a number of serious infections, including infections of the membranes lining the brain (meningitis), lungs (pneumonia), and skin (cellulitis).

  - Three to four doses of Hib vaccine are given before age 18 months.

- *Polio.* A paralyzing disease caused by the poliovirus.

  - Three doses of oral polio vaccine are given before 18 months; a fourth dose at ages 4 to 6 years.

- *Measles, mumps, rubella (MMR).* All of these diseases are caused by viruses. Measles produces a cough, runny nose, red eyes, and a rash. Complications include pneumonia and infection of the brain (encephalitis). Mumps causes infection of the salivary glands (located below and in front of the ear). It can also cause infections of the brain and other organs. Rubella (German measles) causes cold-like symptoms with a rash. If the woman catches rubella early in pregnancy, it can cause abnormalities of many organs in the developing baby.

  - One dose of MMR vaccine is given at age 1; a second dose at ages 4 to 6 years.

- *Varicella (chickenpox).* Chickenpox is caused by infection with a virus, producing fever and an itchy rash that looks like lots of little blisters. Complications include infections of the skin and brain.

  - One dose of varicella vaccine is given after age 1 if your child hasn't already had chickenpox. Another dose at 4 to 6 years is recommended. (If your child has definitely had chickenpox, he or she doesn't need this vaccine.)

- *Pneumococcal vaccine.* Prevents infection with a bacteria called *Pneumococcus,* which can cause meningitis, ear infections, and pneumonia.

  - Four shots of pneumonococcal vaccine are given by age 18 months.

- *Hepatitis A.* Infection of the liver with a virus, which can be passed from person to person.

  - Hepatitis A vaccine is recommended for children ages 1 to 18, beginning at age 1, with a booster shot 6 months later.

- *Influenza.* A virus that sometimes causes severe infections of the respiratory tract (throat, airways, and lungs).

  - A yearly "flu" shot is now recommended for all children between 6 months and 5 years old. It is also recommended for family members and others in close contact with children under 5.

- *Meningococcal vaccine.* Prevents infection with bacteria that can cause meningitis.

  - Recommended for children ages 11 to 12. Also recommended at the beginning of high school and for college freshmen living in dormitories.

- *Human papillomavirus (HPV).* A family of viruses that causes genital warts, a sexually transmitted disease. These viruses are also an important cause of cancer of the cervix (the opening of the womb). Preventing HPV infection significantly lowers the rate of cervical cancer.

  - The new HPV vaccine is now recommended for all girls—three shots beginning at ages 11 to 12.

  - Future recommendation may also include boys.

- *Rotavirus.* This virus is the most common cause of severe diarrhea in children in the United States and worldwide. The new rotavirus vaccine is a live "attenuated" vaccine, which means that the virus has been changed so that it doesn't usually cause disease.

  - Three doses of the oral rotavirus vaccine are given in early infancy.

Additional immunizations may be recommended in special circumstances, such as travel abroad.

 A few children should not be immunized with certain *live* vaccines. Children with cancer or other serious diseases are at higher risk of getting severe disease from the virus used in the vaccine. Fortunately, as long as most other children in the community are immunized, the risk of spreading these diseases is low.

Are immunizations safe?

Yes. Modern vaccines are tested for years before they are used in your child. Once in use, vaccines are continuously monitored to make sure they are safe and effective.

- Getting many vaccinations early in life does not reduce your child's ability to fight off disease. Instead, it protects him or her from the most dangerous childhood diseases.

- It is not true that mercury (thimerosal), which has been used in some vaccines, causes autism or other diseases. Most vaccines no longer contain thimerosal. There is also no scientific evidence that the MMR vaccine causes autism.

What are some possible complications of immunizations?

The doctor will give you information on possible reactions to vaccines every time your child receives an immunization.

- Most complications of vaccines are mild and temporary. By far the most common are mild skin reactions (redness and warmth at the injection area).

- Sometimes children seem to get sick soon after a vaccine. Parents may think this means that the vaccine has caused the disease it was supposed to prevent. Most of the time, however, illness after a vaccine is just a coincidence.

- Rarely, a vaccine is not completely effective. Your child may get the disease he or she has been vaccinated against.

- Allergic reactions to vaccines are rare. If your child has a serious allergic reaction to a vaccine, later doses may be skipped.

What if my child is ill?

If your child is moderately to severely ill at the time of a scheduled vaccination, the dose will be delayed. If he or she is only mildly ill, the dose can be given as usual.

Vaccine recommendations are different for children with certain chronic diseases, such as human immunodefiency virus/acquired immunodeficiency symdrome (HIV/AIDS), absent spleen (asplenia), kidney failure, or diabetes. Additional vaccines may be recommended to prevent diseases that your child's immune system may be unable to fight off.

Children with below-normal immune function (for example, those receiving cancer treatment or infected with HIV) may not receive some of the "live" vaccines containing active germs.

What if my child misses a recommended immunization?

If a recommended vaccine was not given at the scheduled time, your child can receive "catch-up" immunizations.

When should I call your office?

Call our office if:

- You are unsure whether your child's immunizations are up-to-date or you have questions about the latest recommendations.

- You think your child may be having a serious reaction to a vaccine, such as difficulty breathing, severe swelling, or hives.

Where can I get more information?

- The American Academy of Pediatrics' Childhood Immunization Support Program. Online at *www.cispimmunize.org*.

- The National Immunization Program of the Centers for Disease Control (CDC) provides information on vaccine safety. (The CDC is a federal agency that deals with various aspects of infections on the national level.) Online at *www.cdc.gov/nip/vacsafe/vacsafe-parents.htm*.

- You can also call the CDC's Immunization Hotline: 1-800-232-2522 (English), 1-800-232-0233 (Spanish).

Sleep Problems and Bedtime Issues

Children of all ages can have sleep problems. For infants, it can be difficult to establish a good sleep routine. Toddlers and preschoolers may resist going to bed at night. Teens may have different types of sleep problems. Feeling sleepy during the day is a common sign of sleep problems; behavior problems may also occur. Ask your doctor if you have questions or concerns about your child's sleep and bedtime habits.

How much sleep does my child need?

The amount and patterns of sleep vary by age. At all ages, it is normal to wake up briefly during the night, followed by going back to sleep. Although every child is different, the following sleep patterns are typical:

- Newborns sleep up to 16 or 20 hours per day for the first few months. The pattern varies a lot but is generally 1 to 4 hours of sleep followed by 1 to 2 hours of awake time. Most babies settle into a nightly sleep routine by 2 to 3 months.

- Sleep needs slowly decrease with time. By 9 months, most babies are sleeping through the night, plus 2 to 4 hours of nap time per day. Naps usually end by age 5.

- School-aged children sleep 10 hours per night. They may "catch up" on sleep over the weekend. Teenagers should sleep 9 hours per night but often sleep less.

What is a good bedtime routine?

You can develop some regular bedtime routines that will help your child develop healthy sleep habits.

- Share some quiet time with your child in the hour before bedtime. Choose quiet activities like reading or listening to soft music—not rough play, watching TV, or playing video games. Keep the TV out of your child's bedroom.

- A light snack before bed is OK, but avoid heavy meals or caffeine (including cola drinks or hot chocolate).

- Your child's room should be quiet and dark. (A dim nightlight is OK for children who are scared of the dark.) Keep the temperature cool but not cold.

- Make sure your child gets some exercise/outside time during the day. Don't use your child's room for punishment or "time-outs."

- Keep bedtime and wake-up times consistent; too much difference between the two on the weekends can cause problems.

What kinds of sleep problems occur and how are they treated?

Almost all the time, the proper treatment for sleep problems in infants and children is a change in bedtime routines and behaviors.

Medications are rarely used for sleep problems in children (and are probably used more often than they should be in teens or adults).

- Not getting enough sleep, at any age and for whatever reason, can make your child tired during the day. This may lead to fussiness or crying in infants. In older children, it can lead to poor school performance or falling asleep during the day.

- Children who do not get enough sleep can have behavior problems, including lack of attention and hyperactivity. They may act just like a child with attention-deficit hyperactivity disorder (ADHD).

- Every child with daytime sleepiness should be checked for possible sleep-related breathing disorders, such as obstructive sleep apnea (OSA). Loud or persistent snoring is the main symptom of OSA.

Other common sleep problems vary with age:

- *Infants and toddlers.* Some babies and toddlers develop a habit of falling asleep only under certain conditions, such as when being rocked or fed. They may resist going to sleep unless you're there. If they wake up briefly during the night, as is normal, they are unable to go back to sleep without crying or going to their parents' room. This can lead to not enough sleep for both children and parents.

  - If your baby can't or won't go to sleep without a parent there, the best approach is to gradually reduce the amount of time you're present and the routines you've developed (for example, rocking).

  - For younger infants, let your baby cry for a little bit longer each night. For example, the first night, wait 5 minutes before checking the first time; 10 minutes before the second check; and 15 minutes before every check after that. When you check, talk or sing to your baby a little and pat him or her on the back. Try not to pick up or rock the baby; the goal is let your infant soothe himself or herself back to sleep.

  - This approach takes some willpower. For the first few nights, your baby may cry more than ever! Try not to

give in; if you pick up your baby to rock or feed him or her, you may have to start the process all over again.

- Toddlers can take a stuffed animal or other toy to bed. Reward your child for staying in bed, for example, with praise or stickers.

- *Preschoolers and older children.* Some children have difficulty falling asleep. They may resist going to bed or keep getting up after they go to bed. This behavior is sometimes called "curtain calls"—your child keeps asking for "one more glass of water" or "one more story." The most common cause is a lack of consistent limits and a regular bedtime routine. Several steps may be helpful:

  - Establish a regular bedtime routine, as outlined earlier. Set a schedule and stick to it.

  - Don't pay attention if your child stalls or tries to delay bedtime. Don't get mad or yell. Instead, try giving positive rewards for appropriate behavior, for example, praise your child when he or she goes to bed on time without getting up.

  - For older children, learning some simple relaxation techniques may help them calm down and fall asleep.

  - Talk to your doctor if these measures aren't successful in promoting change in your child's sleep habits.

- *Teenagers.* Teens need as much sleep as younger children but often get less. Many teens sleep only 7 hours rather than the 9 hours they need. Part of the reason is that teens stay up later, especially on the weekends when they sleep later in the morning. Teens may also have *insomnia:* sleeplessness is often related to anxiety. This can result in daytime sleepiness, leading to problems at school and in other areas of life.

  - Talk to your doctor to determine the reasons for sleep problems and to decide on proper treatment for your child.

  - Many other types of sleep problems are possible, including:

    - Nightmares and night terrors

    - Narcolepsy (difficulty staying awake during the daytime)

    - Restless legs syndrome (a problem where the person cannot lie still)

When should I call your office?

Call our office if:

- You need help in dealing with your child's sleep and bedtime problems.

- You've made a good effort at changing your child's bedtime routine, but sleep problems continue or get worse.

Smoking: Risks and How to Quit

For parents and teens, smoking leads to serious health problems. Cigarettes and other forms of tobacco use increase your child's risk of many types of cancer, heart and lung diseases, and other serious diseases. Smoking also reduces your ability to play sports and do physical activity and damages your appearance. The people around you can also suffer health effects from your smoking. Cigarettes are addictive, making it very difficult to quit. If you or your child smokes, your doctor can help you quit or direct you to someone who can.

What are the health effects of smoking?

- *Smoking kills people.* It is the most common preventable cause of illness and death. One in five deaths is caused by a smoking-related illness; on average, smokers die 10 years earlier than nonsmokers. Smoking increases the risk of many serious diseases, including:

  - Lung cancer and other cancers.

  - Heart disease, including heart attacks.

  - Other lung diseases, ranging from bronchitis (inflammation of the airways) to emphysema (permanent loss of lung function).

  - Blood vessel diseases (vascular diseases), leading to problems such as stroke and high blood pressure. In men, smoking increases the risk of problems with sexual function (erectile dysfunction).

- *Smoking damages your health now.* Most of the health effects of smoking occur later in life. However, smoking also has harmful health effects in teens and young adults, including:

  - Reduced physical fitness. Even in trained athletes, smoking reduces physical performance and endurance.

  - Problems with lung function, including bronchitis and "smoker's cough," increased phlegm production, wheezing.

  - Smoking has several effects that damage your appearance and attractiveness, including dry skin and wrinkles, voice changes, stained teeth, and other dental problems.

- Although less common, serious health effects can occur even in young people. For example, women who smoke and take birth control pills may be at increased risk of heart attack.

- *Smoking hurts the health of people around you.* Second-hand (passive) smoke causes serious health effects, even in people who don't smoke. This is especially true for children. For women, smoking during pregnancy increases the risk of health problems in the developing fetus. Children exposed to their parents' smoking are at increased risk of sudden infant death syndrome (SIDS), have a higher rate of respiratory infections, and may be at increased risk of cancer.

- *Smokeless tobacco is harmful too.* Chewing tobacco and snuff also increase the risk of health problems, especially mouth and throat cancer and gum (periodontal) disease.

What are the facts on smoking and teens?

- Most smokers start in their teen years. Most teens who smoke continue to smoke as adults.

- *Smoking is addictive.* Once their bodies get used to the nicotine in tobacco, smokers have physical cravings for cigarettes and tobacco. Once they're addicted, smokers tend to increase the amount they smoke.

- The good news is that teen smoking rates have dropped significantly in recent years. However, nearly one fourth of high school students still smoke. So do 8% of middle school students.

- The longer you smoke, the greater the health risks. There is no "safe" number of cigarettes or length of time to smoke. "Low-tar" or "light" cigarettes are no safer than regular cigarettes. No matter how long you smoke, the health risks decrease once you quit.

How can I quit smoking?

Quitting smoking is tough because nicotine is addictive. All smokers should be urged to quit and be offered help in making a plan for quitting. Most states have a "Quitline" that can put you in touch with people who can help you quit. The American Cancer Society can help you find a Quitline in our area; call 1-800-ACS-2345 (1-800-227-2345).

Several approaches can improve your chances of quitting smoking successfully, including medications and behavioral change programs. The results are best when these two approaches are used together.

- *Nicotine replacement therapy.* Different types of medications can provide your body with the nicotine it craves while you're trying to quit.

  - One common form is a nicotine-containing patch that you put on your skin. The patch supplies a steady level of nicotine throughout the day to help you resist cravings. The dose of nicotine in the patch is gradually lowered.

  - Other forms of nicotine replacement therapy are available, such as chewing gum. Some of these products can be bought at a drug store, while others require a doctor's prescription.

  - Talk to your doctor before using any type of nicotine replacement therapy. Pregnant women and certain other people shouldn't use these products. Don't smoke or use any other type of tobacco (including "smokeless" tobacco) while using nicotine replacement.

- *Other medications.* Certain other medications can aid in quitting. For example, the antidepressant drug Zyban (generic name: buproprion) can be helpful. Side effects are possible. These drugs should only be used under a doctor's supervision.

- *Behavioral change programs.* Many types of behavioral change programs are available for people trying to quit smoking. These may include brief follow-up appointments or phone calls, Quitlines, and counseling to help you in quitting or coping with withdrawal. Ask your doctor about resources in our community.

- *Physical withdrawal* is a problem for people trying to quit smoking, even with nicotine replacement therapy.

For some period of time, you may have withdrawal symptoms such as dizziness, headache, and bad mood. These are usually worst in the first two or three days after quitting and gradually get better after that.

- *Psychological withdrawal* is also a problem. For most smokers, quitting smoking is a major habit change. Especially for the first few days, try to avoid situations in which you would previously have smoked, such as being around other smokers. Try to think of alternative activities to do instead of smoking (exercise is a great one). Most important, quitting smoking takes willpower!

- *Most attempts at quitting fail.* That's how addictive smoking is. Don't get too discouraged if this happens; try to learn from the experience. Most people try several times before they finally succeed in quitting smoking.

When should I call your office?

Call our office if:

- You have questions about how to quit smoking.

- You are thinking of taking nicotine replacement therapy or any other medication to help quit smoking.

Where can I get more information?

- Smokefree.gov (*www.smokefree.gov*) provides accurate, up-to-date information and professional assistance to help support the immediate and long-term needs of people trying to quit smoking.

- The American Cancer Society offers a "Guide to Quitting Smoking" and many other helpful resources. On the Internet at *www.cancer.org*, or call 1-800-ACS-2345.

Talking to Your Teen about Sex

With proper information and advice, teenagers can make responsible choices regarding sex. Adolescents are at high risk for harmful consequences of sexual activity, including sexually transmitted diseases (STDs) and unintended pregnancy. Your teen needs accurate information about sex, even if he or she makes the healthy decision to delay or abstain from sexual activity. Teens who are sexually active should use a condom every time they have sex; this reduces the risk of STDs, including human immumodeficiency virus/acquired immunodeficiency syndrome (HIV/AIDS). Your doctor can provide information about more effective options for birth control.

Teens and sex—Why you need to talk

By their early teens, girls and boys are sexually mature. Their bodies are physically capable of having children, and they develop a normal interest in relationships and sex.

Although they are physically mature, adolescent boys and girls are not necessarily mature in other ways. Compared with adults, sexually active teens are at higher risk of problems like unintended pregnancy and sexually transmitted diseases (STDs), including HIV and AIDS. (HIV is the virus that causes AIDS, or acquired immunodeficiency syndrome.)

Myths and incorrect beliefs about sex are common among teens. To make responsible choices, your teen needs accurate information about sex, including issues like abstinence and "safe sex" to reduce the risk of STDs as well as information on birth control.

Sex is a highly personal topic that can be difficult for parents and teens to discuss. This chapter is intended as a starting point for you to discuss sexual issues with your adolescent. Be sure to talk to your doctor if you have questions or specific problems you need to discuss.

What does my teenager need to know about sex?

The truth! Just like when he or she was little and asked you, "Where do babies come from?," your adolescent son or daughter needs accurate information about sex. Around puberty and throughout the teen years, children may hear a lot of inaccurate information about sex. Parents play an important role in providing correct information as well as the guidance and values teens need to become responsible young men and women. Your teen needs accurate information on:

- Preventing STDs, including abstinence and "safe sex."

- Preventing unintended pregnancy (options for birth control).

- Dealing with peer pressure and avoiding risky sexual situations.

When should I talk to my teen about sex? This depends on your child's maturity and other factors. However, it's best to open the conversation before your son or daughter begins encountering situations dealing with sexuality or relationships. Ideally, this should take place before your child and his or her friends start talking about dating or having girlfriends or boyfriends.

Talking about sex is likely to be embarrassing and uncomfortable for both parents and teens. However, it's important to let teens know that they can talk to you openly about this important issue.

What about preventing STDs?

Sexually active teens are at higher risk of STDs compared with adults. This includes not only HIV/AIDS, but also other diseases like syphilis, gonorrhea, and infection with *Chlamydia*, *Trichomonas*, and genital herpes. All teens need information on preventing/reducing the risk of STDs.

- *Not having sex (abstinence)* is the best way to prevent STDs. Teens should know that about half of all high school students do not have sex until they are older. There are many other ways to show affection and love for another person besides having sexual intercourse. Abstinence is a healthy choice for many teens. Delaying intercourse not only prevents the health risks of STDs but also avoids unintended pregnancy and other difficult consequences of becoming sexually intimate before your teen is emotionally and intellectually ready for it.

- *"Safe sex."* Whether they are planning to be abstinent or not, all teens need to know about "safe sex" to reduce the risks of STDs, including HIV and AIDS.

  - Safe sex means using a condom ("rubber") *every time* you have sexual intercourse. It also means not having sex if you don't have a condom.

  - *Limit the number of partners.* The more partners a person has, the higher the risk of contracting or spreading STDs.

  - *Talk to your partners about their sexual status.* Remember that a person can look perfectly healthy and still have an STD. People who inject drugs and men who have sex with other men are at high risk of HIV/AIDS.

- Teens who start having sex at younger ages and those who use drugs or alcohol also seem to be at higher risk of STDs. Both of these factors are related to risky behaviors, such as having a lot of partners and making poor decisions while under the influence of drugs or alcohol.

What about preventing pregnancy?

Your teen needs to understand the consequences of unintended pregnancy. Teen mothers are less likely to finish high school and go to college and also earn less money in their lives. Their children are at increased risk of health problems and problems at school. Teenage boys need to understand that they are financially responsible for supporting their children.

- *Abstinence.* Abstinence (not having sex) is the best way to avoid getting pregnant. Sexually active teens are at a higher risk of unintended or unplanned pregnancy compared with adults.

- *Birth Control.* If your teen is sexually active, he or she needs some form of birth control to avoid unintended pregnancy. "Contraception" is another word for birth control. Teens may get incorrect information about their risk of pregnancy; for example, they may hear that a girl can't get pregnant if she has sex during her period, if she douches after sex, or if the boy "pulls out" early. Teens need to know that *pregnancy is possible any time a male and a female have sexual intercourse!*

  - *Birth control pills* are pills that girls and women take to reduce their risk of pregnancy. They are also called oral contraceptives or sometimes just "the pill." These medications work by changing the woman's hormone levels.

    - Birth control pills can only be prescribed by a doctor. They sometimes have side effects, and they are not safe for some women and girls to take. A woman should never take birth control pills that have not been prescribed for her.

  - *Hormone shots (Depo-Provera).* Generally given once every 3 months. Hormone shots work in the same way as birth control pills but do not have to be taken every day. Again, this form of birth control must be prescribed by a doctor.

  - *Hormone patches.* Worn on the skin.

  - *Hormone implants (Norplant).* Placed under the skin through a small incision.

  - *Emergency contraception (for example, "Plan B").* Hormone pills that can prevent pregnancy if taken within 72 hours after unprotected sex.

  - *Intrauterine devices (IUD).* Devices placed by a doctor within the uterus (womb).

  - *Condoms.* The most important use of condoms is practicing "safe sex" to reduce the risk of STDs. Used properly, they can also reduce the risk of pregnancy. However, there are two things your teen should know:

    - Because they are not always used properly, condoms are *not* a particularly effective form of birth control. Most doctors would recommend some other form of birth control for a sexually active teen.

    - None of the other options for birth control can prevent STDs. Even when using another method for birth control, condoms are still needed to reduce the risk of STDs.

    - Other less-effective forms of birth control include the use of diaphragms (a device the woman places in her vagina before intercourse) and spermicides (substances that work by killing sperm in the vagina.)

What does my teen need to know about healthy relationships?

Try to maintain an open dialogue with your teen about his or her relationships. Especially in older teens who are dating, boyfriend/girlfriend issues have a big emotional impact on their lives.

There are some important issues you should discuss with your teen to promote healthy and safe relationships:

- *Never let anyone pressure you into doing anything you don't want to do.* That's true not just for sex but also drugs, alcohol, cigarettes, and other temptations. Teens should have the willpower to walk away from people who are trying to manipulate them into doing things that don't feel right.

- *Avoid risky situations.* Teens need to watch out for situations in which they might be vulnerable: for example, meeting people from Internet chat rooms, getting into cars with people they don't know, going to parties where alcohol is being served. Set a rule that your teen can call you for a ride at any time, with "few questions asked."

- *Stand up for yourself.* Teens may hear that "everybody's" having sex or fear that they'll lose a relationship if they don't have sex. By talking to your teen and setting a good example, show the importance of maintaining good self-esteem in relationships and other areas of life.

When should I call your office?

This chapter introduces some of the important sex and relationship issues you should discuss with your teen. Call our office if you or your teen has questions or concerns about sexuality, STDs, safe sex, or birth control and related physical and mental health issues.

Where can I get more information?

Teen sexuality is an emotional and sometimes controversial issue. This can make it difficult to find accurate and unbiased information. Here are a few good resources for teens and parents with questions about sexual issues:

- The American Social Health Association provides information on sexual health and STDs. Online at *www. ashastd.org*, or call 1-800-227-8922. A special website for teens can be found at *www.iwannaknow.org*.

- The U.S. Department of Health and Human Services offers information on talking with teens about sex and other topics, emphasizing abstinence. Online at *www.4parents.gov*.

- Planned Parenthood offers information and services related to birth control and sexual health. Online at *www.plannedparenthood.org*, or call 1-800-230-PLAN (1-800-230-7526).

Toilet Training

Toilet training is an important step in your child's development. Children are ready for toilet training at different times. The key to success is waiting until your child is ready, setting up regular toilet times, and praising your child when his or her efforts succeed. Talk to your doctor if you have questions or concerns about toilet training.

When should toilet training start?

There is really no time that is right or "normal" for every child. To toilet train successfully, your child needs to be physically ready. This means knowing when it's time to go, being able to hold it for at least a little while, and being able to let you know when he or she needs to go, even by facial expressions. Often, children who are ready for toilet training simply don't like wet, dirty diapers and want to wear underwear.

For most children, toilet training starts anywhere between 2 and 4 years—many kids aren't ready before age 2. The decision to start toilet training often depends on circumstances such as starting day care. Toilet training should never be forced and should never be a power struggle between parent and child. When starting toilet training, choose a time when things are relaxed—not too many errands to run, no stressful events in the home.

In general, girls tend to be toilet trained earlier than boys. Most children achieve bowel control (controlling bowel movements [BMs]) before they achieve bladder control (controlling urination). As in adults, the frequency of BMs varies in children. They may occur a couple of times a day or once every few days. Either way, BMs should be soft and not uncomfortable to pass.

How should I toilet train my child?

No single approach to toilet training is right for every child. The keys are to establish a regular toilet routine and to be patient!

- Choose a potty chair. Having their own potty chair is more comfortable for children. A potty chair also lets your child's feet touch the floor, which is reassuring.
- Having the child watch parents or siblings go to the bathroom can be helpful.
- Praise your child's efforts at potty training, even if he or she tells you they already went. Don't be negative or angry if your child has occasional "accidents"—they are a normal part of toilet training. If accidents are happening a lot, it may mean that your child isn't ready for toilet training.

- If your child says or shows signs that he or she needs to go to the bathroom, then take him or her to the potty chair. Boys usually learn to urinate sitting down at first.
- Your child should sit on the potty for a few minutes, whether he or she goes or not. Schedule potty trips before and after naps, after meals—every couple of hours.
- Keep the mood positive and light. If your child insists on not sitting on the potty, don't force the issue. This may mean that he or she isn't ready.
- Teach your child how to wipe with toilet paper. Girls should wipe from front to back to avoid spreading stool (BM) to the vagina. Teach your child to wash and dry his or her hands after using the potty.
- When your child is getting the idea, try switching to training pants. These are special underpants that act like diapers in case of accidents.
- Some children are afraid of flushing the toilet. Give your child some time to get used to the idea of moving from a potty seat to the big toilet.
- Toilet training can take weeks or even months. As always, be patient; even in the most difficult cases, toilet training happens eventually!

What kinds of problems can occur?

- Temporary setbacks or "accidents" are a normal part of toilet training. If the parent is patient and accepting, they gradually become less frequent.
- Frequent accidents (wetting or soiling) may mean that your child isn't yet ready for toilet training. If this happens, it's OK to go back to diapers for a little while. Try again when your child shows more signs of readiness.
- Another possible problem is constipation—difficult or uncomfortable BMs. Call our office if this occurs.
- Sometimes children who have been successfully toilet-trained go back to having accidents again. This may be related to some kind of stressful event in your child's life, for example, moving to a new house. It may help to try talking to your child about the issue. Other medical reasons are possible; call our office if the problem continues.
- Some children have physical or medical problems that delay toilet training or make it impossible (for example, various types of developmental delay or medical problems involving the urinary or gastrointestinal system). Your doctor will discuss with you how to handle these situations.

When should I call your office?

Call our office if:

- You have questions about toilet training.

- Your previously toilet-trained child starts having accidents again.

- Your child has difficult or uncomfortable BMs (constipation).

Section II ▪ Allergy

Anaphylaxis

Anaphylaxis is the most serious type of allergic reaction. It can develop suddenly after your child is exposed to something he or she is allergic to. Symptoms include hives (welts), difficulty breathing, and shock (very low blood pressure). If your child has any of the symptoms of anaphylaxis, get emergency help immediately. (Call 911 or another emergency number.)

What is anaphylaxis?

Anaphylaxis is a severe reaction of your child's body to something he or she is allergic to. Certain immune system cells suddenly release substances that can affect almost every organ or body system, including the skin, lungs and breathing tubes, heart and blood vessels, and stomach and intestines.

If your child has had serious allergic reactions in the past, he or she may be at risk of developing anaphylaxis if exposed to the substance causing the reaction. You should have a written emergency plan to follow in case of serious future reactions. You should keep a self-injectable epinephrine kit (EpiPen) handy and know how to use it.

What does it look like?

Symptoms of anaphylaxis may occur within seconds to minutes after your child is exposed to something he or she is allergic to. He or she may not have all of the symptoms mentioned.

Get medical help immediately if your allergic child has any of the following symptoms after being exposed to an allergen (for example, inhaling or eating something, getting a shot, being stung by an insect):

- Tingling or numbness around the mouth.
- Difficulty breathing.
- Coughing or wheezing (high-pitched sounds coming from the lungs).
- Severe swelling, often around the face or hands.
- Tightness in the throat and chest.
- Difficulty breathing or feeling anxious.
- Stomach cramps, vomiting, and diarrhea.
- Itching all over, often accompanied by hives (itchy, red splotches on the skin).
- Pounding heart.
- Fainting.

What causes anaphylaxis?

Anything that your child had an allergic reaction to in the past could cause an anaphylactic reaction if he or she is exposed to it again. Anaphylaxis can even be caused by substances your child has never had a reaction to. The most common allergens are:

- Foods, especially peanuts and shellfish. Allergies to milk and eggs are common causes of anaphylaxis in infants.
- Stings or bites by bees or insects related to bees (wasps, yellow jackets, hornets, and ants).
- Medications, including antibiotics. This is a more likely cause when the medications are injected, rather than taken by mouth.
- Pollen.
- Exercise.

Some causes of anaphylaxis occur in the hospital:

- Latex allergy is common in children who have undergone several surgical procedures, such as those with spina bifida or cystic fibrosis. Outside the hospital, these children may "cross-react" to foods containing proteins related to latex, for example, bananas or kiwi fruit.
- Injected drugs or other chemicals, including dyes used in some x-ray tests.

What puts your child at risk of anaphylaxis?

- If your child has had allergic reactions to these or other allergens, he or she may be at risk of anaphylaxis if exposed again. The risk is higher if your child has had more severe allergic reactions in the past.
- If your child has other allergic conditions, such as eczema, asthma, or hay fever, he or she may be at increased risk of anaphylaxis.

Can anaphylaxis be prevented?

Avoiding allergens is the best way to prevent anaphylaxis. For example:

- If your child is allergic to peanuts or other foods, be careful that he or she avoids those foods.
- If your child is allergic to bees and related insects, wear protective clothing when outside. Immunotherapy (allergy shots) is an effective treatment for allergy to bees and related insects (for example, wasps, yellow jackets, hornets, and ants).

- If your child is allergic to penicillin or other medications, tell all health care providers about this allergy. Get your child a Medic-Alert bracelet or pendant warning about the allergy. Take the same precautions if your child is allergic to latex.

- *Emergency treatment* for allergic reactions can help keep them from becoming more severe. Keep an emergency kit containing self-injectable epinephrine (EpiPen) handy at all times. Learn how to inject this medication to interrupt severe reactions. Older children can learn to do this for themselves.

- Make sure to tell those who care for your child—such as day-care providers and camp counselors—about your child's allergy. They must also know how and when to use the EpiPen. They should call 911 or another emergency number if your child has any symptoms of anaphylaxis.

What are some possible complications of anaphylaxis?

Anaphylaxis is a life-threatening medical emergency. Keeping an EpiPen and knowing how to use it in an emergency may save your child's life.

How is anaphylaxis treated?

- *Emergency treatment.*

  - If your child has symptoms of anaphylaxis, call 911 or another emergency number. Your child needs to go to the emergency room or receive other medical attention immediately.

  - Use injected epinephrine (EpiPen) immediately.

  - Give oral Benadryl (generic name: diphenhydramine) immediately.

- *Additional treatments.* In the hospital, your child may receive other treatments such as:

  - Oral or intravenous steroids and antihistamines. These treatments may be given for a few days to keep allergic symptoms from coming back.

  - Additional epinephrine or other medications needed to interrupt the allergic reaction.

- Necessary treatments to keep the breathing tubes open, possibly including mechanical ventilation (a machine to help your child breathe).

- *Follow-up treatments* may be needed to reduce the risk of future attacks of anaphylaxis. These may include:

  - Evaluation to find out what your child is allergic to, if you don't already know.

  - Preventive measures, such as obtaining an EpiPen and Medic-Alert tag.

  - Education for you and your child in how to avoid allergens and how to recognize and treat early signs of allergic reactions.

  - Immunotherapy (allergy shots) may be helpful if your child is allergic to specific allergens. A visit to an allergist/immunologist (a specialist in treatment of allergic diseases) may be recommended.

When should I call your office?

Anaphylaxis is a medical emergency! If your child has symptoms of anaphylaxis, call 911 or another emergency number. Some of the most serious symptoms are:

- Tightness in the throat and chest.

- Tingling or numbness around the mouth.

- Coughing or wheezing (high-pitched sounds coming from the lungs).

- Severe swelling, often around the face or hands.

- Difficulty breathing or feeling anxious.

Where can I get more information on anaphylaxis?

The Food Allergy and Anaphylaxis Network provides excellent information to help in dealing with the practical and emotional issues surrounding food allergies and other serious allergies. Visit *www.foodallergy.org* or phone 1-800-929-4040.

Asthma

Children with asthma may have repeated attacks of wheezing, coughing, and difficulty breathing. Besides medications for attacks, some children will need to take medication daily to prevent symptoms. You may receive an asthma action plan, including instructions for treating asthma attacks at home. If your child has a severe attack or one that does not get better with treatment, call our office or go to the emergency room.

What is asthma?

Asthma is a chronic disease that involves inflammation (swelling and spasm) of the lung airways, resulting in narrowing of the breathing tubes. This can cause attacks of wheezing (high-pitched sounds coming from the lungs), coughing, and difficult breathing.

The cause of asthma is unknown. It probably involves a combination of inherited and environmental factors. Many factors may trigger asthma attacks, such as colds and other infections, allergies, exercise, tobacco smoke, air pollution, perfumes, and cold or dry air.

Asthma may affect up to 12% of American children, and rates seem to be increasing. About 80% of children with asthma have their first attack before age 6. Childhood asthma is a major health problem, causing frequent emergency room and doctor's office visits and missed school days. However, with proper treatment, few children die from asthma attacks.

- *Wheezing when a child has a cold* is fairly common in young children. Many children with this type of wheezing do not develop asthma.

- *Intermittent asthma* describes asthma attacks that don't happen very often. Your child may need treatment only when attacks occur.

- *Persistent asthma* describes asthma attacks that happen fairly frequently. Your child will probably need daily treatment with some type of asthma control medication.

What does it look like?

- During asthma attacks, your child may have coughing or wheezing (high-pitched sounds coming from the lungs). Asthma can be subtle—you may not even realize your child is having "attacks."

- Tightness of the chest and shortness of breath may occur, especially in older children.

- Symptoms may be worse at night.

- Coughing and/or wheezing with physical activity.

- Coughing without a cold, especially at night.

During *severe asthma attacks,* you may see your child's chest caving in, ribs sticking out (retractions), belly going up and down, and nostrils flaring. *This is an emergency!* Take your child to the emergency room immediately.

What causes asthma?

Asthma is likely caused by a combination of inherited and environmental factors. Once asthma is present, attacks may be triggered by a wide range of factors, including:

- Colds and other infections.

- Allergens to which your child is sensitive.

- Exercise.

- Anything that irritates the airways, such as tobacco smoke, air pollution, perfumes, and cold or dry air.

What puts your child at risk for asthma?

- If you or other members of your family have asthma, your child may be at increased risk.

- Allergies.

- Eczema (atopic dermatitis)—a skin rash caused by allergies.

- Episodes of wheezing.

- Tobacco smoke (secondhand smoke).

- Asthma is more common in boys than in girls.

- Asthma tends to be more severe in African-American children.

Can asthma be prevented?

To reduce the risk of your child's developing asthma:

- Don't smoke during or after pregnancy.

- Breast-feed for at least several months after birth.

- Vaccinations do *not* increase the risk of asthma. Your child should receive all regular childhood immunizations. This includes a yearly influenza vaccine ("flu shot"), unless your child is allergic to egg.

To reduce the risk of asthma attacks:

- Eliminate or reduce exposure to things that trigger asthma attacks—such as allergens and irritants like cigarette smoke, air pollution, or perfumes.

- Follow your child's Action Plan and other recommended treatments. Prompt home treatment can keep asthma attacks from becoming severe.

- Get treatment for diseases commonly seen with asthma, such as hay fever (allergic rhinitis) and sinusitis. Get treatment for gastroesophageal reflux disease (GERD), if present.

- Don't let your child play in damp, moldy places (basements, for example).

- Keep household dust under control.

- If you already have a pet, testing may determine if your child is allergic to it.

What are some possible complications of asthma?

Severe asthma attacks can cause serious complications. These risks are higher if the attack is severe enough to require hospitalization and mechanical ventilation. Teenagers may be at highest risk.

The following situations are emergencies:

- Pneumothorax (air leak from the lungs into the chest), which causes very sharp chest pain.

- Severe blockage of the airways, which can lead to respiratory failure. If your child is having difficulty breathing and speaking or is anxious, go to the emergency room immediately.

In the long term, asthma can lead to chronic lung disease. Proper treatment reduces this risk.

How is asthma treated?

Your child's treatment will depend on the frequency and severity of his or her asthma attacks or symptoms. Depending on their severity, your child may need frequent asthma checkups and tests of lung function.

An Action Plan may be developed if your child's asthma is a significant problem. The plan will tell you how to manage your child's asthma in different situations, including how to handle asthma attacks. Even if attacks are mild, your child may still need treatment.

Your child may receive a peak flow meter. This is a simple device that can tell you how severe an attack is and how treatments are working to keep your child's asthma under control.

- *Intermittent asthma.* If your child has only occasional asthma attacks, he or she will likely receive an inhaler with a "short-acting" beta-agonist drug, such as albuterol. This inhaler helps to open up the breathing tubes. It is used only during asthma attacks. If your child has wheezing and/or coughing several times a week, he or she may have persistent asthma.

- *Persistent asthma.* In addition to a short-acting inhaler, your child will receive a controller medication to prevent attacks. These anti-inflammatory treatments should be used every day, whether or not your child is having trouble breathing. Drug treatments for persistent asthma may include:

- *Inhaled steroids.* Giving steroids through an inhaler avoids many of the side effects of oral steroids. If used in high doses for a long period, inhaled steroids may temporarily slow your child's growth. However, they probably won't affect his or her final height. Taking inhaled steroids can cause yeast (*Candida*) infections in the mouth. Your child should rinse out the mouth after taking inhaled steroids. These are the most effective inhaled drugs for asthma.

- *Leukotriene inhibitors.* These medications, such as Singulair (generic name: montelukast), prevent the release of substances that cause inflammation. They may help to reduce the dose of inhaled steroid your child requires.

- *Long-acting beta-agonists.* These medications, such as Serevent (generic name: salmeterol), help to keep the breathing tubes open for a longer period.

- *Oral steroids.* If more severe persistent asthma develops or if attacks come back, your child may need to take oral steroids. When used for short periods (5 to 10 days), oral steroids don't reduce growth or have other major side effects.

- *Immunotherapy.* A minority of children with asthma, especially those with difficult-to-control disease, may benefit from "allergy shots." This is helpful only if your child is allergic to specific allergens.

When should I call your office?

Call our office any time you have questions about your child's asthma care, including:

- If your child develops new or frequent symptoms of asthma.

- If your child's peak flow is in a range considered dangerous.

The following situations are emergencies. Take your child directly to the emergency room:

- If your child is having difficulty breathing or speaking or is anxious.

- If your child has an asthma attack that doesn't get better with treatment or gets worse despite treatment.

- If your child has retractions (chest caving in, belly going up and down) or symptoms of pneumothorax (sharp, acute chest pain).

Bee Stings and Other Insect Stings

Insect stings are common in children and usually are not serious. However, if your child is allergic to bees and related insects, serious reactions can occur. If your child is allergic to bees, you should keep an emergency kit (EpiPen) handy. Allergy shots can reduce or eliminate bee allergy.

Should I be concerned about bee stings?

Nearly all children get stung by bees or other insects at one time or another. Most often, the sting causes only a minor skin reaction. A cold washcloth and pain reliever are the only treatment needed.

The situation is different if your child is allergic to bees or other stinging insects. If your child has a large skin reaction or a more general bodily reaction to a bee sting, he or she is probably allergic. Your child may need treatment to prevent more serious reactions in the future.

What kind of reactions can occur?

Allergic reactions to bee stings range from minor skin reactions to life-threatening reactions.

- *Minor reactions.* Your child will have a raised, red area around the sting. You may see the insect's stinger in the skin. Minor reactions to bee stings usually go away in a day or less. Sometimes they don't appear for a few hours.

- *Larger skin reactions.* Your child may develop a larger skin reaction over several hours or a few days. The area of swelling around the sting becomes larger. The reaction goes away after a few days.

- *Non–life-threatening reactions.* Your child may develop a more severe skin reaction. This usually starts within minutes after the sting. You may see red splotches spreading around the sting and sometimes on other parts of the body. Swelling and itching may be intense.

- *Life-threatening reactions.* In addition to an intense skin reaction, your child may develop signs of a more serious allergic reaction, such as wheezing (high-pitched sounds coming from the lungs) and/or coughing. This is called anaphylaxis. *This is an emergency.* Call 911 or another emergency number.

What causes reactions to bee stings?

Bees and related insects—including wasps, yellow jackets, hornets, and ants—inject a weak venom (poison) when they sting. For most people, this small amount of venom does no harm.

However, 1% to 4% of people are allergic to bees and related insects (called *Hymenoptera*). If your child has ever had more than a small, local reaction to a sting, he or she is at risk of more severe reactions to future stings.

Mosquitoes, ticks, and other insects can also give painful bites. However, allergic reactions to these insects are not common.

Can reactions to bee stings be prevented?

Some simple steps can reduce the risk of bee stings *for all children*:

- Don't bother bees or other insects. Most will only sting if disturbed. (Yellow jackets are more aggressive, however.)

- Wear protective clothing, including shoes and long pants, when walking in grass or through fields.

- Using insect repellants containing a chemical called "DEET" is effective against tics and mosquitoes, but not bees.

- Avoid things that may attract bees, such as perfumes or bright-colored clothing.

If your child is allergic to bees, other preventive steps are needed:

- If your child has had anaphylaxis or other serious reactions to bee stings, you should keep an emergency kit containing self-injectable epinephrine (EpiPen) handy at all times. You will be taught how to inject this medication to interrupt severe reactions. Older children can learn how to do this themselves.

- Make sure to tell those who care for your child, such as day-care providers and camp counselors, about your child's bee allergy. They must also know how and when to use the EpiPen.

- Typical insect repellants don't work against bees and other stinging insects.

What are some possible complications of bee allergy?

- Even if your child has a minor reaction, the area around a bee sting or bite can become infected. Simple treatments may reduce this risk. Try to stop your child from scratching the area.

- Although death caused by allergy to bees and related insects is rare, it is a risk. Keeping an EpiPen and knowing how to use it in an emergency may save your child's life.

How are bee stings treated?

If your child is not allergic to bees:

- Place a cold washcloth on the area. Pain relievers may be helpful.

- If the stinger is present, scrape it out. Don't pull on it or use tweezers—this may cause more venom to be injected.

- Apply a paste of meat tenderizer and water to help reduce swelling.

If your child is allergic to bees:

- If your child develops a large area of swelling, redness, or a rash, or develops wheezing or difficulty breathing, go to the emergency room immediately.

- If your child has previously had serious allergic reactions to bee stings, you should keep an EpiPen handy at all times. If he or she seems to be having another allergic reaction, use the EpiPen immediately. Then call 911 or another emergency number.

- If your child has serious reactions to bee stings, allergy shots (venom immunotherapy) are helpful.

  - In this treatment, your child receives a series of shots of venom from *Hymenoptera* (bees and related insects—wasps, yellow jackets, hornets, and ants). Over a long time, the dose is gradually increased until your child is no longer allergic.

Treatment is highly effective in reducing the risk of future serious allergic reactions. A specialist in allergic diseases (an allergist/immunologist) can tell if venom immunotherapy is a good option for your child.

When should I call your office?

Call our office if:

- Your child has any symptoms of a serious allergic reaction to a bee or insect sting (red splotches, intense itching and swelling, noisy breathing). *This is an emergency!*

- If the sting does not feel better after home care or doesn't clear up within 2 or 3 days.

- If the sting becomes red, swollen, warm, and tender a few days after the sting. These may be signs of infection.

- If your child develops a fever.

Food Allergies

Many babies and older children have allergies to foods, such as milk, eggs, and peanuts. If your child has had severe reactions to foods, you need to be careful to avoid repeated exposure to that food. Rarely, allergic reactions to foods may be life-threatening, requiring immediate emergency care.

What are food allergies?

Food allergies occur when your child becomes hypersensitive to specific foods. They affect about 6% of children from birth to age 3. Many children "outgrow" food allergies, but others remain allergic throughout their lives.

Reactions occur within minutes to hours after your child eats the food to which he or she is allergic. The reactions can sometimes be serious, sometimes even life-threatening. If your child has serious reactions to specific foods, you must be very careful to avoid those foods.

Not all reactions to food are allergic reactions. For example, some people cannot tolerate milk because of lactose intolerance, but they are not allergic to milk.

What do they look like?

Food allergies may cause several different types of reactions:

- *Gastrointestinal reactions.* These may include vomiting, diarrhea, and bloody stools (most common in infants who are allergic to cow's milk–based or soy-based baby formulas). Older children may experience itching, tingling, and swelling of the lips, mouth, and throat.

- *Skin reactions.* These may include an itchy rash (eczema, atopic dermatitis) or hives and swelling (urticaria and angioedema).

- *Respiratory reactions.* These range from mild to severe:
  - Typical symptoms of hay fever, such as stuffy nose and sneezing (allergic rhinitis). These usually occur with other allergic symptoms, such as hives.
  - Wheezing (high-pitched sounds coming from the lungs), difficulty breathing, tightness of the throat.
  - Symptoms of *anaphylaxis*. This is a severe allergic reaction that includes difficulty breathing, chest and throat tightness, hives, and fainting.

What causes food allergies?

Food allergies are caused by specific foods to which your child has become allergic. The following allergens (things you are allergic to), along with wheat and fish, account for about 90% of food allergies in infants, children, and teenagers:

- *Cow's milk or soy milk.* These allergies usually develop in infants fed baby formula. Milk allergy almost always appears before the child is 1 year old.

- *Egg.* Usually appears by age 18 months.

- *Peanut.* Usually develops after infancy.

- *Cross-reactive allergens.* If your child reacts to one type of allergen, he or she may also react to certain related food allergens. For example, a child who has hay fever caused by birch pollen may also be allergic to fruit from plants in the birch family, such as apples or cherries.

How are food allergies diagnosed?

It can be difficult to tell what food your child is allergic to, or if he or she has any allergy at all. Other types of reactions to foods are possible, such as various types of food intolerance. Options for identifying the cause of food allergy include:

- Keeping detailed information about what types of foods your child has eaten before reactions occur. For example, has he or she had similar reactions previously when eating the same food? Avoiding the suspected food for a while and then trying it again may provide useful information but should be done under a doctor's orders.

- Skin tests may be helpful. However, sometimes the results will suggest that your child is allergic to a type of food that does not cause reactions.

- Special blood tests (RAST) or other tests are sometimes performed. Some children may need to see an allergist/immunologist (a specialist in treating allergic diseases) to make the diagnosis. It's important to make sure you have identified the true source of the allergy before making major changes to your family's diet and lifestyle.

What are some possible complications?

- Serious, life-threatening reactions can occur, although rarely.

- Children with food allergies often have other types of allergic reactions as well.

- Trying to avoid common foods that are served frequently can be very difficult and stressful for your family, so it's important to find out exactly what food your child is allergic to.

What puts your child at risk for food allergies?

- If your child has had allergic reactions to a certain type of food, he or she may be at risk for more serious reactions if exposed again. The risk is higher if your child has had more severe allergic reactions in the past.

- If your child has other allergic conditions—such as eczema, asthma, or hay fever—he or she may be at increased risk of food allergies.

Can food allergies be prevented?

- It is unknown whether food allergies can be prevented. Some experts think that if allergies run in your family, delaying introduction of allergenic foods until your baby is older may help to reduce the risk of food allergies. However, this theory is unproven.

- Breast-feeding for the first several months may help to reduce the risk of allergies.

How are food allergies treated?

- The best way to manage your child's food allergies is to avoid the foods that cause reactions.

- If your child has had *anaphylaxis* and other serious reactions to foods, you should keep an emergency kit containing self-injectable epinephrine (EpiPen) handy at all times. You will be taught how to inject this medication to interrupt severe reactions. Older children can learn how to do this themselves.

- Make sure to tell those who care for your child—such as day-care providers and camp counselors—about your child's food allergy. They must also know how and when to use the EpiPen. They should call 911 or another emergency number if your child has trouble breathing or any symptoms of anaphylaxis.

- If your child develops a large area of hives or swelling or develops wheezing or difficulty breathing, call our office or go to the emergency room.

- Various medications may be used to treat the symptoms of allergic reactions to foods:
  - Beta-agonist drugs, such as albuterol, to open up blocked breathing tubes. This medication is inhaled (breathed in) and is often used to treat asthma attacks.
  - Epinephrine and other emergency treatments for anaphylaxis and other serious reactions.
  - Antihistamines.

Many children eventually "outgrow" their food allergies. This is most likely if your child is allergic to milk, soy, or eggs. It is also more likely if the allergy develops early and the food is eliminated from the diet. If your child is allergic to peanuts or fish or if the allergy develops later, he or she is less likely to outgrow it.

When should I call your office?

Call our office if:

- Your child has any symptoms of a serious allergic reaction to foods (red splotches, intense itching and swelling).

- Your child develops wheezing or difficulty breathing. Use the EpiPen, if available. Then go to the emergency room or call 911 or another emergency number. *This is an emergency!*

Where can I get more information on food allergies?

The Food Allergy and Anaphylaxis Network provides excellent information to help in dealing with the practical and emotional issues surrounding food allergies. Visit *www.foodallergy.org* or phone 1-800-929-4040.

Hay Fever (Allergic Rhinitis)

Like adults, children can sniffle and sneeze because of allergies. Effective treatment includes medications and steps to avoid allergens. Hay fever and eczema (atopic dermatitis) in young children are risk factors for asthma.

What is hay fever?

Hay fever includes a runny nose, stuffy nose, sneezing, and other symptoms caused by allergies.

- In about 20% of cases, allergic rhinitis is *seasonal.* Your child will have symptoms only during certain times of the year, when whatever he or she is allergic to is present (for example, specific types of pollen).

- In another 40%, the problem is *perennial.* Your child will always have symptoms, because the allergen is always present (for example, if you have pets).

- In the remaining 40%, the problem is *mixed.* Symptoms are always present but worse at some times of the year than others.

What does it look like?

- Stuffy, runny nose.

- Itchy nose and eyes (allergic conjunctivitis).

- Sneezing.

- Headaches.

- Instead of blowing his or her nose, your child may sniff and snort.

- Young children may rub their noses upward with the palm of the hand. This habit—sometimes called the "allergic salute"—may cause a crease over the bridge of the nose.

- Your child may breathe with his or her mouth open and have dark circles under the eyes.

What causes hay fever?

Some of the most important allergens to which your child has become allergic are:

- Pollens. If your child is allergic to *tree pollen,* symptoms will appear or worsen in the spring. *Grass pollen* levels are high in early summer, while *weed pollen* levels peak in late summer. Symptoms of pollen allergy may disappear in the fall, after the first frost occurs.

- Molds, outdoor or indoor.

- Pets, especially cats and dogs. Because pet fur is carried on clothing, it may be found even in pet-free areas, such as at school and day care.

- Household pests, especially house dust mites and cockroaches.

What are some possible complications of hay fever?

- Chronic sinusitis: infection or inflammation of the sinuses (the spaces behind the nose).

- Ear problems, including congestion behind the eardrum.

- Nosebleeds, caused by frequent nose blowing and irritation.

What increases the risk of hay fever?

- If parents or other family members have allergies, your child is more likely to have hay fever.

- Poor housing conditions, such as dampness or cockroaches, increase the risk of problems related to allergies.

Can hay fever be prevented?

- There is no proven way to avoid developing allergies. Babies who are breast-fed may be at lower risk of allergies.

- Avoiding allergens is the best way to reduce symptoms of hay fever.

How is hay fever treated?

- Avoid allergens.

  - Skin tests or blood tests may be done to find out what your child is allergic to, if necessary. Once you have this information, you can take steps to reduce exposure to that allergen. For example:

    - Special pillow and mattress covers can reduce exposure to house dust mites. Wash sheets and blankets in hot water every week.

    - When your child is indoors, reduce pollen exposure by keeping the air conditioning on. Special air filters may help to lower indoor mold levels.

- Medications can reduce symptoms of hay fever.

  - Antihistamines. These drugs help block the effects of substances that produce allergy symptoms. Newer antihistamines avoid the drowsiness caused by older antihistamines. Most, like Claritin (generic name: loratadine) or Allegra (generic name: fexofenadine), are taken orally. A nasal antihistamine is also available.

- Decongestants. Decongestants such as Sudafed (generic name: pseudoephedrine) can help to reduce stuffy nose. Decongestants are available without a prescription and come in oral and nasal spray forms. Don't give your child nasal sprays for more than a few days.

- Nasal steroids. If your child's symptoms are severe or do not improve, stronger medications called steroids may be used. These medications, such as fluticasone and budesonide, can safely reduce allergic inflammation in the nose.

- Other medications. Singulair (generic name: montelukast) can also reduce hay fever. This drug is also used to treat asthma.

- Some medications are most effective if started a week or two before the start of pollen season. If your child has hay fever, try to use the lowest dose that controls symptoms.

- If your child's symptoms do not get better with treatment, we may recommend a visit to a specialist in allergic diseases (an allergist/immunologist). This specialist may recommend further treatments, such as immunotherapy (allergy shots) to reduce your child's allergies.

When should I call your office?

Call our office if:

- Your child's allergic symptoms don't get better with treatment, or if they get worse.

- Your child develops signs of asthma, such as wheezing (high-pitched sounds coming from the lungs) or coughing.

- Your child develops signs of sinusitis (such as fever, headache) or if he or she simply isn't feeling well.

Hives

Hives (urticaria and angioedema) are a common and uncomfortable skin reaction. They are usually caused by viruses or allergies, but many other causes are possible. Hives usually improve with simple treatments. If hives last for several weeks, they may be a sign of another disease.

What are hives?

Hives are raised bumps or welts that appear on the skin or lips and mouth. They range in size from pinpoint to inches and are usually itchy. Hives are also called *urticaria*.

Hives are caused by the release in the skin of a substance called histamine—the same substance responsible for many allergic reactions. They are often caused by allergens, but many other causes are possible. *Angioedema* is larger areas of swelling—for example, of the lips or hands.

Hives usually appear suddenly. They may swell and join together, forming large, red, swollen areas. Because they appear and grow so quickly, hives can be frightening for you and your child. Although they may be a sign of a serious reaction, hives usually disappear within a few hours or days.

What do they look like?

- Hives first appear as small, raised bumps or welts. They may occur suddenly and can be very itchy.

- Hives can occur anywhere on the skin or all over the body.

- Hives may swell, forming large pink or red areas. The wheals may then join together to form even larger areas called angioedema.

- Hives and angioedema may change shape, disappear, and reappear unpredictably. These changes can occur in a matter of minutes or hours.

- Hives can appear anywhere on the body. The face, tongue, hands, feet, and genital area are most commonly affected.

What causes hives?

- There are many possible causes of hives. The most common are:

  - Allergic or other types of reactions. These may be caused by drugs, foods, pets, bee stings, or anything else your child is allergic to.

- Infection with a virus or bacteria.

- Sometimes hives are a sign of another disease. Or they may result from physical causes, such as exposure to cold, pressure, sunlight, or even water. However, these other causes are rare, especially in children.

- Often, no specific cause of hives is identified.

What are some possible complications of hives?

- Hives can be a warning sign of a serious allergic reaction.

- Rarely, hives do not go away on their own or with simple treatments. If hives last for several weeks, further tests may be performed to try to identify the cause.

Can hives be prevented?

- If your child is allergic—for example, to foods or pets—avoiding those allergens will help to reduce the risk of hives.

- In the rare cases in which hives result from physical causes—such as cold or sunlight—avoiding those causes will reduce the risk of hives.

- Otherwise, hives are a common but unpredictable problem.

How are hives treated?

For most common causes of hives in children, only simple treatments are needed. Even without treatment, the hives may go away on their own.

- The main medications used are antihistamines, such as Benadryl (generic name: diphenhydramine). To avoid the side effect of drowsiness, you may prefer to give your child one of the newer antihistamines, such as Claritin (generic name: loratadine) or Allegra (generic name: fexofenadine).

- If one of the less common causes of hives is found, we may recommend other medications.

- If hives are caused by allergies, you should try to prevent your child from being exposed to whatever he or she is allergic to.

- If your child's hives are part of a serious allergic reaction (difficulty breathing or *anaphylaxis*), emergency treatment is needed.

When should I call your office?

Call our office if:

- Your child develops hives that do not go away on their own or do not improve with simple treatments.

- Your child develops any of the symptoms of a serious allergic reaction (such as tingling or numbness around the mouth, coughing or wheezing, severe swelling, or tightness in the throat and chest). Call 911 or another emergency number. *This is an emergency!*

Section III ▪ Behavior—Psychology

Adjustment Disorder

Adjustment disorders are emotional or behavioral reactions to some type of change in your child's life, such as a death or divorce. Some children become sad and withdrawn while others become angry and difficult. The problems usually get better in a short time. Talking with a mental health professional and exploring other forms of support may be helpful.

What is adjustment disorder?

Adjustment disorders arise from some type of change in your child's behavior related to a recent stressful event. It may be a major life event, such as a death in the family, or something relatively minor, such as moving or starting at a new school. The behavioral or emotional reactions vary widely. Your child may become depressed, angry, withdrawn, disobedient, or a mix of these.

By definition, adjustment disorders do not last any longer than a few months. If the problems linger, your doctor may recommend further evaluation for another problem such as anxiety or depression. During times of stress, counseling can be very helpful for children and families.

What does it look like?

Your child's reaction to a stressful event may take many forms, such as:

- *Depressed behavior.* Your child may act very sad and withdrawn. He or she may cry a lot, have trouble sleeping, feel hopeless.

- *Anxious behavior.* Your child may seem tense, nervous, and worried. Sometimes depressed and anxious feelings occur together.

- *Angry behavior.* Your child may begin disobeying rules at home and at school. He or she may skip school, get into fights, or get into trouble with the police.

- Many other behavior changes or emotional reactions are possible, including an illness that cannot be explained by anything physical. Because reactions vary so widely and the stressful event triggering the reaction may not be recognized, it can be hard to figure out why your child's behavior has changed.

What puts your child at risk of adjustment disorder?

- Adjustment disorders are common in children and teens (in adults as well). We all have stresses and changes in our lives to which we must adapt and adjust.

- More serious or sudden life changes are more likely to cause a reaction. Losing someone or something that was very important to your child may provoke a strong response.

- Your child and family's unique situation and resources will affect how you and your child react to stress and change.

Can adjustment disorder be prevented?

There's no way to prevent stressful life events or to predict how we'll react to those changes. If your child has a strong support system—for example, at home, at school or church, or among friends—he or she may be better able to cope with life changes.

How is adjustment disorder treated?

- The first goal is to find out what stressful event might be causing your child's adjustment disorder. Although this is sometimes obvious, at other times it is not.

- We may recommend an appointment with a mental health professional, such as a psychologist. This person can help to determine whether your child is having an adjustment disorder or whether some other diagnosis (for example, anxiety or depression) is more appropriate. Sometimes having a chance to talk with a mental health professional about life problems and stresses can be very helpful. The appointments may involve you, your child alone, or other members of your family.

- Talking with your child about the stressful event or life change is helpful. You can provide support and encouragement to help your child adapt to and cope with the stressful situation.

- If marital problems are an issue, marriage counseling for the adults may be helpful. If there has been a death in the family, grief counseling may help your child and family to adjust.

- Medications such as antidepressants are usually not needed for children or adolescents with adjustment disorders. However, depending on your child's situation, short-term treatment with one of these medications might be helpful.

- Follow-up visits are important to make sure your child's adjustment disorder is resolving. If your child is having continued symptoms of depression or anxiety, it's important to get proper evaluation and treatment.

When should I call your office?

Call our office if:

- Your child's emotional or behavioral changes do not begin to improve or if they get worse. Symptoms of adjustment disorders usually resolve within 3 to 6 months.

- You and your family are having a hard time dealing with some type of life change or stressful situation. Mental health resources are available and can be very helpful in dealing with such situations.

Anxiety

Everyone feels nervous and anxious sometimes, especially in stressful situations. However, when fears and anxiety interfere with your child's home, school, and social life, they become a problem in need of attention. Several types of anxiety disorders are common at different ages in children and teens. Evaluation and treatment, often involving a mental health professional, can be helpful.

What is anxiety?

Anxiety can take several forms in children. Some types of anxiety are normal in children at certain ages: for example, babies become anxious when separated from their parents, while toddlers are often afraid of the dark. Anxiety is also very common in children in unfamiliar situations, such as starting school.

Anxiety becomes a problem when it starts interfering with your child's normal activities. For example, school-age children may worry about being separated from their parents and refuse to go to school. Older children may worry about bad things happening or making mistakes, and these fears may make it difficult for them to perform normal and expected activities. If anxiety is overshadowing other aspects of your child's life, it may be helpful to seek mental health care evaluation and treatment.

What does it look like?

- Anxiety is anxiousness, fears, and worries that are on your child's mind a lot of the time. Every anxious child's situation is different, depending on his or her specific circumstances and age. Nervousness and anxiety may start after holidays or around the time of a divorce or separation.

- Common symptoms include:

  - Nightmares, especially about being separated from parents.

  - Complaints of not feeling well or being emotionally upset.

  - Panic attacks.

- *Separation anxiety* may develop in younger children. Your child may be:

  - Very clingy—afraid to be separated from his or her parents.

  - Worried about something bad happening to himself or herself or to his or her parents.

  - Afraid of leaving home; he or she may be reluctant or even refuse to go to school.

- *Social anxiety* may occur in older children, associated with a lot of worries about not being accepted at school or in other social situations. Some children become socially isolated, causing even greater distress and making anxiety worse.

- *Generalized anxiety* is a problem in which anxiety or worries are a main feature of everyday life. Your child may:

  - Have a lot of unrealistic worries about things that might go wrong.

  - Be very critical of himself or herself and embarrassed about things that happened in the past.

  - Feel like he or she is incompetent—"no good at anything."

  - Feel vaguely ill a lot of the time, be very self-conscious, and need a lot of reassurance. He or she may find it very difficult to stop worrying and relax, even for a short time.

- Some specific anxiety disorders are *panic disorder,* involving periods of intense fear or discomfort (panic attacks); *obsessive-compulsive disorder,* which results in repetitive thoughts and routines; and *post-traumatic stress disorder*, in which disturbing thoughts are related to a specific, traumatic event.

- Every anxious child is different. Your child may have different symptoms, or any combination of these. *The main thing to remember is:* If anxiety is interfering with your child's normal activities, it's a good idea to talk to the doctor or another professional.

What causes anxiety?

There may be no specific cause. Anxiety disorders are common in children as well as adults. However, your child's anxiety may be related to some stressful event in his or her life, for example, marital problems in your family.

What are some possible complications of anxiety?

- Anxiety can cause serious interference in your child's life, such as panic attacks or refusing to go to school.

- Anxiety sometimes occurs together with other mental health disorders, such as depression and drug or alcohol abuse.

Can anxiety be prevented?

Everyone must deal with some anxiety in his or her life. Recognizing that your child's anxiety is interfering with his or her normal activities and getting help may reduce this interference.

How is anxiety treated?

- If anxiety is interfering with your child's normal activities, we may recommend a visit to a child and adolescent psychiatrist or another mental health professional. This specialist can perform an evaluation to understand and, if necessary, recommend treatment for your child's anxiety.

- Several treatments for anxiety may be helpful, depending on your child's situation. Options may include:

  - *Psychotherapy or counseling.* Talking with a mental health professional can be very helpful in understanding what is causing your child's anxiety and helping him or her to deal with it.

  - One helpful type of therapy is called *cognitive behavioral therapy.* The goal is to help your child to look at his or her anxieties more realistically and learn more effective ways of dealing with them.

- Your mental health provider may recommend counseling or therapy for your child alone. Sometimes family therapy is recommended.

- *Medications.* Medications may be helpful, particularly if your child's anxiety seems severe or is causing a lot of disruption in his or her life.

- *School involvement.* If your child's anxiety is causing problems at school, your child's care may be co-coordinated with school personnel. These may include teachers, counselors, social workers, or others.

- At home, you can provide support and reassurance while helping your child to find effective ways of dealing with his or her anxieties.

When should I call your office?

Call our office if your child's anxiety gets worse, if it doesn't seem to improve after starting treatment, or if it returns after treatment. Your doctor or mental health professional can inform you about the expected results of treatment.

Attention Deficit–Hyperactivity Disorder (ADHD)

> Attention defiit–hyperactivity disorder (ADHD) is common, affecting up to 12% of school-aged children. Children with ADHD have difficulty paying attention and controlling their behavior, leading to problems at home and school. Medications and other treatments can help to lessen these problems.

What is ADHD?

ADHD is a behavioral disorder consisting of difficulty paying attention and controlling impulses and being overactive. The result is problems with school work, trouble getting along with friends and family, and low self-esteem. Children with ADHD may have other emotional, behavioral, language, and learning disorders.

What does it look like?

Children with ADHD have problems in three key areas:

- *Inattention.* They may be easily distracted and have trouble paying attention. They may lose or forget things, or they may not seem to listen or follow instructions.
- *Impulsivity.* Children with ADHD may have trouble controlling themselves. They may interrupt others frequently or have trouble waiting their turn.
- *Hyperactivity.* They are overactive and have trouble sitting still or being quiet. They may leave their seats in the classroom or talk too much.

Your child's main problem may be hyperactivity or inattention or a combination of these. The inattentive behavior seems more commonly found in older children and in girls. Other characteristics of ADHD are:

- Symptoms occur before age 7.
- Symptoms occur at home and school and other places.

Your doctor may have you and your child's teacher fill out questionnaires (such as the Conner's scale) to aid in making the diagnosis of ADHD.

What causes ADHD?

There is no single, known cause of ADHD. Both inherited and environmental factors probably contribute.

- ADHD may occur from injury to the brain caused by head trauma, premature birth, lead poisoning, and other risks.
- High stress or parenting difficulties may contribute to your child's problems but do not cause ADHD.

What puts your child at risk for ADHD?

- Male sex—ADHD is diagnosed three to four times more often in boys.
- Having an affected sibling.
- Other behavioral or mental health problems, including conduct disorder, anxiety, depression, and learning disorders.

Can ADHD be prevented?

There is no known way to prevent ADHD. Getting treatment and learning how to live with ADHD may lessen its impact.

What are some other problems associated with ADHD?

- Many children with ADHD have continued symptoms through adolescence and into adulthood. Attention problems become more of an issue in older children, leading to health and social problems.
- Without treatment, ADHD may increase your child's risk of experiencing later problems such as injuries, disappointments at school and work, and risky behaviors.
- Taking medications for ADHD does *not* lead to addiction. In fact, children who receive medication may be less likely to abuse drugs or alcohol.

How is ADHD treated?

Psychosocial treatments. Learning about ADHD's many effects on your child's behavior, school life, and family life is the first step in treatment. Sometimes this means finding ways of adjusting the home and school environments to better meet your child's needs. Key goals include:

- Improving relationships with family, teachers, friends, and classmates.
- Reducing behaviors that cause problems while increasing your child's ability to do necessary tasks at home and school.
- Working to improve your child's self-esteem.

Behavior management. Training in behavior management is an important part of getting your child's ADHD symptoms under control. It also helps address problems with relationships and self-esteem.

- One of the keys is parental consistency, that is, making sure your child knows the consequences of his or her actions, both positive and negative. Both parents should respond to situations in the same way.

- Your child should receive rewards for good behavior (positive reinforcement) and face consequences for not meeting behavior goals (negative reinforcement).

- We may recommend a visit to a mental health provider if your child has more severe ADHD or associated conditions such as depression or anxiety.

- Other forms of therapy may help with other behavior or mental health problems, such as depression or anxiety.

School interventions. Some simple changes in school routines are helpful to children with ADHD:

- Having your child sit at the front of the class may limit distractions while increasing supervision.

- Ask your child's teacher to repeat instructions, if possible.

Medications. Stimulants and other types of medications can help in treating ADHD. Medications for ADHD do not change your child's personality or cause addiction. In most cases, proper medications help to reduce the behaviors that cause problems for your child.

- Children respond differently to the various medications used to treat ADHD. It may take a few tries to find the best medication for your child.

- Stimulants are the most commonly used type of medication. They reduce major ADHD symptoms in about 80% of children.

- Side effects are usually mild and don't last very long. When they occur, we may lower the dose or try a different drug. Common side effects include:

  - Loss of appetite.

  - Weight loss.

  - Trouble sleeping.

  - Although uncommon, tics may develop. (Tics are repetitive body motions, such as eye blinking or making certain sounds.)

- Other types of drugs may also be helpful. For example, antidepressants may be useful if your child has depression along with ADHD.

- A relatively new, nonstimulant drug called Strattera (generic name: atomoxetine) may be recommended. It has fewer side effects than stimulants but may be less effective.

- Your child will be followed up at regular intervals to check for side effects and monitor the effectiveness of treatment.

- *Developmental testing.* Because some children with ADHD have associated learning disabilities, your doctor may suggest developmental testing.

When should I call your office?

Your child should be seen on a regular basis to check for side effects and monitor improvement in ADHD symptoms. Between appointments, call our office if:

- Your child's ADHD symptoms get worse or don't get better with treatment.

- Your child develops new symptoms, including possible drug side effects.

Bipolar Disorder

> People with bipolar disorder have cycling episodes of "mania" (overexcitedness, overactivity) and depression. The cycles may occur very rapidly, especially in children. Long-term treatment, including medications, can help to stabilize your child's mood and permit a normal, productive life.

What is bipolar disorder?

Bipolar disorder is a type of mental illness. Your child may have periods in which he or she is very "high," with excited behavior, constant talking, and unrealistic plans. These are followed by periods in which he or she is very "low": depressed and sad, with low energy. An old term for this condition is "manic-depression."

The pattern varies for every patient—your child may have other symptoms as well. Fortunately, medications known as mood stabilizers are very helpful for bipolar disorder. Getting treatment will help your child feel better and improve his or her performance in school, relationships, and other important areas of life.

What does it look like?

- Mood swings that are often rapid and unpredictable.

- During manic episodes, your child may act excited and energetic. He or she may talk rapidly and constantly, sometimes without making sense. Your child may make grand plans and talk as if he or she is very important. Other symptoms may include spending sprees, sexual promiscuousness, or hallucinations (seeing or hearing things that aren't there).

- During depressed episodes, your child may be sad, listless, and hopeless. He or she may have trouble sleeping, yet stay in bed all day. Your child may worry a lot about problems, real and imagined, and neglect school and other activities or responsibilities.

- Some children have angry or aggressive behavior. They may be diagnosed with other disorders, such as attention deficit–hyperactivity disorder (ADHD) or conduct disorder.

- Behavior problems can lead to trouble at school and in relationships. Children may abuse drugs and alcohol and get in trouble with the police.

What causes bipolar disorder?

The cause is unknown. If you or others in your family have had anxiety or depression, your child may be more likely to develop mood disorders.

What are some possible complications of bipolar disorder?

- Bipolar disorder can be difficult to manage for your child and those around him or her. It can lead to problems in school, relationships, and other areas of life.

- If it is severe or left untreated, bipolar disorder can lead to serious consequences, such as job and relationship difficulties, legal troubles, or suicide.

Can bipolar disorder be prevented?

There is no way to prevent bipolar disorder.

How is bipolar disorder treated?

- Getting the correct diagnosis is an important first step. Evaluation by a psychiatrist or other mental health professional is essential in recognizing and getting effective treatment for bipolar disorder.

- A child and adolescent psychiatrist or other mental health specialist will probably direct your child's treatment. This professional has the training and experience to recommend the best care for your child's situation.

- Treatment usually includes mood-stabilizing drugs. These medications can help to make your child's mood swings less severe, allowing him or her to get back to normal activities.

- The most common medication is lithium carbonate. It can have a number of side effects, so your child will need follow-up blood tests.

- Other drugs, including Tegretol (generic name: carbamazepine), Depakene (generic name: valproic acid), or Lamictal (generic name: lamotrigene) may be used. These also carry a risk of side effects and require close monitoring.

- Your child may have to continue taking mood stabilizers or other recommended medications indefinitely. Going off medications can cause a return of bipolar symptoms or a relapse. If a relapse occurs even when your child is taking medication, a change in treatment may be needed.

- Psychotherapy or counseling from a mental health professional can help your child to cope with daily stresses and aid in keeping bipolar symptoms under control.

When should I call your office?

- During treatment for bipolar disorder, call your mental health provider if your child seems to be having mood swings—feeling either too high or too low.

- Call your mental health provider if your child develops any medication side effects, such as a rash, confusion, drowsiness, or behavior changes.

- If you cannot reach your mental health provider and you're concerned about these or other problems, call our office.

Bullying

Bullying is a common problem for school-aged children. All kids get picked on sometimes, but bullying that happens repeatedly can have a real impact on your child's life. There are things you, your child, and your child's school can do about bullying. Children who are bullies may have even greater problems and may need help in stopping their aggressive behavior.

What is bullying?

Bullying is aggressive or hostile behavior that is repeated and intentional. Bullying happens when stronger kids pick on weaker kids. When it is severe and relentless, bullying can affect your child's school performance, self-esteem, and other areas of life.

The child who is doing the bullying has problems too. Bullying can be a sign of trouble at home or of emotional problems such as depression. Some of these kids may be bullied or abused themselves.

If your child is being bullied, the best thing he or she can do is avoid and ignore the bully as much as possible. If bullying becomes a frequent or severe problem, make sure your child knows to tell you, a teacher, or another trusted adult. Schools may also have methods to address the issue.

What does it look like?

- Bullying can be physical (hitting, shoving, stealing) or verbal (taunting, threatening). Today, bullying can even take place on the Internet: in e-mail, instant messages, or chat rooms.

- The child who is being bullied may act passively—not standing up for himself or herself. Others may get angry or react in other ways that only encourage the bully.

- Your child may not tell you about the bullying. He or she may be embarrassed or may feel that telling an adult would be "tattling." You may notice unexplained bruises, changes in mood or behavior, or missing articles of clothing or other belongings.

- Bullied children may be afraid to walk their usual route to school or go to the bus stop. They may seem depressed or anxious. Bullying sometimes contributes to problems with refusing to go to school.

- If your child has been bullying others, you may hear complaints from the school or from other parents. Parents of bullies are often unaware of their child's behavior.

What causes bullying?

It's hard to say why some kids like to push others around. Some bullies have problems at home, while others are bullied or abused themselves. Kids who are weaker or more vulnerable in some way make tempting targets for bullies.

What are some possible complications of bullying?

- Being bullied may contribute to emotional problems in your child, for example, feelings of depression or anxiety. School performance and self-esteem may be affected. In severe cases, being bullied can really interfere with your child's daily activities.

- Bullying can be an early sign of more serious behavior problems. Kids who are bullies may be at increased risk of problems such as conduct disorders and drug or alcohol abuse, especially in later years.

What increases your child's risk of bullying?

- Up to one fourth of kids say that they are bullied at least sometimes. Bullying is very common around age 8 or 9 but can occur in later years as well.

- Both boys and girls can be bullied. Boys are more likely to bully other kids in physical ways, whereas girls are more likely to be verbal bullies.

- Bullies tend to pick victims who are smaller, weaker, or more vulnerable. Shy children or those with few friends are more likely to be bullied.

What can be done about bullying?

If your child is being bullied:

- Ask your child to tell you about the problem. Let your child know that he or she can discuss the problem honestly and that you are taking it seriously.

- *Don't* tell your child to fight back. *Do* tell him or her to ignore the bullying or avoid the bully as much as possible. He or she should walk away from the bully or ask for help from a teacher or other adult.

- Tell your child not to react to the bullying by getting angry, crying, or acting scared—that's just the kind of reaction the bully is trying to get. It may help just to say, "Leave me alone" and walk away.

- Talk to your child's teacher or school principal about the problem. More and more schools are realizing that bullying is an important problem that has to be dealt with. Many schools have started programs to monitor and prevent bullying and aggressive behavior.

- It may help to talk to the parents of the child who is doing the bullying. Often they are unaware that their child is acting like a bully.

If your child is a bully:

- It is important to get help for the children who are bullies. Bullying can be a sign of problems at home or an early sign of more serious behavior problems.

When should I call your office?

Call our office if:

- Your child is having frequent feelings of depression or anxiety or if he or she refuses to go to school.

- You need help dealing with a serious bullying problem.

- Your child has been bullying other children or engaging in other types of aggressive or hostile behavior (such as fighting or stealing).

Conduct Disorder

Children with conduct disorder behave in various unacceptable ways—from lying and fighting to violent criminal offenses. Conduct disorder can obviously cause a lot of trouble for your child and family. It may also be linked to other problems, such as learning disabilities and drug and alcohol abuse. Evaluation and treatment can help to reduce your child's conduct problems.

What is conduct disorder?

Conduct disorder is a term used to describe the problems of children and teens with repeated, serious forms of antisocial behavior. Although all children break rules now and then, children with conduct disorder repeatedly get into trouble for things like stealing, lying, damaging property, and assaulting other people. Conduct disorder may occur in association with other problems, such as attention deficit–hyperactivity disorder (ADHD) or bipolar disorder.

Over time, especially in the teen years, children with conduct disorder may commit more serious offenses and get into legal trouble. If your child has this type of problem, it's important to get him or her evaluation and treatment. Especially with treatment, most children with conduct disorder grow up to be responsible adults.

What does it look like?

Children with conduct disorder may act in many different unacceptable, antisocial ways:

- They break rules and get into trouble at school and at home. Your child or teen may skip school, stay out at night, or run away.
- Your child may act aggressively, including bullying and fighting with others. He or she may shoplift, set fires, or harm animals.
- Children and adolescents with conduct disorder may commit serious criminal offenses.
- Your child may have additional psychological problems, including depressed or anxious mood, inattentiveness and/or hyperactivity, or drug and alcohol abuse.

What causes conduct disorder?

Many factors may be involved, including genetics, medical problems, and family difficulties.

What are some possible complications of conduct disorder?

- Behavior and discipline problems can make your child's home, school, and social life very difficult.
- The more serious offenses committed by children and teens with conduct disorder can obviously lead to severe legal consequences.
- Some youngsters with conduct disorder continue to have social and behavioral problems as adults.

How is conduct disorder treated?

If your child has a history of repeated aggressive, destructive behavior, we may recommend evaluation by a mental health professional.

The goal of psychological evaluation is not to "label" or stigmatize your child. Rather it's to understand the factors contributing to your child's behavior problems and to find the best way of addressing them.

- *Psychotherapy* may be helpful. Psychotherapy works through helping your child to understand the reasons why he or she acts in certain ways through building a trusting relationship with the therapist. However, for children with conduct disorder, it may be difficult to develop a trusting relationship with a therapist.
- *Group therapy* is sometimes more useful for adolescents with conduct disorder because they are more likely to respond to other teens with similar problems than to a therapist. For younger children with conduct disorder, anger management techniques may help.
- Some important techniques for treatment of conduct disorder are:
  - *Parent management training.* This form of therapy seeks to teach parents how to interact with their child in ways that will help to avoid unacceptable behaviors.
  - *Cognitive-behavioral therapy.* This form of therapy focuses on problem-solving skills. The goal is to help your child to be aware of the causes and consequences of problems and to focus on developing new ways of dealing with situations.
  - *School interventions.* Your child's school may also be involved in the management of conduct disorder. Comprehensive approaches involving all aspects of your child's life may be more likely to succeed. If your child has a learning disability, special education may be needed.

- *Medications* may be part of your child's treatment but should not be the only treatment. Medications have little effect on aggressive or hostile behavior problems, but they may help in managing other problems sometimes associated with conduct disorder, for example, attention deficit–hyperactivity disorder or depression.

Treatment for conduct disorder is a long-term process. Your doctor can help to put you in touch with mental health professionals and services that can help to understand and reduce your child's behavior problems.

When should I call your office?

Call our office if your child develops a pattern of antisocial or destructive behavior.

Depression

As in adults, depression can happen in adolescents and children. Your child may feel sad most or all of the time, which interferes with his or her everyday activities. Depression in children is sometimes related to a certain life event, but not always. Effective treatments for depression in children are available.

What is depression?

Depression is feelings of sadness and hopelessness that are present much of the time and interfere with daily activities. Everyone feels sad now and then, including children. However, if your child is sad most of the time, is not engaging in usual play or other activities, and is having other problems such as sleeplessness or loss of appetite, he or she may have some form of depression.

If your child has symptoms of depression, it is important to get medical help. Your doctor or mental health professional can evaluate your child and recommend appropriate treatment, which may include psychotherapy, medication, or both. Treatment can help your child recover from an episode of depression and get back to his or her normal mood and activities.

What does it look like?

- Feelings of sadness or hopelessness. Depressed children may seem more irritable than sad.
- Loss of interest in activities your child used to enjoy. For example, rather than playing with friends, your child may become withdrawn.
- Frequent crying, often for no reason.
- Low energy—feeling tired all the time.
- Doing worse or poorly in school.
- Sleeping too little or too much.
- Eating too little or too much; losing or gaining weight.
- Feeling worthless and/or feeling guilty for no or little reason.
- Some depressed children act passively or are clingy; others are aloof or withdrawn.
- Thinking or talking about death or suicide.
- Other symptoms are possible: as happens in adults, depression may take many different forms in children.

What causes depression?

There is no single cause of depression. Genetic factors, social factors, and life experiences probably all play a role.

What are some possible complications of depression?

- Suicide, particularly in depressed adolescents. If your depressed teen talks about committing suicide, call your mental health professional or doctor's office immediately!
- Especially when it is not treated, depression can become a chronic or recurrent problem that interferes with all aspects of life: job, family, relationships.

What puts your child at risk of depression?

- Depression is common, occurring in up to 2.5% of children and 8% of teens.
- In teens, it is more common in girls than in boys.
- Depression often occurs with other mental health disorders, including anxiety, behavior disorders, learning disorders, or substance abuse.
- If you or others in your family have had depression, your child may be at higher risk.
- Depression may follow some type of loss in your child's life, for example, a death or family disruption.

Can depression be prevented?

There is little that can be done to prevent depression in children.

How is depression treated?

- If depression is suspected, we may recommend evaluation by a mental health professional, such as a child and adolescent psychiatrist or psychologist. Having such a professional meet and talk with your child can help in assessing whether your child is depressed, how severe the depression is, and what factors may be contributing to it.
- Depression may be classified in different ways:
  - *Major depression:* episodes of severe depression, sometimes bad enough to require psychiatric hospitalization.
  - *Dysthymia:* depression that is less severe but sometimes more persistent.
  - *Bipolar disorder:* depression alternating with episodes of overexcitedness and overactivity (formerly called "manic-depression").
  - Even if your child does not fall into any of these categories, depression can be an important problem requiring evaluation and treatment by medical or mental health professionals.

- *Hospitalization* is sometimes needed for children or adolescents who are very depressed, especially if they have attempted suicide, have serious thoughts about committing suicide, or have other severe symptoms.

- *Medications* are an important part of treatment for depression. Your doctor or mental health professional can prescribe drugs to help reduce your child's feelings of sadness or helplessness.

  - Especially for teens with depression, it is important to balance the expected benefits of antidepressant drugs with the potential risk of suicide. Depending on the medications used, it may take several weeks before your child's depression starts to improve.

  - Your child will be monitored closely while receiving antidepressant medications.

- *Psychotherapy* is often helpful for depressed children. Talking to a mental health professional can help your child understand factors affecting his or her feelings and how to manage depression in everyday life.

- If other mental health problems are present (for example, anxiety or drug or alcohol abuse), these will need to be evaluated and treated as well.

- Treatment may also include family therapy, parent management training, and involvement in your child's school. Specific treatments depend on many factors, including the severity of your child's depression, the situation at home, and other accompanying problems.

- Your child should receive follow-up exams or sessions to see how his or her depression is responding to treatment. Depression can be a chronic or recurrent problem, especially without proper treatment and follow-up.

When should I call your office?

- Call your mental health provider if your child's symptoms of depression get worse, if they don't start getting better with treatment, or if they return after treatment.

- If you cannot reach your mental health provider and you're concerned about these or other problems, call our office.

- If your depressed teen talks about committing suicide, call your mental health professional or doctor's office immediately. If you cannot reach anybody, take your child to the emergency room.

Divorce

Having parents get divorced or separated is usually a difficult experience for children. They react to divorce in different ways: younger children may become depressed, while older children may become angry. The best ways to help your child adjust after a divorce are to make sure he or she remains involved with both parents and to avoid conflict with your ex-husband or ex-wife.

How do I deal with divorce?

Going through a divorce or separation is a very hard time for your family. When considering divorce, all parents worry about how it will affect their children. Your child's reactions will depend on many factors, including his or her age and temperament and how well the family was functioning before the split. Another key factor is the parents' ability to focus on their child's reactions during this sad and stressful time.

Divorce can have harmful effects on children. However, there are ways of helping your child adapt to the change. Probably the most important thing is to avoid putting your child in the middle of any family conflicts. You should also allow your child to maintain contact with both parents, if possible. If needed, your doctor's office can put you in touch with mental health professionals and others who can help your family.

How do children react to divorce?

Every child is different, but children of certain ages tend to react in different ways:

- Very young children (5 or under) may become distressed, sad, or irritable. Behavior problems are common; for example, your child may start "acting like a baby" (sometimes called *regression*).

- In school-aged children, reactions may range from indifference to depression to anger. Most children cling to the hope that the divorce or separation won't really happen. Your child may feel guilty, as if the breakup were his or her fault. Children may try to protect their parents by blaming themselves. Behavior problems or symptoms of illness may be an attempt to keep the parents together.

- Older children and teens are usually angry. They may feel disillusioned and let down by one or both parents. Conflict at home, poor school performance, drug or alcohol abuse, and other behavior problems are common in these children.

What is the long-term impact of divorce on children?

Divorce can obviously have negative effects on children. Some remain unhappy and dissatisfied with their family lives in the years after divorce. In adulthood, some children of divorce are reluctant to form intimate relationships because they fear repeating their parents' experience.

However, other children and families adapt well to divorce. Although divorce is sad, some children and families find they do better without the frequent conflicts that led to the split. The parents' reactions—both when the breakup happens and in the months and years afterward—have a major impact on the children's responses.

How can I help my child adjust after divorce?

- The initial separation is often the hardest time for children as well as for parents. Both you and your child are likely to feel loss, sadness, anger, and distress.

- Try to continue your child's usual routines—including school and friendships—as much as possible. Keep consistent expectations for good behavior, chores and responsibilities, and discipline.

- Allow your child to talk about his or her feelings. Make sure your children know that the divorce is not their fault and that there is nothing they can do to bring their parents back together.

- Parents should take care of themselves as well. Pay attention to your health, and keep in touch with your social support system such as friends and extended family.

- Don't criticize or complain about your spouse in front of your child. Even though you're angry, it is harmful to insult the other parent or to expect your child to take sides.

- The best thing you can do to promote healthy adjustment is to allow your child to maintain contact with the other parent and to avoid conflict with your ex-spouse. Siblings and other family members are also an important source of support.

- Remember that divorce is an ongoing process. As your child grows and develops, the impact of your family situation will change as well.

- Counseling can be very helpful. Our office can put you in touch with mental health professionals for your child or yourself.

When should I call your office?

If your family is experiencing separation, divorce, or other problems, talking to your doctor may be helpful for recommendations on the care and services that are best for your child and family.

Drugs and Alcohol: Use and Abuse

Many teens try alcohol, drugs, or both at some time. It's important to talk openly with your child about substance use, including the consequences of breaking rules regarding drugs and alcohol. He or she also needs to know about the serious dangers of substance abuse and addiction. If you have concerns about your child's drug or alcohol use, make sure to discuss them with your doctor.

How do I deal with my child's drug and alcohol use?

Experimenting with drugs or alcohol is very common during adolescence—perhaps even normal. Still, using drugs or alcohol always carries a risk of harm, especially in younger teens and when driving is involved. Driving under the influence of alcohol or drugs is a very serious health risk to both your child and others.

When drug or alcohol use becomes frequent or affects your child's daily functioning, it becomes a problem that needs treatment. Substance abuse is not an isolated problem but is part of larger issues related to your child and family. Your doctor is an important source of information, evaluation, and treatment for problems related to drug and alcohol abuse.

What do drug and alcohol abuse look like?

For most parents, discovering that their child has been using drugs or alcohol comes as an unpleasant surprise. Your child may have behavior changes or a sudden drop in grades at school. Other signs may include:

- Missing school.

- Having a lot of accidents or injuries, especially car accidents.

- Having physical complaints and symptoms with no apparent explanation.

The changes you notice may depend on what substance(s) your child has been using. With all of these substances (except marijuana), overdoses can be fatal.

- *Alcohol.* Your child may seem giddy, groggy, or talkative. Slurred speech and stumbling are common. If he or she becomes very drunk, your child may pass out. Alcohol abuse is still the biggest substance abuse problem.

- *Marijuana.* Your child may act giddy and elated. He or she may seem scattered and have difficulty concentrating and remembering. Appetite is increased and inhibitions are decreased. Your child may seem lazy and uninterested in his or her usual activities, especially with long-term marijuana use.

- *Hallucinogens.* Such drugs include LSD ("acid"), MDMA ("ecstasy" or "X"), and PCP ("angel dust"). These drugs alter perceptions and awareness. Your child may lose his or her sense of reality, seeing or hearing things that aren't there (hallucinations). Some types of hallucinogenic drugs may cause seizures or stroke.

- *Cocaine.* Cocaine may be sniffed or smoked ("crack"). Your child may seem giddy and overactive. Widened pupils and fast heartbeat are common. Seizures, bleeding in the brain, heart attack, and other serious medical complications may develop.

- *Amphetamines.* Amphetamines are also known as methamphetamine or "speed." Your child may seem agitated, overexcited, restless, or talkative. As the drug wears off, he or she may "crash," suddenly becoming depressed. With long-term use, personality changes, weight loss, and medical complications may occur. Medical risks include convulsions/seizures and abnormal heart rhythms.

- *Opiates.* For example heroin, which may be sniffed, injected, or taken in other ways. It causes an intense "high" at first, then grogginess and sleepiness. Heroin is highly addictive; addicts who cannot get the drug experience intense withdrawal symptoms. Medical complications are common, including coma and apnea (not breathing).

- *"Date rape" drugs.* Drugs such as Rohypnol or GHB may be given to an unsuspecting person as part of a sexual assault. The victim may not remember anything about the attack afterward. Alcohol may also act as a "date rape" drug.

What increases the risk of drug and alcohol abuse?

- A number of factors are involved in the development of abuse. Genetic factors may play a role; for example, alcoholism runs in families. Other contributors may include family problems and other stressors, depression, the availability of drugs, and peer pressure.

- Certain other conditions are linked to substance abuse, including conduct disorder, attention deficit–hyperactivity disorder (ADHD), and personality disorders. Children who start using drugs in their early teen years may be more likely to have substance abuse problems in adulthood.

What are some possible complications of drug and alcohol abuse?

There are too many complications to list. Drug and alcohol abuse cause serious health, family, and social problems. Consequences range from difficulties in home and work life, to legal problems, to life-threatening medical complications.

Can drug and alcohol abuse be prevented?

- To reduce your child's chances of developing a substance abuse problem, provide a supportive environment that allows your child to build positive life attitudes, behaviors, and relationships.

- Talk openly with children about drugs and alcohol, even before the teen years. Encourage healthy after-school activities, such as sports.

- In a way that is appropriate for your children's ages, keep an eye on their activities: who their friends are, where they go after school, what time they get home at night. Even for older teens, parents need to set rules for expected behavior and enforce consequences for rule breaking.

- Talk to your child about the dangers of alcohol and driving. Make sure he or she knows never to get in a car with anyone who has been drinking or is on drugs. Establish a rule that he or she can call you for a ride at any time, with "few questions asked."

What should I do about my child's drug or alcohol use?

- If you have concerns about substance abuse by your child or adolescent, make sure to mention them to your doctor. He or she can talk to you and your child and assess the severity of the drug or alcohol use. This may include blood or urine tests for drugs or alcohol. For older teens, drug testing without the patient's permission is generally not recommended, except in certain situations (for example, repeated injuries or accidents).

- The way to deal with drug or alcohol use depends on many factors, including the age of the child, his or her situation at home or at school, what substances are being used, and how often.

- The severity of the drug or alcohol abuse is the main factor to consider in treatment. We may recommend a treatment program for substance abusers or referral to a specialized counselor. These programs can fully assess your child and recommend the most appropriate level and intensity of treatment.

- Treatment may start with a brief intervention, offering information and advice to your teen about the need to make good decisions about drugs and alcohol. This is most appropriate if substance abuse is a new or short-term problem.

- Teens with more severe problems may need more intensive treatment. A stay in the hospital or other special treatment center may be needed for "detoxification." This is especially important if substance abuse has caused medical or psychological problems.

- Patients with serious substance abuse often need long-term rehabilitation. This includes medical follow-up as well as psychosocial support to deal with drug or alcohol dependence and related issues. Family therapy or group therapy—sometimes including other teens with substance abuse problems—can be helpful.

- After treatment, there is always the danger of a relapse. Follow-up with a professional or with a "help" group such as Alcoholics Anonymous is invaluable for helping substance abusers to stay sober over the long term.

When should I call your office?

- Call our office if you have any concerns related to drug or alcohol use by your teenager or younger child. Recognizing and dealing with the problem as early as possible can help to minimize the damaging effects on your child's life.

- After your child has had treatment for substance abuse, call our office if he or she shows any signs of using drugs or alcohol again (relapse).

- If your child shows signs of serious drug or alcohol intoxication or medical complications (such as unconsciousness, seizures, difficulty breathing, and so forth) seek medical care immediately. *This is a potential emergency.*

Eating Disorders

Eating disorders are fairly common in teens, especially girls. These children have unrealistic expectations of how their bodies should look. Patients with anorexia nervosa avoid food because they think they're fat, even though they're really too thin. However, even a child who is normal weight or overweight can have an eating disorder. Poor nutrition can lead to serious health problems. With treatment, including nutritional therapy and counseling, many patients with eating disorders recover.

What are eating disorders?

Patients with eating disorders have abnormal eating habits related to unrealistic fears of being fat. The two main eating disorders are *anorexia nervosa,* in which patients eat little or no food, and *bulimia nervosa,* in which they eat heavily then make themselves vomit (throw up) or engage in other abnormal behaviors to avoid gaining weight.

Eating disorders can lead to serious complications. In severe cases, the patient can starve to death. Recovery usually requires medical, nutritional, and mental health treatment.

What do they look like?

In both anorexia nervosa and bulimia nervosa, your child develops abnormal eating behaviors because she or he fears getting fat.

Anorexia nervosa. Your child severely limits the amount she eats, especially foods she considers fattening. Symptoms include:

- Intense fear of getting fat, even after losing weight.

- Unrealistic view of her body: "feels fat," even if she looks skinny to others.

- Refusal to gain weight, even normal weight for growth.

- If beyond puberty, child stops having menstrual periods.

- Other symptoms may include:

  - Exercises excessively.

  - Never admits to being hungry, yet is preoccupied with food. Eating behaviors may seem unusual.

Bulimia nervosa. Patients with bulimia nervosa are not necessarily underweight but are overly concerned about body weight and shape. They also have a sense of losing control over their eating habits. Your child may "binge and purge"—this means eating a lot all at once, then getting rid of the food by vomiting or other ways, such as enemas, fasting, or exercise.

- Eating binges occur over a short period, often in secret. During these times, your child may fear she won't be able to stop eating.

- After bingeing, your child may make herself vomit, often by sticking a finger down her throat. Some patients with bulimia use laxatives. Others switch between periods of bingeing and periods of eating hardly any food.

- Your child's weight may go up and down. Patients with bulimia are usually not as thin as those with anorexia.

What causes eating disorders?

Many factors may contribute to eating disorders, including the family environment and the child's personality characteristics. Our culture's preoccupation with being thin and dieting plays a role. Eating disorders seem to run in families.

What are some possible complications of eating disorders?

Eating disorders can cause many serious health problems. Almost any organ in the body may be affected. Some of these complications, but not all, resolve when the patient starts eating normally again.

- Heart rate and blood pressure abnormalities.

- Dental problems caused by vomiting: cavities or erosion of tooth enamel.

- Sleep problems.

- Changes in normal hormone levels, leading to lack of menstrual periods in girls.

- Slow growth or no growth.

- Kidney problems.

- Difficulties thinking and concentrating.

- Abnormal changes in body chemistry (electrolytes), sometimes related to drinking a lot of water or abusing laxatives.

- Weakening of the bones, which may lead to fractures.

- In severe cases, death may occur, often related to electrolyte problems in the blood. Suicide occasionally occurs, most often with anorexia nervosa.

What puts your child at risk of eating disorders?

- If your child is preoccupied with how her body looks, and especially with the fear of being fat, she may be at increased risk of anorexia or bulimia.

- If you or others in your family have had eating disorders, your child may be at higher risk.

- Eating disorders are much more common in girls, but boys can have them too.

- Eating disorders are most common in the teen years but may start in childhood and last into adulthood.

- Eating disorders were once thought to occur mainly in higher income groups. However, they are now known to occur in all races and income levels.

Can eating disorders be prevented?

- Get regular medical checkups for your child to ensure that he or she is growing and gaining weight normally.

- It may help to discuss unrealistic expectations about how the body should look with your child. As a society in general and as parents, we should not focus too much on appearance, particularly on being thin.

How are eating disorders treated?

If we suspect your child has anorexia or bulimia, we will recommend a visit to a specialized team for evaluation and treatment. Eating disorders can be difficult to diagnose and treat. Your child may deny there is any problem and resist attempts to change her eating habits.

Treatment for eating disorders will probably include:

- *Nutrition therapy,* especially *re-feeding.* Your child may be treated in the hospital for a while to ensure proper nutrition under medical supervision.

- *Psychotherapy* with a psychiatrist, psychologist, or other mental health professional.

- *Behavior modification* and *nutritional rehabilitation.* Your child should receive long-term follow-up to help change her attitudes toward food and eating and to stop unhealthy eating habits.

Other treatments may be recommended, depending on your child's situation. For example, antidepressant medications are helpful if your child is depressed.

When should I call your office?

Any child with an eating disorder should receive regular medical follow-up. During treatments, call your child's therapist if:

- The eating problems don't seem to be getting better, or if they return after treatment.

- You have other concerns about mental health issues.

Our office will continue to oversee your child's overall health. Call if you have any health questions, or in an emergency if your child's therapist is unavailable.

Nightmares and Night Terrors

Nightmares are very common in children. Your child awakens suddenly, scared by a "bad dream." Reassure your child by reminding him or her that the dream wasn't real and that everything is all right. Night terrors are less common but also usually are harmless. Your child suddenly screams, often without waking up. Afterward, he or she doesn't remember the event.

What are nightmares and night terrors?

Nightmares are just bad dreams—everyone has them now and then. Nightmares may seem very real, especially to younger children. Just telling your child that the nightmare was "just a dream" and that he or she is safe and protected may calm him or her down enough to return to sleep.

Night terrors, sometimes called sleep terrors, are different. Your child cries out in the middle of the night as if terrified. However, he or she does not seem very responsive and may not even wake up. When your child finally does wake up, he or she doesn't remember any bad dream.

Both nightmares and night terrors might be helped by providing a relaxing bedtime routine. If these or other sleep problems become a frequent event, be sure to discuss them with your child's doctor.

What do they look like?

Nightmares:

- Scary or vivid dreams that cause your child to awaken suddenly.

- Most common around ages 3 to 5 but can occur in older children.

- Most commonly occur very early in the morning (4:00 to 6:00 a.m.), when your child is sleeping relatively lightly. This kind of sleep is called rapid-eye movement (REM) sleep. However, nightmares can occur at other times.

- Your child will probably recall the dream very clearly. The dream may involve something disturbing experienced that day. Your child may have the same dream repeatedly.

- Because nightmares are so scary, it may be difficult for your child to settle down and go back to sleep.

Night terrors:

- Your child suddenly screams and sits up in bed. He or she may seem very agitated—sweating, heart racing, pupils wide.

- Even though his or her eyes are open, your child may actually still be asleep. It may be several minutes before he or she finally wakes up.

- When your child does awaken, he or she doesn't remember any bad dream. As a result, getting back to sleep after night terrors may be less difficult than after than nightmares.

- These episodes are most common in preschool and older children.

Sleepwalking occurs when your child gets out of bed and moves around, even though he or she is still asleep.

What causes nightmares and night terrors?

- Occasional nightmares are normal. Night terrors are less common, but they still occur in many children. Night terrors may run in families.

- Usually there is no specific cause. Nightmares are often related to something your child experienced during the day. Scary movies or TV shows commonly cause nightmares.

- Certain medications may lead to nightmares.

- If nightmares or night terrors occur frequently, they may result from something that's bothering your child. Be sure to discuss this with your doctor.

How can nightmares and night terrors be prevented?

- Having a stable, relaxing bedtime routine may be helpful. Put your child to bed around the same time every night. Don't let him or her get overtired. Allow some time for the excitement of the day to wind down before bedtime.

- Don't let your child see movies or TV shows that are scary or violent.

- Nightmares sometimes reflect a problem or worry in your child's life. If you can figure out the source of the worry, it may help to talk to your child about it.

What can be done about nightmares and night terrors?

- Nightmares and night terrors rarely signal a serious problem. Usually no special treatment is needed, except for comforting your child.

- If nightmares or night terrors persist or are very frequent, call your doctor's office. Rarely, they are a sign of some problem affecting your child's life.

Nightmares:

● Hug and comfort your child. Let him or her talk about the bad dream.

● Reassure your child it was just a dream. Point out familiar things in the bedroom. Remind your child that you are nearby and he or she is safe and protected.

● Try to distract your child by talking about other things—maybe something fun that's coming up the next day. It may take a little while before your child is able to stop thinking about the bad dream.

● It's best not to let the child stay up or sleep in your bed. If you do, it may be harder to get him or her back to bed after the next bad dream.

Night terrors:

● Don't panic! Night terrors can be pretty alarming for parents, but they are usually harmless to the child.

● Attempt to wake your child gently. He or she may not respond, at least at first.

● When your child does awaken, he or she will probably remember little or nothing about the event. It proba-bly won't be difficult to get him or her to go back to sleep.

Sleepwalking:

● Like night terrors, sleepwalking is usually harmless. The problem is that your child may be injured when he or she gets out of bed while still asleep. You may need to put some safety measures in place to prevent such injuries. For example, you may have to put a gate in the doorway to your child's room, especially if there are stairs.

When should I call your office?

Call our office if:

● Nightmares or night terrors are a frequent or persistent problem.

● Night terrors or frequent nightmares occur in an older child or adolescent.

● Nightmares or night terrors appear related to some specific traumatic event in your child's life or if they seem to be related to medications he or she is taking.

Obsessive-Compulsive Disorder

Children with obsessive-compulsive disorder have repeated thoughts and rituals that are upsetting or get in the way of everyday activities. For example, if children are obsessed with worry about germs, they may constantly wash their hands. Specialist evaluation and treatment can reduce your child's obsessive-compulsive behavior.

What is obsessive-compulsive disorder?

Obsessive-compulsive disorder (OCD) is a relatively common mental health problem in children and teens. Your child may have obsessive worries (cannot stop thinking about them) and compulsive rituals (cannot stop doing them). The worries and rituals are disturbing, take up a lot of time, and interfere with home and school activities.

Obsessive-compulsive disorder can be an upsetting problem for your child and family. Your child probably would like to stop the compulsive behavior but cannot control it. Effective treatments for OCD are available. Your doctor can put you in touch with mental health professionals who can diagnose and treat this problem.

What does it look like?

- *Obsessions* are specific, repeated thoughts that your child just cannot keep out of his or her mind. For example, he or she may constantly worry about germs and dirt, or that an intruder will break into your home.

- *Compulsions* are specific, repeated behaviors that your child enacts to deal with his or her worries. For example, if she is worried about germs, your child may wash her hands constantly. If your child is worried about intruders, he may continually check that all windows and doors are locked.

- Your child's worries are usually unrealistic and illogical. The compulsive behaviors may go on in an endless cycle because your child may fear that something terrible will happen unless he or she does certain things.

- Rituals may occur when your child is under stress or when some life change occurs.

What causes obsessive-compulsive disorder?

The exact cause of OCD is unknown. It seems to be related to abnormal activity in certain parts of the brain. Since OCD runs in families, genetic factors are likely involved.

In about 10% of children with OCD, the problem may be related to infection with a certain type of bacteria called group A streptococci. This type of OCD may occur suddenly and is sometimes accompanied by nervous tics (specific, repeated muscle movements).

What are some possible complications of obsessive-compulsive disorder?

There are no medical complications of OCD. However, it can cause serious interference with your child's schoolwork and activities and social life. Effective treatment can help to lessen the impact of OCD on your child's life.

What puts your child at risk of obsessive-compulsive disorder?

- If you or someone else in your family has had OCD, your child may be at increased risk.

- Infection with group A streptococci (rarely).

- Usually starts in adolescence, but sometimes earlier.

Can obsessive-compulsive disorder be prevented?

There is no known way to prevent OCD.

How is obsessive-compulsive disorder treated?

- If your child has symptoms of OCD, we will probably recommend a visit to a child and adolescent psychiatrist or other mental health professional. This specialist can evaluate and recommend the best treatment for your child.

- Medications are an important part of treatment for OCD. Antidepressants or other drugs may be recommended. It may take several weeks for these drugs to have their full effect. When OCD is related to infection with group A streptococci, antibiotics may be used.

- Psychotherapy may be recommended. Psychotherapy works by helping your child to understand the reasons why he or she acts in certain ways and by building a relationship with the therapist.

- Cognitive-behavioral therapy can help your child look at his or her fears more realistically and learn more effective ways of dealing with them.

- For many patients with OCD, a combination of medications and psychotherapy gives the best results.

- Treatment usually doesn't "cure" OCD completely. However, it can reduce your child's obsessive fears and compulsive behaviors and allow him or her to get on with life. Having OCD is nothing to be ashamed of—it is a fairly common and treatable mental health disorder.

When should I call your office?

- Children with OCD should receive regular mental health follow-up visits.

- Call your mental health provider if the obsessive worries or compulsive rituals don't seem to be getting better or if they return after treatment.

- If you cannot reach your mental health provider and you're concerned about these or other problems, call our office.

Panic Attacks and Panic Disorder

> Panic attacks are very upsetting for your child and family. Your child may have episodes of intense fear causing physical and psychological reactions. Your child may even fear that he or she is going to die, which makes the panic even worse. Effective treatments are available that can help keep panic attacks from interfering with your child's life.

What are panic attacks?

Panic attacks are sudden, repeated episodes of intense fear or discomfort. In addition to being upsetting for your child, the attacks cause physical symptoms, such as a racing heartbeat and a feeling that it's hard to breathe. These symptoms make your child's sense of panic even greater.

Panic attacks that occur frequently enough to interfere with your child's life are called *panic disorder*. In extreme cases, he or she may develop a fear of being in places where escape is difficult or impossible, such as in public. This condition is called *agoraphobia*.

Professional evaluation and treatment are essential and can help to lessen the impact of panic attacks and panic disorder.

What do they look like?

- Panic attacks may occur suddenly and unpredictably. It is often unclear what triggers them.

- Your child feels intense fear or discomfort. Often, he or she feels that something is going to go terribly wrong, or that he or she is dying.

- Physical symptoms occur, including:
  - Pounding heartbeat (palpitations).
  - Sweating, shaking, dizziness.
  - Shortness of breath; your child may feel like he or she cannot breathe.

- The physical and psychological symptoms set up a vicious circle: your child feels like she cannot breathe, which makes her feel like something bad is going to happen, causing her to panic even more.

- If your child has repeated panic attacks, he or she may be afraid to be away from home and may refuse to go out, even to attend school.

What are some possible complications of panic attacks?

- Panic attacks can interfere with school and other activities, especially if your child becomes fearful of going out.

- People with panic disorder may have other psychiatric disorders as well, such as anxiety, depression, and drug or alcohol abuse.

What puts your child at risk of panic attacks?

- Attacks most commonly start between ages 15 and 19.

- They may be more likely to occur in teens with other psychiatric disorders, including anxiety and depression, drug or alcohol abuse, or phobias (irrational fears).

Can panic attacks be prevented?

There is no known way to prevent initial panic attacks. However, effective treatments may help to prevent future attacks.

How are panic attacks treated?

Even for doctors, it can be difficult to determine that your child is having a panic attack. For example, shortness of breath may lead to tests for asthma and other breathing disorders. After a medical examination, your doctor may be able to reassure you and your child that there is no physical problem causing shortness of breath, racing heartbeat, or similar symptoms.

We may recommend a visit to a child and adolescent psychiatrist or other mental health professional. This specialist will perform a thorough evaluation and recommend a plan to treat your child's panic attacks.

- Several types of treatment can help teens (and adults) with panic attacks and panic disorder:
  - Medications, including antidepressants. These drugs may help make panic attacks less frequent.
  - Counseling or psychotherapy may help your child to reduce stress and other factors that trigger panic attacks, as well as learn new ways of interrupting panic attacks when they start.
  - A combination of medications and psychotherapy is most helpful for many patients.

- Panic attacks may lessen over time, especially with good medical follow-up and mental health care.

When should I call your office?

If your child's panic attacks continue or seem to get worse after the start of treatment, call your mental health provider. (If your child has been prescribed antidepressant medications, it may be a few weeks before they take full effect.) If you cannot reach your mental health provider and you're concerned about panic attacks or other problems, call our office.

Phobias

Fears are a normal part of growing up. At specific ages, children are normally afraid of certain things. Phobias are extreme and persistent fears that make your child anxious fairly frequently and interfere with his or her usual routines. Simply talking to your child about his or her fears can help to reduce them. If phobias are causing a lot of disruption in your child's life, mental health treatment can be helpful.

What are phobias?

All children have some fears. Certain fears seem to be normal at specific stages of your child's development. For example, babies and toddlers are commonly afraid of strangers or of being separated from their parents. Preschoolers tend to be afraid of imaginary things, like monsters. Older kids may have more realistic but unlikely fears, such as natural disasters.

When your child becomes preoccupied by a specific fear or it starts interfering with his or her usual activities, the fear becomes a phobia. In many cases, your child will respond to reassurance that he or she is safe and protected. Irrational fears usually go away after a while. More severe phobias can disrupt your child's life, leading to refusal to attend school or other problems. If this is the situation, your doctor may recommend evaluation and treatment by a mental health professional.

What do they look like?

- Phobias are not just fears. They are fears that are greater than they should be—out of proportion to whatever is causing them. If they continue, phobias can interfere with your child's activities.

- Fear of strangers or unfamiliar situations may lead your child to become very shy, making it difficult for him or her to make friends. Sometimes, children with these *social phobias* refuse to go to school. In severe cases, children with social phobias may refuse to leave home at all. This is called *agoraphobia* and may occur with panic attacks.

- Fear of the dark or fear of being alone may interfere with sleep. Your child may refuse to go to bed or to stay in bed. These fears may be normal at certain ages. However, when they become extreme and persistent, they are phobias.

- Your child may develop irrational fears of specific things, for example, dogs, insects, heights, flying, or being in closed spaces. He or she may avoid any situation in which there is a chance of encountering the feared object.

What causes phobias?

- It is unclear why normal childhood fears sometimes develop into phobias. They may arise from early, unpleasant experiences or may reflect an insecure attachment to parents.

- Phobias may be a reaction to a stressful situation in your family. For example, your child may become fearful around the time of a divorce or separation, after moving to a new home, or when a parent becomes ill.

What are some possible complications of phobias?

- Phobias can make it difficult for your child to have the normal experiences and opportunities of childhood, such as making friends and trying new things. More severe phobias can interfere with school attendance and disrupt your family's life.

- Phobias are sometimes part of other problems related to anxiety, such as panic disorder.

What puts your child at risk of phobias?

A history of anxiety in your child or family may make your child more likely to have irrational, disruptive fears.

Can phobias be prevented?

Reassure your child that he or she is safe from harm. Avoid exposing him or her to frightening things, including scary movies or TV shows.

How are phobias treated?

In most cases, simply continuing to reassure your child can do a lot to reduce his or her fears.

- Let your child know that he or she is safe and protected.

- Help your child find ways of dealing with the fear. For example, provide a nightlight for children who are afraid of the dark.

- Be sympathetic, and let your child know that his or her fears are normal. Especially with older children, point out when what they fear is very unlikely to happen.

- As much as possible, put limits on the extent to which fears disrupt your child's activities. For example, be understanding that your child is anxious about going to school, but don't let him or her simply stop going to school.

If your child's fears seem more severe, or if they are interfering with his or her normal activities, your doctor may recommend a visit to a child and adolescent psychiatrist or other mental health provider.

- Childhood fears and phobias often improve a lot with relatively simple treatments. They don't necessarily mean that your child has a serious mental disorder.

- Psychotherapy can help your child to understand what's causing his or her fears and to see them more realistically.

- If fears are very specific, a process called *desensitization* may be recommended. In this form of therapy, your child is gradually exposed to whatever it is he or she fears and taught ways of dealing with the fear. The goal is that, over time, your child will be better able to tolerate the feared object.

- Medications are generally not helpful for children with phobias. However, if depression or panic attacks are present, antidepressants or other medications may be a helpful part of treatment. It may take several weeks before these medications begin to take effect.

When should I call your office?

Call our office if:

- Your child develops fears that interfere with his or her usual activities or cause a lot of distress.

- Your child's phobias don't seem to be getting better by talking about them or after starting treatment.

- Your child's phobias seem to be getting worse, or he or she is having panic attacks.

☐ Suicide ☐

Suicide is the third most common cause of death of adolescents and young adults. Teen suicide rates have increased dramatically over the years. If your teen has attempted or talked about suicide, it is very important to take the situation seriously. Evaluation and treatment by a mental health professional are needed to assess your child's risk of attempting suicide.

Adolescent suicide—what do we know about it?

Suicide and suicide attempts are relatively common among teenagers and young adults. Many thousands of young people in the United States attempt suicide each year, and about 2000 succeed. Certain factors increase the risk of teen suicide, especially previous suicide attempts, depression, and drug and alcohol abuse.

By far most adolescents survive the suicide attempt. Although most teens who make one suicide attempt don't try again, they are at increased risk of future attempts. Professional mental health evaluation and treatment are the best ways to reduce this risk.

What increases your child's risk of suicide?

The three main risk factors for adolescent suicide are:

- Previous suicide attempts.
- Depression and other mood disorders.
- Drug or alcohol abuse (especially alcohol).

If any of these three risk factors are present—especially in combination—contact our office. All are serious problems that should be evaluated by a mental health professional.

Certain other factors are related to higher suicide risk in teens:

- Suicide attempts occur in all races and social classes. Native-American boys seem to have the highest risk. Suicide rates among African-American boys are increasing.
- Girls carry out more suicide attempts, but boys are more likely to actually kill themselves. This may be because boys are more likely to use violent methods, especially guns. Taking a lot of pills is the most common form of attempted suicide—fortunately, it is also one of the least likely to succeed.
- Gay or bisexual teens have a higher suicide rate than straight teens.

- Having a gun at home is a major risk factor for successful suicide. This is so even if the guns are unloaded and locked up. We recommend removing all guns from the home, especially if your child has risk factors for suicide.
- Past mental health or behavioral problems, such as foster home or group home placement, physical or sexual abuse, or psychiatric illnesses put a child at increased risk.
- Genetic factors may play a role.

What leads to adolescent suicide attempts?

It can be difficult for adults, especially parents, to understand why a teenager would attempt to commit suicide. Suicide attempts by teenagers are influenced by cultural factors, mental health disorders, stressful life events, or personal problems, such as:

- Fights with parents, or parents' marital problems.
- Trouble at school—discipline problems or flunking.
- Breaking up with a boyfriend or girlfriend.
- Feeling isolated from peers.
- "Cluster suicides" may occur; news reports about teen suicides sometimes seem to prompt other suicide attempts.

How can doctors help after adolescent suicide attempts?

- When a teen (or an adult) attempts or talks about suicide, it may be viewed as a "cry for help." People only attempt suicide when they are feeling desperate. It is important for your child to understand that the "cry for help" has been heard and that he or she will be helped.
- If your child has made a suicide attempt, has talked seriously about suicide, or seems to be at high risk of suicide:
  - *We will recommend that your child see a psychiatrist or other mental health professional as soon as possible.* This expert will perform a thorough evaluation of your child's suicide risk and recommend further action.
- To be on the safe side, psychiatric hospitalization is sometimes recommended after suicide attempts. It allows time for the situation to calm down and permits a full medical and mental health evaluation.
- In other situations, management outside the hospital may be the best option. Even if your child seems to be at relatively "low risk" for a successful suicide attempt, the situation should be treated seriously. Seeing a crisis counselor may help your family to deal with the situation and to figure out what the next step should be.

● It is very important to get follow-up care for your child and family. Follow-up sessions should include education about adolescent suicide and its treatment and the warning signs of repeat suicide attempts.

What are the warning signs of adolescent suicide?

Although each case is different, certain warning signs should raise concern about possible suicide attempts.

❗ ● *Any time your child talks about committing suicide, wishing he or she was dead, etc., seek help immediately.* Statements about killing oneself should always be taken seriously.

Other possible warning signs include:

● Sudden behavior changes. Even suddenly acting cheerful after a long period of depression may be a warning sign of a suicide attempt.

● Statements of hopelessness ("Nothing matters anyway").

● Talking a lot about death and dying.

● Obtaining a gun.

● Giving away or throwing away possessions.

● Serious trouble with parents or at school.

It's important for parents to keep a dialog open with children and teens. Make it easy for them to talk about problems. If your child seems to have emotional problems, such as anxiety or depression, be sure to mention it to the doctor. On a broad scale, it would be helpful for schools to encourage teens to recognize suicide risk.

📱 When should I call your office?

Call our office if:

● Your child talks about committing suicide, or any of the warning signs occur. Seek help as soon as possible. Contact your mental health provider, or call our office.

● *Your child has made or is planning a suicide attempt. Get help immediately!* Our office can provide you with a local suicide hotline number, or call the National Hopeline Network at 1-800-SUICIDE (1-800-784-2433). **❗**

Temper Tantrums

Temper tantrums are a common problem in toddlers, and one that can be difficult for parents to handle. It is important to remain calm and keep your own anger under control when handling your child's temper tantrums. Children usually outgrow temper tantrums after age 3.

What are temper tantrums?

Temper tantrums are common in toddlers, especially between 18 months and 3 years. Tantrums may be triggered by a number of things, most often anger or frustration at not getting something your child wants. They may also be influenced by overtiredness, hunger, or attention seeking.

Temper tantrums can be very challenging for parents to handle. If you give in to your child's demands or if you get angry yourself, your child will learn that throwing tantrums gets a response. Responding calmly and with control is the best way to handle tantrums. You'll be glad to hear that problems with temper tantrums eventually go away!

What do they look like?

- A tantrum includes any kind of inappropriate behavior that your child uses to express anger or frustration. When upset, your child may cry, scream, or hold his or her breath. The behavior may seem way out of proportion to your child's disappointment.

- During the toddler years (the "terrible twos"), tantrums can become a frequent problem. Sometimes it may seem as if your child has a tantrum anytime he doesn't get what he wants.

- Tantrums have a definite effect on parents. You may feel angry, embarrassed, and overwhelmed by your child's behavior. Understanding why young children have tantrums and forming a rational plan for dealing with them can reduce a lot of the negative impact of tantrums.

What causes temper tantrums?

As toddlers grow, they want to be more independent, but they're too young to really make many decisions for themselves. They're also not intellectually mature enough to understand the reasons for things, or why they have to wait for some things. They lack the language skills to express their frustration in words. It's also hard for them to control powerful emotions, especially if they are feeling tired or hungry.

All of these factors contribute to temper tantrums as a way for young children to express frustration and anger. Handling tantrums in a "calm, cool, and collected" way helps to prevent them from turning into a regular habit.

What are some possible complications of temper tantrums?

- The main risk of tantrums is that your child will somehow be hurt while he or she is out of control. You may need to take steps to ensure your child's safety until the tantrum has passed.

- Sometimes children hold their breath so long that they faint. Although these "breath-holding spells" are scary, they don't really cause any harm.

- If these severe types of tantrums become a frequent occurrence—or if they are accompanied by other problems like head banging or very aggressive behavior—you should discuss the problem with your doctor.

What puts your child at risk of temper tantrums?

Children with certain medical conditions, disabilities, or developmental problems may be more likely to have tantrums.

Toddlers may be more likely to have temper tantrums in certain situations:

- When feeling tired, hungry, or sick.

- At times of stress or changes at home; for example, when a new baby comes home.

- When usual routines are disrupted.

Can temper tantrums be prevented?

There are things you can do to help keep temper tantrums to a minimum:

- Establish routines and stick to them as much as possible. Tantrums may be less likely if your child knows what to expect during the day.

- Be firm but flexible. Make clear to your child what kind of behavior you expect from him or her, but try not to be too strict.

- Allow your child to make choices when possible. This helps children feel like they have some control over their day.

- Avoid overstimulation and frustration if possible. Know when your child is starting to have enough excitement for one day. Provide him or her with age-appropriate activities; toddlers sometimes get frustrated when they can't do things older kids are doing.

- Make sure your child gets enough sleep and don't let him or her get too hungry.

What's the best way to handle tantrums?

- Handling tantrums in a "calm, cool, and collected" way is the best way to shorten and reduce the number of tantrums.

- Turn away for a minute or two. This gives your child time to recover, while allowing him or her to see that the tantrum isn't getting the desired response.

- Try not to get angry. Don't hit or spank your child. If you react with anger, your child will get the message that out-of-control emotions are an acceptable way to respond to frustrating situations. If you're having trouble staying calm, leave the room for a few minutes. *The most important thing is to show your child the ways of controlling anger that you want him or her to use.*

- Don't give your child what he or she wants to make the tantrum stop. If you do, your child will get the message that tantrums work!

- If tantrums are relatively minor, you can often just ignore them. You may be able to distract your child with a toy or by making funny faces. Saying positive things and giving your child a chance to calm down may be helpful. If that doesn't work, then turn away until the tantrum has passed.

- If your toddler is holding his or her breath, you can usually just ignore it. Even if he or she passes out, there is rarely any harm done. But be sure to mention this behavior to your doctor.

- For more severe tantrums, you may need to take steps to ensure that your child doesn't hurt himself or others or doesn't destroy property. If the tantrum is happening in a public place, take your child somewhere more private (for example, to a car or restroom) until he or she calms down. If it seems like there is a danger of physical harm, you may have to hold or restrain your child until he or she calms down.

- After the tantrum has passed, don't punish your child. However, when your child is calm, you should explain that his or her frustrations are understandable, but that tantrums and other kinds of out-of-control behavior are not acceptable. If hunger or sleepiness seems to have contributed to your child's tantrum, give him or her a snack or a nap.

- Fortunately, temper tantrums usually become less frequent after age 3. The tantrums should stop by age 4. By this time, your child will have more control over his or her day and more ability to communicate his or her feelings.

When should I call your office?

Call our office if:

- Your child is still having temper tantrums at age 4 or older. A more in-depth discussion of parenting may be needed.

- Your child is having severe temper tantrums that pose a risk of harm to himself or herself or others, or if he or she is having destructive tantrums.

- Your child is holding her breath during tantrums, particularly if she passes out.

- Your child's tantrums are accompanied by head banging, physical symptoms such as headaches, or other changes in behavior.

Section IV ▪ Blood Disorders

Blood Clots (Thrombotic Disorders)

> Problems related to abnormal blood clots are rare in healthy children. However, children with certain diseases or injuries are at risk of developing blood clots, causing complications related to reduced blood flow. Some of these complications are very serious, including strokes, which may cause damage to the brain. Several inherited diseases also can cause abnormal blood clotting. Children who are at risk of complications related to abnormal clotting may need anticoagulant (blood-thinning) medications.

What kinds of problems can be caused by blood clots?

Blood clotting is the normal process in which blood cells stick together to stop bleeding. When abnormal blood clots develop, they may result in serious complications. The clot may block or severely reduce blood flow to an organ, such as the brain or kidney; or to one of the limbs, usually the leg.

Problems resulting from clots within a blood vessel are called "thrombotic disorders." Other problems occur when a clot breaks free and moves through the blood vessels ("thromboembolic disorder"). Both types are rare in healthy children. However, they can occur in children with many types of illnesses or injuries, or in children with medical monitoring equipment in place. Other children have inherited conditions causing abnormal blood clotting.

Thrombotic disorders can cause many complications, including strokes when a clot blocks the blood flow to the brain. If your child has a blood-clotting abnormality, anticoagulant medications (sometimes called blood thinners) can help to reduce the risk of serious complications. Your child needs close medical follow-up while taking these drugs.

What are the conditions causing blood clots, and what do they look like?

Inherited clotting disorders. These are genetic (inherited) problems with one of the substances (proteins) controlling the clotting system in our blood.

- Infants with some genetic blood-clotting abnormalities develop serious complications soon after birth. Depending on the severity of the disorder, these complications can be fatal if they are not treated promptly.

- If the clotting disorder is less severe, it may lead to clot-related complications later in childhood, or even in adult-

hood. For example, girls with certain clotting disorders may not experience problems until they become pregnant or start taking birth-control pills.

Acquired clotting disorders. A number of diseases and conditions can lead to problems with blood clots. Some examples are:

- Tissue injury from trauma, burns, or other causes. Severe injury to the brain or other organs damages the blood vessels, causing clots.

- Severe infections.

- "Indwelling" catheters. Clots can occur with devices, such as intravenous (IV) tubes that are placed in the patient's blood vessels for monitoring and treatment during an illness.

- Cancers.

The *signs* and *symptoms* of clotting disorders vary, depending on where the clot is located—whether it is in an artery (vessel taking oxygen-containing blood from the heart) or vein (vessel carrying blood back to the heart and lungs to obtain oxygen), and how badly it is interfering with the blood supply to an organ or body part.

- For example, a clot in the artery supplying a limb will cause the limb to be cold and pale, with no pulse. If the clot is in a vein, the limb will be swollen and painful.

What increases your child's risk of abnormal blood clots?

- If you or others in your family have any genetic disease causing abnormal blood clotting, your child may be at higher risk. Genetic counseling may help you to understand this risk.

- Many different medical conditions and certain medical procedures can lead to blood clots.

How are abnormal blood clots treated?

For some clots, no treatment is necessary.

Thrombolytic drugs. These drugs may be used to help dissolve abnormal clots and restore blood flow to the affected organ or body part.

- Thrombolytic therapy is only helpful if the clot is relatively recent: less than 3 to 5 days old.

- This type of treatment is most effective when the thrombolytic drug can be delivered right to the site of the clot.

- Thrombolytic therapy may be used for clots blocking the blood flow to the lungs, a blocked leg vein, or a blocked catheter. These medications are used less often in children. Close monitoring in the hospital is needed both during and after the attempt at thrombolytic therapy.

Anticoagulant therapy. Anticoagulant drugs, or blood thinners, decrease the blood's ability to form clots. This gives the body a chance to dissolve clots and prevents new clots from occurring.

- If your child's increased risk of clots is likely to be only a temporary problem (for example, after an infection or injury), anticoagulants may be used for only a short time. If the increase in clot risk is related to a genetic disease or other permanent condition, long-term anticoagulant therapy may be needed.

- The two main types of anticoagulant drugs are heparin and warfarin, although other medications such as aspirin are used for certain conditions. While taking any anticoagulant drug, your child will need close medical monitoring. There can be an increase in the risk of bleeding complications from their use. Your doctor will let you know what monitoring tests are needed and how often they should be done.

- *Many factors can affect your child's level of anticoagulation.* For example, if your child is taking warfarin, the blood-thinning effect may be affected by various medications. Aspirin, antibiotics, laxatives, vitamin E, and other medications may increase the anticoagulant effect, increasing the risk of bleeding. Other medications, such as vitamin K and birth control pills, may decrease the anticoagulant effect, thereby increasing the risk of clots.

- *Even minor bleeding can lead to problems if your child is taking anticoagulants.* During treatment, your child will have to avoid some sports and other activities. Make sure to inform your dentist and any other health care professionals that your child is taking anticoagulant medications and is at risk of bleeding complications. Special preparations may be needed before dental and medical procedures, especially surgery. Teachers and the school nurse should be informed as well.

- Your doctor will also tell you what to do if your child has an episode of bleeding while taking anticoagulants. For example, for patients taking warfarin, vitamin K can be used to treat bleeding problems.

When should I call your office?

During anticoagulant treatment, your doctor will give you specific instructions on monitoring, prevention of complications, and what to do in case of an emergency. Get medical help immediately if your child develops symptoms of either blood-clotting problems or excessive bleeding.

Enlarged Lymph Nodes

Lymph nodes are found around the neck, underarms, groin, and many other areas of the body. They play an important role in the immune system. Lymph nodes often become swollen during minor infections, such as colds. Enlargement and swelling may also mean that the node itself is infected, or it may be a sign of another disease. An examination will help the doctor decide whether your child needs further evaluation to determine the cause of enlarged lymph nodes.

Why do lymph nodes become enlarged?

Lymph nodes are normally small structures containing cells that are part of the immune system. These cells help to control infections caused by bacteria and other germs. They also react to other foreign substances in our bodies. The lymph nodes and their cells can become enlarged for a number of reasons:

- *Infections* are by far the most common cause, for example, a simple cold.

  - When infection is in one part of the body, lymph node enlargement usually occurs in that area only; for example, with an abscess or "boil" (localized area of infection and pus, usually tender).

  - Other infections cause more widespread lymph node enlargement. Infectious mononucleosis ("mono") causes lymph node enlargement in many areas, including the neck, armpits, and groin. Infections or abscesses may develop within an enlarged lymph node, causing redness and tenderness.

- Any foreign substance that produces inflammation or stimulates the immune system—even bug bites—can cause enlarged nodes.

- *Other causes* of enlarged lymph nodes are much less common:

  - Cancer cells that develop in or spread to the lymph nodes.

  - Diseases affecting the immune system.

What do they look like?

- Enlarged lymph nodes produce a round swelling underneath the skin. Generally, lymph nodes are considered enlarged if they are bigger than 1 centimeter (2/5 of an inch).

- Lymph nodes are found in many different areas of the body. Some common sites of enlarged nodes are:

  - In the neck area. This is very common when your child has a sore throat.

  - In the underarm area.

  - In the groin.

  - Many other locations are possible, including areas where nodes cannot be seen or felt (such as the head, chest, abdomen, pelvis, chest, and limbs).

- Your child may have enlargement of just one node, of several nodes in a particular area (regional), or of nodes all over the body (generalized).

- Nodes that are soft, not tender or red, and easy to move are often seen with simple viral infections (like a cold).

- When nodes are tender and the skin over them is red and warm, they may be infected (adenitis). This most often occurs in the neck.

- Lymph nodes "suspicious" for possible malignancy (cancer) or other serious conditions are often firm, "matted down," and not easy to move. Nodes in certain locations, for example, just above the collarbone, may also prompt the doctor to check for more serious disease.

How are enlarged lymph nodes managed?

Examination is the important first step in determining the cause of enlarged lymph nodes.

- Most of the time, lymph nodes are enlarged because of viral infections, such as a cold. It may take a few months for the nodes to shrink back to their usual size.

- If the node itself is infected, your child will be treated with antibiotics. If an abscess is present, the doctor may need to perform a simple procedure to drain it.

- If the nodes appear abnormal, are in unusual locations, or don't get smaller with time, various tests are done to find the cause.

When should I call your office?

Call our office if enlarged lymph nodes don't start to reduce in size after a few weeks.

Iron-Deficiency Anemia

Iron-deficiency anemia is a relatively common problem, usually occurring when your child's diet does not provide enough iron. It is most common in children ages 1 to 2. Iron-deficiency anemia can also occur in adolescents—especially girls—because of additional blood loss during their periods. In most cases, the anemia clears up quickly once your child is given extra iron.

What is iron-deficiency anemia?

Our bodies need iron to produce a substance called hemoglobin, which allows red blood cells to carry oxygen. If iron levels aren't high enough, the body can't make enough hemoglobin. Anemia means low levels of red blood cells or hemoglobin. When the problem is caused by a lack of iron, it's called iron-deficiency anemia.

The most common cause is not enough iron in the diet. Children ages 1 to 2 are most commonly affected. In this age group, it can be hard to provide enough iron through a good diet. Losing blood from our bodies can also cause iron-deficiency anemia, as the body needs extra iron to make up for the blood loss. This may occur in teenage girls whose menstrual periods are heavy or last a long time. It can also occur in children with digestive problems, if they are losing blood in their stools.

Some children and teens may have low iron levels but not low enough to cause iron-deficiency anemia. They still may need treatment. Whatever the cause, your child's red blood cell and hemoglobin levels should return to normal soon after more iron is added to the diet. If not, further tests and treatment may be needed.

What does it look like?

- Iron-deficiency anemia may not cause any symptoms. It may be recognized during routine blood tests. Symptoms are usually present only when the hemoglobin level drops pretty low.
- Skin may appear pale (pallor).
- Your child may be easily tired or irritable. He or she may have difficulty concentrating or have a poor appetite.
- If the anemia is severe, your child may be very pale or be out of breath after just light activity.
- Even without anemia, low iron levels may have mild effects on attention and learning.

What causes iron-deficiency anemia?

- The most common cause is not enough iron in the diet. This is most common in infants and toddlers ages 9 to 18 months.
- Infants drinking large amounts of cow's milk (greater than 20 to 24 ounces per day) may be at increased risk. Infants who are fed only breast milk can also be at increased risk. Beginning at about 6 months of age, breast-fed babies should receive additional iron in the form of iron-rich foods or liquid iron if necessary.
- Risk is increased for premature infants, who have less iron in their bodies at birth. They also grow quickly and need more iron.
- In teens, prolonged or heavy menstrual periods may cause anemia.
- Rarely, unrecognized bleeding may cause anemia. This is most often related to problems in the digestive system.

What are some possible complications of iron-deficiency anemia?

After proper levels of iron are added to the diet, there are usually no further problems.

Can iron-deficiency anemia be prevented?

Make sure your child's diet contains enough iron:

- Breast-fed babies should receive extra iron starting at about 6 months of age.
- Bottle-fed babies should receive iron-fortified formula until 1 year of age.
- When your baby starts solid foods, give him or her iron-fortified cereals.
- Limit intake of cow's milk to less than 24 ounces per day.
- For older children, give foods that are high in iron. These include red meats, fish, egg yolks, beans, and leafy vegetables. If you don't feel your child is getting enough iron in the diet, it's reasonable to give an iron supplement or multivitamin. It's especially important to make sure your child gets enough iron during periods of rapid growth, during athletic training, or after the start of menstrual periods.

How is iron-deficiency anemia treated?

- Treatment includes iron supplements, usually given in drops (for infants), tablets, or pills. Your doctor can recommend the best iron dose for your infant or child. Your child's anemia should start to improve within a few days.

- We may recommend that your child continue taking iron for a few months. Iron and hemoglobin levels should be rechecked to make sure they are going up.

- *Very* rarely, children with severe anemia may need a blood transfusion.

When should I call your office?

Call our office if you are having trouble using iron supplements or increasing the amount of iron in your child's diet, as recommended.

Sickle Cell Disease and Sickle Cell Trait

> Sickle cell disease is an inherited blood disease most common in African Americans. Over time, serious complications can occur. Treatment focuses on preventing complications and keeping your child as healthy as possible. Sickle cell trait is different from sickle cell disease! People with this trait rarely have any health problems but may benefit from genetic counseling.

What is sickle cell disease?

Children with sickle cell disease have abnormal red blood cells with a "sickled" or crescent-moon shape. They have *anemia,* which means they have low amounts of hemoglobin, or red blood cells, in their blood.

These problems occur when your child inherits abnormal types of hemoglobin, which carries oxygen in the blood. The most common form of sickle cell disease is sickle cell anemia. Other abnormal hemoglobins can be inherited along with the "sickled" hemoglobin, causing other forms of sickle cell disease.

The sickle cells block small blood vessels, causing damage when blood cannot get to parts of the body. This leads to attacks of pain and other symptoms and complications. Sickle cell disease is a lifelong problem. It is more severe in some children than others.

What is sickle cell trait?

Sickle cell *trait* is much more common than sickle cell disease and generally does not cause any health problems. It occurs in 8% to 10% of African Americans. Children who are born with sickle cell trait live a normal lifespan and do not have sickle cell disease. They should receive regular medical attention, just like other children. Genetic counseling will help you to understand your family's risk of passing on sickle cell disease and sickle cell trait to future generations.

Complications are rare. People with sickle cell trait should make sure they stay well hydrated (drink lots of fluids) and avoid becoming overheated. Sickle cell trait can result in decreased ability of the kidneys to concentrate urine, which may lead to blood in the urine. There may be an increased risk of sudden death during exercise. None of these problems has been well studied. However, as mentioned, children with this trait rarely have such problems.

What causes sickle cell disease and sickle cell trait?

- Sickle cell disease is caused by abnormal (mutated) genes. To have sickle cell anemia, your child must inherit two sickle cell genes—one from each parent. If your child just inherits one sickle cell gene, he or she will have sickle cell trait (which rarely causes problems).

- If both parents have sickle cell trait, the risk of sickle cell anemia is 25% for each child. If one parent has sickle cell trait and the other has no abnormal hemoglobins, the chance of sickle cell trait is 50% in each child.

- Sickle cell disease is most common in African Americans, affecting about 1 in 625 newborns.

What kinds of health problems are caused by sickle cell disease?

- *Pain* is the most noticeable symptom:
  - Every child is different—some have more frequent and severe episodes of pain than others.
  - He or she may have occasional attacks of severe pain. These attacks, called *sickle cell crises,* may require hospital treatment. There is no way to predict how often your child will experience sickle cell crisis.
  - Pain usually occurs in the arms and legs in younger children, and in the head, chest, abdomen, or back in older children.

- *Hand-foot syndrome (*also called *acute sickle dactylitis)* may be the first sign of sickle cell disease. The hands and feet become painful and swollen. The blood vessels become blocked, causing damage to the bones.

- *Acute chest syndrome* is an occasional problem. Damage to the lungs occurs when blood vessels become blocked by sickle cells, causing attacks of chest pain. Acute chest syndrome often causes problems getting enough oxygen into the blood. In children, it often is seen along with infection of the lungs (pneumonia). This can be a very serious complication.

- *Anemia.* Low hemoglobin levels cause your child to become easily tired.

- *Infections.* Patients with sickle cell anemia are at increased risk of serious infections with bacteria.

- *Splenic sequestration* is an uncommon but serious complication. The spleen is an organ that filters blood, removes damaged red blood cells and certain germs, and contains cells important for immune system function. It is located on the left side of the upper abdomen. It is usually under the ribs, but when enlarged it can be felt in the abdomen.

- The spleen can fill up with blood and become quickly enlarged. This can cause your child to become anemic quickly and is a very serious situation. Your child will need a blood transfusion as soon as possible.

- *Strokes* occur in up to 10% of children with sickle cell disease. This happens when sickle cells interfere with blood flow to parts of the brain, causing damage to those areas.

- *Priapism.* This is an abnormal erection of the penis that can be painful and last a long time.

- *Aplastic crisis.* The body isn't making enough red blood cells. This causes your child to become very anemic. Aplastic crisis is usually caused by infection with a specific virus (Parvovirus).

- Over time, sickle cell disease can cause damage to many parts of the body, including the heart, kidneys, and eyes. It also may result in poor growth.

How is sickle cell disease diagnosed?

A simple blood test called *hemoglobin electrophoresis* determines whether your child has sickle cell disease or trait. Most states test all newborns at birth.

How is sickle cell disease treated?

Treatment focuses on preventing complications and treating your child as soon as possible when problems occur.

- *Infections.* Your child will receive vaccinations to help prevent infections. At least for the first 5 years, your child will take an antibiotic, such as penicillin.

  - When infections occur, they will be treated aggressively (quickly). This is because sickle cell patients have reduced ability to fight infections.

- *Pain crisis.* Pain crises are usually treated with strong pain medications, such as narcotics. Lots of fluids are needed to help prevent sickle cells from plugging blood vessels. Patients with severe pain crises often need hospital treatment.

- *Acute chest syndrome.* This is often treated with oxygen and blood transfusion.

- *Strokes.* Blood transfusion is needed to lower the number of sickle cells in the blood.

- *Priapism* (prolonged erections). If the problem doesn't clear up with pain medications and fluids, blood transfusion is needed.

- *Splenic sequestration.* This condition requires prompt blood transfusion.

- *Drug therapy.* Treatment with a drug called hydroxyurea, which decreases the amount of sickle hemoglobin in the blood, can be helpful for some patients.

- *Bone marrow transplantation* may cure the disease for some patients. However, there are many problems involved in performing this procedure. It usually requires a family member with "matched" bone marrow.

When should I call your office?

Call our office if any of the following occurs:

- Pain that seems like your child's "usual" pain but does not improve with medications and extra fluids.

- Fever of 101°F (38.5°C) or higher.

- Chest pain.

- Enlargement of the spleen. (Parents are taught how to feel the abdomen for an enlarged spleen.)

Sickle cell disease is a serious and complicated condition. Call your doctor's office if you have questions about this disease or about your child's treatment.

Section V ▪ Cancer

Hodgkin's Disease

Hodgkin's disease is a relatively common form of cancer in children and teens. The first symptom is usually painless swelling of the lymph nodes in the neck that does not clear up with time. With modern treatments, Hodgkin's disease is curable in most young patients.

What is Hodgkin's disease?

Hodgkin's disease is a kind of cancer called a lymphoma, which means a cancer of the lymph tissue (lymph nodes). The lymph nodes, which are spread throughout the body, play an important role in the immune system. Hodgkin's disease can spread rapidly to neighboring lymph nodes. The outlook for patients with Hodgkin's disease is best when it is diagnosed early.

It's devastating to hear that a child has any form of cancer, and treatment of your child for Hodgkin's disease will be a difficult time for your family. A specialist in cancer treatment (oncologist) will perform further tests and recommend the best treatment for your child. Fortunately, with modern chemotherapy and other treatments, there is an excellent chance of curing your child's cancer.

What does it look like?

- The first symptom is usually swollen lymph nodes in the neck and shoulder area (less often, in the groin or underarm area). Chest x-rays often show involvement inside the chest.

- Swollen lymph nodes are a very common sign of minor illnesses, such as colds or other infections. The doctor may be concerned if your child has swollen lymph nodes without any other symptoms of illness.

- The swollen nodes may feel firm and are usually not painful.

- Many other symptoms are less common but possible, depending on where the lymphoma spreads. These may include difficulty breathing (from chest involvement) or problems related to the liver, kidneys, or bone marrow, where different types of blood cells are made.

- Other symptoms may include fever, weight loss, and night-time sweating.

- Because Hodgkin's disease interferes with the functioning of the immune system, your child may have frequent or unusual infections.

What are the causes and risk factors for Hodgkin's disease?

- The exact cause of Hodgkin's disease is unknown. Infection with a common virus called Epstein-Barr virus may play a role. (This is the same virus that causes infectious mononucleosis, or "mono.")

- The risk of Hodgkin's disease is increased for patients with any type of immunodeficiency: conditions that reduce the body's ability to fight infections.

- If anyone in your family has had Hodgkin's disease, your child may be at higher risk. Under age 10, boys are affected more often than girls.

What are some possible complications of Hodgkin's disease?

- Depending on where the disease appears, it may cause problems in many different organs and organ systems, including the heart and lungs, liver, blood and bone marrow, or kidneys.

- It may cause frequent infections, including unusual infections such as tuberculosis or infections caused by fungus.

- Like any cancer, Hodgkin's disease can spread to other parts of the body. Although treatment is effective for most children and teens, there is a risk of death. Even if the initial treatment is successful, there is a risk that the cancer may come back (relapse).

How is Hodgkin's disease diagnosed and treated?

Hodgkin's disease is diagnosed by a relatively minor surgical procedure called a *biopsy*. A sample of a lymph node is taken to the laboratory to check for cancer cells.

- Once the diagnosis of Hodgkin's disease is made, your child's care will probably be managed by an oncologist (cancer specialist). Your child may be treated by a team that includes other health care professionals, such as nurses and a psychologist.

- The first step in treatment is *staging*. Various tests are done to find out how far your child's cancer has spread, including examination, blood tests, x-rays, or other imaging studies. Stage I is the earliest stage, meaning the disease is less advanced. Stage IV is the most advanced, meaning that the cancer has spread widely throughout the body.

Treatment decisions depend on the stage of your child's cancer, his or her age, and the symptoms.

- The usual treatment for Hodgkin's disease is *chemotherapy.* Chemotherapy drugs kill cancer cells by interfering with their metabolism.

  - Chemotherapy drugs are very effective at killing cancer cells. However, they also cause side effects, for example, reduced immune function, nausea and vomiting, liver and gastrointestinal problems, skin irritation, and hair loss. Your child will be monitored carefully during treatment to minimize these toxic effects. Side effects usually go away after treatment.

  - Your child may need several courses of chemotherapy to eliminate as much of the cancer as possible. Cancer specialists have worked to design new treatment programs to reduce the dose and shorten the time of chemotherapy as much as possible without sacrificing the effectiveness of the medication.

- Treatment may also include *radiation therapy,* depending on the extent of the disease. This involves special x-ray beams aimed at the cancer cells to destroy them.

  - The dose of radiation is kept as low as possible to prevent side effects, such as skin rashes. Other side effects depend on what area is treated; for example, lung function, heart function, or bone growth may be affected if these areas receive radiation.

With modern treatment, the chances of eliminating Hodgkin's disease are excellent. Only your cancer specialist can provide precise estimates, which depend upon a number of things, including the stage of disease (how far it has spread). The chances in general of disease-free survival are over 90% for children with early Hodgkin's disease and over 70% for those with more advanced disease.

Even if the cancer is eliminated, however, there is a chance it could come back (relapse). Your child will need early and continuous long-term follow-up and testing to detect relapsed Hodgkin's disease as early as possible. If a relapse does occur, most patients respond to further treatment.

Having a child diagnosed with any form of cancer is a devastating event for your family. The health care team will provide both medical and psychological support for your child and family.

When should I call your office?

Call our office or your cancer specialist if you have any questions about Hodgkin's disease or about your child's treatment.

Leukemia

Leukemia is a group of related diseases resulting in rapid growth of abnormal cells in the bone marrow, where different types of blood cells are made. The various leukemias are the most common cancers in children. Examination of a bone marrow sample is needed to make the diagnosis and to find out exactly what type of leukemia your child has. With modern treatments, many types of leukemia can be cured.

What is leukemia?

Leukemia is a group of diseases in which the body's bone marrow makes too many of an abnormal type of white blood cell. The bone marrow is where many types of cells are made, including red blood cells (which have hemoglobin to carry oxygen), platelets (which help stop bleeding), and white blood cells. The white blood cells are important to the immune system because they help to fight infections.

In leukemia, one abnormal type of white blood cells is produced more rapidly. This interferes with the bone marrow's ability to make other cells, including red blood cells, platelets, and normal white blood cells that fight infection. The most common form of childhood leukemia is acute lymphoblastic leukemia (ALL). The symptoms of leukemia may seem relatively mild at first, but the disease can progress rapidly. Eventually, leukemia lessens your child's ability to fight off infections.

It's devastating to hear that a child has any form of cancer, and treatment for leukemia will be a difficult time for your family. A specialist in cancer treatment (oncologist) will perform further tests and recommend the best treatment for your child. Your child's treatment team will probably also include other health care professionals, such as nurses and a psychologist. Your child will receive chemotherapy and other treatments, like radiation, if needed. Depending on factors such as the type of leukemia, the age of the patient, and the number of leukemia cells in the blood, most children with leukemia are cured.

What does it look like?

The symptoms of leukemia vary, depending on the type of leukemia. The early symptoms are often relatively mild. Symptoms can develop rapidly, although sometimes they occur gradually over several months:

- Weight loss.
- Fatigue (low energy).
- Low-grade fever.
- Bone or joint pain.

- Pale appearance, usually caused by anemia, that is (low numbers of red blood cells or hemoglobin levels).
- Easy bruising or bleeding caused by low levels of platelets in the blood.
- Infections, such as sores in the mouth and sometimes more serious infections such as pneumonia.

Many other symptoms are possible, depending on the type of leukemia and how long it has been present.

What are some possible complications of leukemia?

- Problems with bleeding or infections.
- Like most cancers, leukemia can be fatal without effective treatment. Even if initial treatment is successful, there is a risk that the leukemia will come back.
- Treatments for leukemia have many possible side effects.

What puts your child at risk of leukemia?

Many risk factors for leukemia in children have been identified, including:

- Exposure to radiation.
- Exposure to various drugs.
- Genetics—in twins, if one twin develops leukemia, the other will be at higher risk.
- Various genetic diseases, including Down syndrome.
- Occurs most frequently in children ages 2 to 6 years and is slightly more common in boys than girls.

How is leukemia diagnosed and treated?

Often simple blood tests show typical abnormalities of leukemia and problems with your child's bone marrow. However, to diagnose leukemia, the doctor needs to obtain and examine a sample of your child's bone marrow. This is done through a relatively minor surgical procedure.

Once your child has been diagnosed with leukemia, his or her care is managed by a specialist, such as an oncologist (cancer specialist). Doctors and nurses with various types of skills and experience also may be involved in your child's treatment.

Additional tests are needed to find out exactly what kind of leukemia your child has. These tests are very important for making decisions about your child's treatment. The main types of leukemia in children are:

- *Acute lymphoblastic leukemia (ALL).* More than three fourths of childhood leukemias are ALL. ALL responds very well to chemotherapy. Over 80% of children with ALL are still alive after 5 years.

- *Acute myelogenous leukemia (AML).* This is the second most common type of childhood leukemia. About 10% of children with leukemia have AML. It also responds well to treatment.

- *Less common types of leukemia* include chronic myelogenous leukemia (CML) and juvenile chronic myelogenous leukemia (JCML). Together, CML and JCML account for 3% to 5% of childhood leukemias.

- Up to 9% of children with leukemia have some other type that does not meet any of these criteria.

Depending on what type of leukemia your child has, along with other factors, the oncologist and other members of the treatment team will design a treatment program that is best for your child. The right kind of treatment has a major impact on the outcome of children with leukemia.

Leukemias are generally treated with *chemotherapy.* Many children with ALL are treated as part of national or international studies of leukemia treatment. Over the years, these studies have led to major advances in leukemia treatment. Usually, treatment is given in three stages:

- *Remission induction.* In this stage, the goal is to eliminate all leukemia cells from your child's bone marrow.

- *Central nervous system therapy.* In this stage, your child will receive additional chemotherapy, with the goal of keeping the cancer from coming back. This type of treatment greatly reduces the risk that leukemia will reappear in your child's brain or spinal cord.

- *Maintenance therapy.* In the final stage, treatment may continue for a few years. Maintenance therapy is also designed to keep the cancer from coming back.

Chemotherapy consists of drugs that are very effective in killing cancer cells. They can also have a lot of side effects, including reduced immune function, nausea and vomiting, liver and gastrointestinal problems, skin irritation, and hair loss. The side effects usually go away after treatment.

- More serious side effects of chemotherapy are possible. Your child will be monitored carefully during treatment to minimize these toxic effects.

- Bone marrow transplantation is sometimes part of treatment for leukemia, especially for children with AML or CML. The results are best when your child has a sibling whose bone marrow is a good "match" for your child's.

With modern treatment, the chances of eliminating ALL and other leukemias are good. Only your cancer specialist can provide precise estimates. Bone marrow transplantation may offer the best chances of cure for children with AML or CML.

Even if the leukemia is eliminated, there is a chance it could come back (relapse). Your child will need long-term follow-up and testing to detect relapsed leukemia. If your child does have a relapse, further treatment can still be effective.

Having a child diagnosed with any form of cancer is a devastating event for your family. The health care team will provide both medical and psychological support for your child and family.

When should I call your office?

Call our office or your cancer specialist if you have any questions about leukemia or about your child's treatment.

Section VI ▪ Dental

■ Dental Trauma ■

If your child has a tooth broken or knocked out because of an injury, go to the dentist as soon as possible. Take the tooth or tooth fragment with you, if possible. Some simple steps can help to protect your child from dental injuries.

What is dental trauma?

Injuries causing damage to the teeth and the tissues around the teeth are common in toddlers, children, and teens. Prompt action can save a lost or broken tooth. It is essential to see the dentist as soon as possible.

What does it look like?

- Injuries to the teeth or mouth are usually obvious. Something happens to chip or break a tooth, to loosen a tooth, or to knock the tooth out entirely. The injury may cause a lot of pain, often with bleeding.

- Sometimes dental injuries happen as part of more serious trauma, such as a car accident or a blow to the head.

What causes dental trauma?

The main causes of dental injuries vary with age:

- Toddlers: Most commonly injured in falls.

- School-aged children: Most commonly injured in bicycle or playground accidents.

- Teenagers: Frequent causes include sports injuries, car accidents, and fights.

Can dental injuries be prevented?

- Children and teens participating in contact sports (especially football) should wear a mouth guard.

- Front teeth that protrude (stick out) are more easily harmed. Discuss this situation with your child's dentist or orthodontist, who may suggest some protective measures.

- In the car, make sure your child always wears a seatbelt. Babies and toddlers should always ride in car seats.

- Childproof your home to remove possible causes of falls, such as wires or other obstructions that could cause your child to trip and fall.

What are some possible complications of dental trauma?

- Loss of teeth.

- Change of color of teeth.

- Injuries to primary ("baby") teeth can cause damage to the developing permanent tooth underneath.

How is dental trauma treated?

If your child has a primary (baby) tooth knocked out:

- Call your dentist's office. Even though it's a primary tooth, the dentist may want to check for possible damage to the underlying permanent tooth. Usually, it's not necessary to replace lost primary teeth.

If your child has a permanent tooth knocked out:

- Find the tooth.

- Rinse the tooth. Do not scrub it, and do not touch the root. After plugging the sink, hold the tooth by the crown (the biting surface) and rinse it under running water.

- Gently place the tooth back in the socket. Don't worry if it doesn't go all the way back in. If it isn't possible to put the tooth back in, put it in a clean container with cold milk.

- Go to the dentist immediately. Have your child hold the tooth in place with a finger if possible.

If your child has a chipped or fractured tooth:

- Rinse the mouth with water.

- Go to the dentist immediately. If you can find the tooth fragment, take it with you.

What will the dentist do?

- If possible, the dentist will try to replace or repair the missing or fractured tooth. Give the dentist as much information as possible about how your child's injury occurred. Treatment decisions will depend on how much damage the injury did to the teeth, gums, and jaw.

◑ When should I call your office?

If your child has an injury to the teeth or mouth, call or visit your dentist's office.

Preventive Antibiotics for Children with Heart Disease

Children with certain heart diseases are at risk of infective endocarditis, a serious infection of the heart valves or the inside lining of the heart. To prevent this infection, your child may need to take antibiotics before certain dental and medical procedures, especially surgery. Make sure to tell your child's dentist and other health care professionals if your child has any form of heart disease.

Why does my child need preventive antibiotics?

Patients with certain types of heart disease are at increased risk of a serious infection of the heart called *infective endocarditis*. This occurs when the valves of the heart or the inside lining of the heart becomes infected with bacteria. The infection can cause destruction of the heart valves and other life-threatening complications.

To prevent infective endocarditis, antibiotics are recommended before certain dental, medical, and surgical procedures in children with heart disease. This includes routine professional dental cleanings. For this and most other procedures, your child needs only a single dose of amoxicillin or another antibiotic a short time before the procedure.

Whether or not your child needs antibiotics depends on his or her level of risk and the specific procedure being performed. Make sure your child's dentist and other health care providers are aware of your child's heart disease.

How do dental procedures lead to infections?

During surgery and certain types of dental and medical procedures, the body's normal bacteria get into the bloodstream. This is called "bacteremia" and in healthy people, it usually does not cause problems.

However, in children with heart disease, there is an increased risk that the bacteria will travel through the bloodstream to cause infective endocarditis. This occurs when bacteria infect the heart valves (usually abnormal valves) or the inside lining of the heart (called the "endocardium"). Giving preventive (also called "prophylactic") antibiotics before surgical or dental procedures reduces that risk.

Recommendations for preventive antibiotics vary, depending on:

- Whether your child is at high risk or moderate risk.

- Whether the procedure being performed carries a high risk of causing bacteria to move into the bloodstream.

For example, procedures with a high risk of bacteremia include teeth cleaning, tooth extractions (pulling teeth), tonsillectomy (surgery to remove the tonsils), and some surgeries involving the intestines.

- Other procedures have a low risk of bacteremia and don't require antibiotics, for example, orthodontic (braces) adjustments or placing ear tubes.

Most cases of infective endocarditis are not caused by dental or medical procedures! Other sources of infection are more likely. Your doctor may make further recommendations for preventing infections, possibly including the use of preventive antibiotics.

What types of health problems require preventive antibiotics?

Heart disease is the most common reason for giving preventive antibiotics before dental or surgical procedures in children.

- *High-risk conditions.* Some types of heart disease carry a higher risk of infective endocarditis:

  - Any type of surgically replaced heart valves (including artificial and animal valves).

  - Major heart defects (such as transposition of the great arteries or tetralogy of Fallot).

  - Major heart surgery, especially if artificial or reconstructed "shunts," vessels, or heart valves were placed.

  - Previous infective endocarditis.

- *Moderate-risk conditions.* For other types of heart disease, risk of endocarditis is still elevated, although not as high as in children with major heart defects and/or reconstructive surgery:

  - Less severe heart defects, such as patent ductus arteriosus, ventricular septal defect, and others. If your child has had surgery to correct these defects, he or she is no longer at increased risk.

  - Heart valve damage caused by rheumatic heart disease.

  - Hypertrophic cardiomyopathy, a condition in which the heart muscle is thickened and does not function properly.

- *Low-risk conditions.* Children with these conditions are at no higher risk than children without heart disease:

  - Surgery for less severe heart defects (see above).

  - "Innocent" heart murmurs.

- Rheumatic heart disease, if it did not cause valve damage.

What types of procedures require preventive antibiotics?

Dental procedures. Any procedure causing bacteria in the bloodstream (bacteremia) could cause infective endocarditis in a high-risk or moderate-risk child. The most frequent source of risk is dental procedures. This is because dental care is performed routinely and because bacteremia can result from the normally harmless bacteria that are present in the mouth.

Preventive antibiotics are only needed for certain dental procedures that have a higher risk of bacteria in the bloodstream. Usually, this means procedures in which significant bleeding is expected. For example:

- Professional dental cleanings (cleanings performed by a dentist or dental hygienist, not routine brushing and flossing).

- Dental surgery, including extractions (pulling teeth) and treatment for gum disease (periodontal disease).

- Replacing teeth that have been knocked out.

- Initial orthodontic treatment (placing bands, though not brackets).

- Certain types of local anesthetic injections.

- Other types of dental surgery, such as implant placement or root canal (endodontic) surgery. (These are uncommon in children.)

Preventive antibiotics are *not* needed for other routine dental procedures, including:

- Personal brushing and flossing.

- Filling cavities and other "restorative" procedures.

- Primary teeth ("baby teeth") coming out.

- Taking x-rays, fluoride treatments, and many other procedures commonly done in the dentist's office.

Other procedures. Other, less common medical procedures carry a risk of bacteremia and may require preventive antibiotics:

- Certain types of surgery, such as tonsillectomy and some surgeries involving the intestines.

- Certain diagnostic or treatment procedures involving the respiratory, gastrointestinal, or urinary system (for example, cystoscopic examination).

Always tell your child's doctors and other health professionals about his or her heart condition and ask whether antibiotics are needed before procedures.

How are preventive antibiotics given?

- In most cases, your child will need only a single dose of antibiotics, given a short time before the procedure.

- The typical treatment for dental procedures is one dose of amoxicillin, given 1 hour before the procedure.

- A different antibiotic will be given if your child is allergic to penicillin. The antibiotic may be given in oral form (a pill) or by injection (a shot).

- For procedures involving the intestines or bladder, the antibiotic instructions are different for patients with "high-risk" conditions.

- Between dental visits, follow good dental hygiene to keep your child's teeth as clean as possible. Daily brushing and flossing are the most important steps.

When should I call your office?

Call our office, or your dentist's office, if you have any questions about preventive antibiotics for your child. Make sure all health care professionals are aware of your child's heart condition.

Tooth Decay and Dental Care

Regular visits to the dentist are very important for children. Don't put your baby to bed with a bottle, because this can cause tooth decay. Regular brushing and dental visits can help keep your child's teeth as sound and strong as possible.

What is tooth decay?

Tooth decay—also called cavities or dental caries—is the main dental problem in children. Certain bacteria in the mouth use sugars to make acids, which can eat away at the outer surface (enamel) of your child's teeth. Some sugars like sucrose (used in candy) are worse than others in causing tooth decay. The longer the sugars are in contact with bacteria in the mouth, the greater the chance of decay.

To prevent cavities, make sure your child gets enough fluoride, which is usually present in water. Your child should brush his or her teeth with a fluoride-containing toothpaste and be careful about drinking and eating too many sweets. Regular dental visits are important to prevent tooth decay and to make sure the teeth are developing normally. Dentists can also detect and treat other problems of the teeth and gums.

What does it look like?

- You may see small pits or holes ("cavities") on the surface of your child's teeth. However, cavities are difficult to see when they are very small. That's why regular dental checkups are so important: to detect tooth decay at an earlier, more treatable stage.

- Infants and toddlers sometimes develop severe decay of many teeth at once. This condition is sometimes called "baby bottle" tooth decay because it usually results from prolonged contact between sugary liquids (including milk) and the teeth. It is especially common in babies who are put to bed with a bottle of milk or juice.

What are some possible complications of tooth decay?

- If untreated, tooth decay can cause pain (toothaches), development of an abscess (localized area of infection), and destruction of your child's teeth. Childhood dental problems can be very painful as well as difficult and expensive to treat.

- If tooth decay causes a severe abscess of the primary teeth ("baby teeth"), it can cause problems with the way the permanent teeth come in.

What puts your child at risk of tooth decay?

- Not brushing the teeth and not visiting the dentist regularly.

- Eating or drinking a lot of sugary foods or liquids. This includes milk, if it's allowed to stay in contact with the teeth for a long time. Some special risk factors are:
  - Putting your baby or toddler to bed with a bottle of juice, milk, or other sugary liquid. The sugar stays in contact with your child's teeth for a longer time, promoting tooth decay. This can also happen in breast-fed babies, if they're allowed to use the breast as a "pacifier."
  - Eating a lot of sticky sweets, especially hard candies.
  - Acidic foods and liquids can also contribute to tooth decay.
  - Low-income children and children from poor countries have higher rates of tooth decay. This may be related to eating behaviors and lack of dental hygiene.

Can tooth decay be prevented?

Yes. There are several things you can do to reduce your child's risk of tooth decay:

- Make sure that he or she gets enough fluoride. In many communities, fluoride is added to the drinking water. You can find out about fluoride in your community's water by calling your local health department. If your home has well water, it may need to be tested for fluoride. If the fluoride level is too high, staining of the teeth may occur. If the level is not high enough, your doctor or dentist may prescribe additional fluoride.

- Have your child brush regularly. Use a fluoride-containing toothpaste. Your child should brush at least twice daily, as soon as he or she is old enough to do so. Young children need supervision to make sure they brush well and don't swallow too much toothpaste. Don't put any more than a pea-sized amount of toothpaste on your child's toothbrush.

- Fluoride toothpaste is generally not used until your child is old enough to rinse out the mouth. For babies, simply wipe the teeth with a piece of gauze at least twice per day.

- Flossing. Older children should learn to floss the teeth every day.

- Visit the dentist regularly. Your child should go to the dentist when recommended, usually every 6 months for teeth-cleaning and examination.

- Don't put your baby or toddler to bed with a bottle, and don't let infants and toddlers use "sippy cups" for prolonged periods of time.

- Reduce your child's intake of sugary foods and drinks, especially sticky sweets. Have your child brush his or her teeth after eating these foods.

How is tooth decay treated?

- Fillings. If your child has tooth decay or cavities, the dentist can remove the infected areas and fill the cavity with special materials.

- Sealants. The dentist may recommend placing sealants to protect the surface of your child's teeth. These sealants are very effective in preventing cavities in the molar teeth.

- Other treatments. If tooth decay becomes severe or advanced, your dentist may recommend other treatments, including placing crowns (caps) on teeth, giving antibiotics, or performing surgery.

What are some other common dental problems in children?

Gum disease (gingivitis). Inflammation (swelling, redness) of the gums can occur, causing bleeding and bad breath. Like tooth decay, gum disease happens when your child's teeth and mouth aren't kept clean. Proper brushing and flossing are usually all the treatment that is needed. Visits to the dentist are essential to treat and prevent gingivitis.

More advanced gum disease, called *periodontitis,* can cause tooth loss. This disease affects the periodontium, which includes not just the gums but also the bones that hold the teeth, ligaments, and other structures. Periodontitis is generally rare in children, unless they have other medical problems. However, it can sometimes occur in otherwise healthy children and teens.

When should I call your office?

Call our office if:

- You need help finding a dentist for your child.

- You have any questions about your child's dental care.

- You can't reach your dentist.

If your child has a toothache, call your dentist and visit as soon as possible. In the meantime, put an ice pack on the sore area.

Section VII ▪ Development

■ Autism ■

Children with the developmental disorder autism have difficulty communicating and interacting with others. They may insist on certain rituals or repeated behaviors and get upset when their routines are disrupted. The cause of autism is unknown, and it is not related to anything the parents have done wrong. Although autism is a difficult behavioral disorder, in recent years there have been great gains in its treatment.

What is autism?

Doctors still have many questions about autism. It is a "pervasive developmental disorder," which simply means that it affects your child's development in many different ways. Children with autism have a hard time communicating and interacting with others. They follow repeated behaviors or rituals and withdraw from normal interactions with other people. Autistic children also may be developmentally delayed (slow). However, because of their communication problems, it is hard to measure their intelligence accurately.

Finding out that a child has autism is a very difficult event for your family. Autistic children need a lot of care and attention. Current treatments can really improve the educational and social functioning of children with autism, especially if they are started early.

What does it look like?

Every child with autism is different—some are more severely affected than others. Parents usually suspect a problem with their child's behavior around the first year. You may notice symptoms such as:

- *Slow language and social development.* Your child may seem withdrawn, "off in his own world." Your child may not make eye contact nor pay attention when you call his or her name. At first you may think there's a hearing problem. In addition, your child may not meet expected stages of development; for example, not pointing to things or not showing the usual baby talk or babbling by age 1. (Children with a related, less-severe disorder called Asperger's syndrome don't have such severe language disorders.)

- *Ritualistic behaviors.* Your child may follow odd behavior routines, such as rocking back and forth. Rather than playing pretend games with toys, he or she may insist on lining them up in a certain way. Autistic children may insist on having consistent rituals and get upset if there is any change in their routine. (Most children also like having consistent rituals and routines but not to the same extent as autistic children.)

- *Intelligence problems.* Some children with autism seem slow, but it is difficult to assess their true intelligence. Social and communication problems may make it impossible for autistic children to learn in a regular classroom. In educational and social situations, they may focus in on small details while missing "the big picture." Although it is true that some autistic children have one isolated, remarkable talent, this is uncommon.

What causes autism?

- The cause of autism is unknown. Possible contributors include genetic factors or some type of brain injury.

- Autism is *not* caused by bad parenting or by a reaction to childhood vaccines.

What are some possible complications of autism?

Children with autism need special education and training programs to maximize their behavioral, social, and intellectual abilities. Delays in diagnosis and treatment may lead to worse outcomes.

What puts your child at risk of autism?

- Boys are affected three or four times more often than girls.

- Autism is more common in children with other neurologic disorders, especially those with seizures. Some rare genetic disorders (fragile X syndrome and tuberous sclerosis) are common in autistic children.

Can autism be prevented?

There is no way to prevent autism.

How is autism treated?

Getting diagnosis and proper treatment for autism is a detailed process. Intensive therapy, beginning as early as possible, can improve your child's language capacity and social functioning. Expert evaluation by a child and adolescent psychiatrist or other specialist is needed.

- *Special education approaches* are needed, even if your child's intelligence and language skills are near normal. Most experts feel that children with autism do best in a structured program specially geared to the needs of children with this disorder.

- Educational interventions should begin as soon as your child's autism is diagnosed, preferably before age 3. At first, the emphasis is on efforts to enhance your child's behavior and communication skills.

- As your child grows, his or her school should provide individualized special education programs. The focus should be on learning social and communication skills. Your child will receive help with educational areas in which he or she is delayed, along with encouragement to pursue areas of strength.

- Older children receive practical help with skills they will need to live as independently as possible.

- *Other treatments* may be helpful, depending on your child's situation:

  - *Psychotherapy* is particularly helpful for autistic children and teens with higher intelligence but poor social skills.

  - *Medication* may help reduce depression, problems with poor attention or hyperactivity, obsessive-compulsive behavior, and other psychiatric symptoms.

  - *Social skills training* appears helpful for older children with autism or Asperger's syndrome.

  - *Unproven therapies.* A number of treatments claim to bring improvement in autism. Some of these, such as specific types of nutritional or vitamin therapy, have not yet been proved beneficial by scientific research. Other approaches, such as facilitated communication, have not been shown to be effective.

It's a good idea to be skeptical of claims about autism treatments. At the very least, what works for one child may not be the best treatment for your child. Intensive research into the causes and treatment of autism is continuing.

- *What is my child's prognosis?* No one can predict your child's final social, educational, and occupational outcomes. Some children with autism grow up to live self-sufficient lives, especially if their speech skills are relatively good. Prompt diagnosis, early treatment, and regular follow-up will help to maximize your child's functioning.

When should I call your office?

- All children with autism should receive regular follow-up evaluation and treatment from mental health and educational specialists. Our office will continue to coordinate your child's medical care.

- Call our office if you have questions about your child's disorder or need help in accessing community resources.

Where can I get more information?

A good place to start is the Centers for Disease Control and Prevention's (CDC's) Autism Information Center: *www.cdc.gov/ncbddd/dd/autism.htm.*

Fetal Alcohol Syndrome

Fetal alcohol syndrome is a developmental disorder that occurs when mothers drink alcohol while pregnant. Effects vary but include abnormal facial features, growth problems, and nervous system abnormalities, including mental deficiency. Even without the full syndrome, significant alcohol-related effects can be present. Completely avoiding alcohol during pregnancy avoids the risk of these birth defects.

What is fetal alcohol syndrome?

Fetal alcohol syndrome is a specific pattern of birth defects related to drinking alcohol while pregnant. These children often have a typical pattern of facial abnormalities, nervous system defects that may include reduced intelligence, and poor growth patterns. Other fetuses affected by the mother's drinking have *alcohol-related neurodevelopmental disorders,* with a similar but less severe pattern of abnormalities.

Children with fetal alcohol syndrome and fetal alcohol effects will likely have lifelong disabilities, requiring early intervention and special education. These effects are most likely in mothers who drank heavily during their pregnancy. However, they can also occur when there has been moderate or only occasional heavy drinking. There is no amount of alcohol that is "safe" to drink during pregnancy.

What does it look like?

The major features of fetal alcohol *syndrome* are abnormalities of the face and central nervous system and slowed or retarded growth:

- *Face.* A typical pattern of small eye openings, flat cheekbones, and an underdeveloped upper lip.

- *Nervous system.* Small head, reduced intelligence (sometimes fairly severe), or delays in normal development milestones.

- *Growth.* Low birth weight and/or slow growth after birth.

- *Other birth defects* may be present as well, such as heart defects and minor bone and joint abnormalities.

Children with fetal alcohol *effects* have a similar but usually less severe pattern of defects. They may not have significantly reduced intelligence but may have learning disabilities, including attention deficit–hyperactivity disorder, behavioral problems, or poor social skills. These conditions are termed alcohol-related neurodevelopmental disorders (previously called "fetal alcohol spectrum").

What causes fetal alcohol syndrome?

- Drinking alcohol while pregnant is the only cause.

- "Full-blown" fetal alcohol syndrome is more common with very heavy drinking during pregnancy. However, even moderate drinking can cause serious birth defects.

What are some possible consequences of fetal alcohol syndrome?

- Fetal alcohol syndrome causes lifelong disabilities. They may range from severe mental deficiency to relatively normal intelligence but with school and behavior problems. Later in life, children with alcohol-related birth defects are at increased risk of delinquency, alcohol and drug abuse, and mental health problems.

- Many other complications are possible, including serious medical conditions.

Can fetal alcohol syndrome be prevented?

- Not drinking during pregnancy completely eliminates the risk of fetal alcohol syndrome and related effects.

- Fetal alcohol syndrome can occur even with moderate drinking. *There is no amount of alcohol considered "safe" during pregnancy.*

- If you are already drinking during pregnancy, stopping now may reduce the risk of harming your baby.

How is fetal alcohol syndrome treated?

- The first step is diagnosis. Expert evaluation by a geneticist (a specialist in genetic diseases) or other expert is needed. Unfortunately, fetal alcohol syndrome and related disorders often go unrecognized. This is especially true of the milder abnormalities that occur in infants with alcohol-related neurodevelopmental disorders.

- Your child should receive a thorough evaluation, not just for diagnosis but also to help determine the best treatment plan. The goal will be to reduce the impact of your child's disabilities while making the most of his or her growth and development.

- In the case of other developmental abnormalities, education is probably the most important part of care:

  - *Early intervention* should start as soon as your child's alcohol-related abnormalities are diagnosed. Every state has an early intervention program. Early intervention experts will assess your child and develop an Individualized Family Support Plan (IFSP), based on your child's development, need for support, and goals for independence.

- *Special education* services are also available in every state. You are entitled to evaluation and educational services for your child. Based on the results, an Individualized Education Program (IEP) can be developed to meet your child's educational needs.

- Professionals from many different areas may play a role in your child's care. For example, a psychologist, speech/ language pathologist, physical or occupational therapist, and/or social worker may be able to offer valuable help to your child and family.

When should I call your office?

Call our office if you have any questions about your child's testing, treatment, or educational intervention.

If you are pregnant or thinking of becoming pregnant and are having trouble controlling your drinking, call our office or your own doctor immediately. Getting help now may reduce the harmful effects of alcohol on your baby.

Learning Disabilities

Learning disabilities can slow your child's progress in school. One common problem is dyslexia, a specific reading disability. Attention deficit–hyperactivity disorder (ADHD) may also be seen as a learning disability. Your child should receive assessment and an individualized educational plan to help deal with his or her learning disability.

What are learning disabilities?

Learning disabilities are disorders affecting specific abilities needed for school performance, such as reading, doing math, movement skills, or attention and focusing. Such problems don't mean that your child isn't smart; learning disabilities usually occur in children with normal intelligence.

Every child learns differently. A learning disability may be present if your child is having problems with schoolwork. Learning disabilities can be linked to social, behavioral, and self-esteem problems as well.

Every child suspected of having a learning disability should have a professional assessment, including an Individualized Educational Plan (IEP). Children with learning disabilities may be helped a lot by some relatively simple steps, such as additional help in certain areas or special adjustments in the classroom. Our office can help put you in touch with the educational resources your child needs and by providing additional follow-up.

What are the types of learning disabilities?

Every child with learning disabilities is different. Some common learning disabilities are:

- *Dyslexia.* A specific reading disability. Your child may read very slowly and inaccurately. He or she may have difficulty "decoding" and recognizing words and reading print. Yet he or she may learn very well when material is read aloud.

- *Dyscalculia.* A specific math disability. Your child has trouble with math calculations; he or she can't seem to memorize math facts or remember the steps needed to solve problems. Some children with language disabilities or attention problems have trouble learning math as well.

- *Dysgraphia.* A specific writing disability. Your child's writing may be difficult to read and his or her handwriting messy. Your child may have difficulty organizing and expressing ideas. Spelling may be difficult as well.

- *Dyspraxia.* A specific disability of fine muscle control. Your child may have difficulty using a pencil or scissors, tying shoes, or typing on a keyboard. Other children have problems with large muscle control, such as catching or throwing a ball.

- *Attention deficit–hyperactivity disorder (ADHD).* Not a specific learning disorder but causes many problems in school (and at home). Your child may have difficulty paying attention, sitting still, or controlling impulses.

Learning disabilities may affect many other areas as well, such as memory, language, or social skills. Children may have more than one type of learning disability. Problems in one area (such as reading) may cause problems with many different school subjects.

In addition to school problems, learning disabilities can affect other areas of your child's life. "Feeling like a failure" may make your child anxious or depressed. Feelings of low self-esteem and not having control over his or her life are common.

What causes learning disabilities?

Usually, no specific cause of learning disabilities is identified. Genetic, medical, environmental, social, and cultural factors may all play a role.

What are some possible complications of learning disabilities?

Without educational interventions, children with learning disabilities can fall behind in school. In the long term, failure and frustration can lead to problems with self-esteem and motivation.

What puts your child at risk of learning disabilities?

Learning disabilities are common. The U.S. Department of Education estimates that about 5% of all children in public schools have a learning disability. Possible risk factors include:

- Genetics. Reading disabilities seem to run in families.

- Preterm birth and other events around the time of birth.

- Medical conditions, such as lead poisoning, infections, or brain injury.

How are learning disabilities evaluated?

If a learning disability is suspected, your child should undergo a complete evaluation, including:

- A physical examination, to make sure there are no contributing medical problems.

- Developmental evaluation, to assess your child's level of development for his or her age.

- A mental health evaluation, to identify any family or psychological issues that may be contributing to your child's problems at school.

Depending on the nature of your child's educational problems, various other specialists may be involved, for example, a speech and language pathologist, an occupational therapist, a neurologist, or a social worker.

Evaluations conducted by schools are usually very helpful. However, they are sometimes limited by budgetary, personnel, and other constraints. If you have concerns about the adequacy of your child's evaluation, make sure to discuss them with your child's doctor.

How are learning disabilities treated?

Educational interventions are probably the most important aspect of care:

- *Early intervention* can lessen the impact of learning disabilities on your child's school performance and other areas of life.

- *Special education* services are also available in every state. You are entitled to evaluation and educational services for your child. Based on the results, an Individualized Education Program (IEP) can be developed to meet your child's educational needs.

- *Having a learning disability doesn't mean your child isn't smart.* It also doesn't mean that he or she is lazy. It simply means that he or she has problems with specific learning skills. Your child's educational program should help to deal with his or her educational weaknesses while maximizing strengths. Recommendations may include:

- *"Bypass" strategies* to limit the impact of your child's learning disability. For example, children with writing difficulties may be allowed to make oral rather than written reports. Children with attention problems may be seated closer to the teacher.

- *Remediation strategies* to strengthen the "weak links" in your child's learning process. This may include tutoring in specific areas like math or reading or more general areas such as study skills. Working on these areas with your child at home can be very helpful. For children with dyslexia (reading disorder), special instruction in phonics may help.

- *Developmental therapies.* These include speech and language therapy for children with language disorders or occupational therapy for certain kids with writing problems.

- *Increasing strengths.* The plan should include opportunities for your child to develop areas that he or she is strong in, not just focusing on weaknesses.

- *Counseling* may help your child in dealing with stress and other issues related to the learning disability. It may include your child alone or your entire family.

- *Medications* may be part of the treatment plan, for example, if your child has attention problems.

- *Diets, exercise programs, and other alternative treatments* are sometimes recommended for children with certain learning disabilities. Although some parents strongly believe in these alternative treatments, most have not been proved effective in scientific studies. Be wary before investing too much time and money in unproven treatments.

When should I call your office?

Call our office if you have concerns about your child's school performance or about the evaluation and treatment of his or her learning disabilities.

Stuttering

Stuttering is a problem in which your child's speech is interrupted by pauses or repeated sounds. It commonly occurs around the time your child's language skills are developing most rapidly. Stuttering may get worse in situations that are stressful for your child. Stuttering usually clears up within a few months. If it doesn't, speech therapy may be helpful.

What is stuttering?

Stuttering is a common speech problem. Your child may repeat or have trouble making certain sounds, especially at the beginning of words. If your child starts feeling nervous about his or her speech problem, it may seem to get worse. Stuttering is sometimes known as "stammering."

Stuttering is most common in toddlers and preschoolers, who are at a stage where they are gaining language skills very rapidly. It is almost never a sign of serious disease or mental health problems.

Most children stop stuttering within a few months. In others, the problem goes on longer. If stuttering becomes a lasting problem for your child, speech therapy can be helpful.

What does it look like?

- The normal flow of your child's speech is broken up or interrupted. He or she may pause frequently when speaking or repeat sounds several times, especially at the beginning of words. Your child just seems to have a hard time "getting the words out."

- Stuttering may be more noticeable when your child is feeling stressed, excited, or just self-conscious about stuttering. In other situations, he or she may have no problem speaking smoothly and fluently.

- In some children you may notice other movements of the face, as if he or she is really struggling to speak. These "struggle behaviors" may include rapid eye blinking, trembling of the lips or jaw, and other movements of the face and upper body.

What causes stuttering?

- Most of the time, stuttering is a "developmental" issue—just a step in your child's language development process. Children with this form of stuttering usually outgrow it.

- Stuttering can be related to psychological or emotional issues. However, most of the time the emotional issues are caused by the stuttering, not the other way around! Feeling anxious about stuttering tends to make the problem worse.

- Other causes—such as brain injuries or serious mental illness—are rare.

What are some possible complications of stuttering?

- Stuttering is rarely a sign of any serious abnormality or illness.

- Stuttering can be an embarrassing problem for your child. Unfortunately, children who stutter are sometimes teased. Besides this type of social problem, there are no real "complications" of stuttering.

What increases your child's risk of stuttering?

- It is most common between the ages of 2 and 6.

- It is more common in boys than in girls.

How is stuttering treated?

- Most of the time, no treatment is needed. Most children "outgrow" stuttering within a few months, as their language skills continue to develop.

- Meanwhile, several steps can help reduce the pressure on your child when he or she is speaking:

  - Provide a relaxed environment. Encourage your child to take his or her time when speaking. Let your child know that you are listening. Speak in a slow, relaxed manner yourself.

  - Don't criticize, tease, or punish your child for stuttering.

  - Don't focus too much attention on the stuttering or act as if it's a major problem. However, if your child brings up the subject, talk openly about it.

  - Be wary of programs or "cures" for stuttering advertised on the Internet or elsewhere. Some have not been scientifically tested; others use medications or electronic devices that can have side effects. It's a good idea to talk to your doctor before starting your child on any kind of treatment program.

- If your child is still stuttering after 6 months, we may recommend further evaluation or treatment. Evaluation may also be recommended for children whose stuttering is accompanied by "struggle behaviors."

- A specialist (called a speech-language pathologist) can provide expert testing, diagnosis, and treatment of stuttering. A speech specialist can teach your child helpful approaches to speaking more fluently.

- Treatment may also address some of the psychological or emotional side effects of stuttering, such as fear of speaking in front of people.

- Most children can be helped with treatment and follow-up. Stuttering in adulthood is relatively rare.

When should I call your office?

Call our office if:

- Your child's stuttering doesn't improve within 6 months or if it seems to be getting worse.

- Your child's stuttering is accompanied by "struggle behaviors" such as eye blinking or other facial movements.

- You have questions about treatments for your child's stuttering.

Section VIII ▪ The Ear

Earwax Problems

Earwax, also called cerumen, is a normal substance that helps protect the ear canal. If too much earwax builds up, it can block the ear canal, causing ear discomfort, reduced hearing, and other symptoms. Excessive earwax can usually be removed by using special drops. If necessary, it can be done by a doctor. Don't try to remove wax from your child's ear by inserting anything in the ear, including cotton swabs.

What kinds of problems are caused by earwax?

The build-up of too much earwax can block the your child's ear canal. This is sometimes called "impaction." Removing the excessive earwax promptly relieves symptoms such as feeling "clogged-up," reduced hearing, and discomfort or pain. Earwax can be removed by using eardrops available at the drugstore or, if necessary, in the doctor's office.

Other ways of trying to remove earwax can lead to problems. Putting cotton swabs (Q-Tips) or other objects in the ear can cause pain or bleeding or puncture holes in the eardrum or lead to an infection of the ear canal (otitis externa).

What do they look like?

If your child has earwax blocking the ear canal, you may notice that she or he has:

- Decreased hearing.
- A "clogged" feeling in the ear—discomfort; pain is uncommon. Young children may hold or pull on their ears.
- You may be able to see earwax inside the ear canal.

What causes problems with earwax?

Some people just produce more earwax than others. Although earwax blockage is a common problem for some people, others rarely or never have this problem.

Can earwax problems be prevented?

- If your child has a lot of earwax build-up, using special eardrops on a regular basis may help to prevent problems.
- Follow the doctor's instructions on removing earwax. Especially in babies, never insert cotton swabs or anything else in the ear to attempt to remove earwax.

How are earwax problems treated?

- Earwax removal kits are available at drugstores. Tilt your child's head sideways and then place drops in the ear. Let the drops remain in the ear for several minutes; they will help dissolve the wax. This procedure can be repeated for a few days, if needed. If excessive earwax is still present, call our office.
- In the doctor's office, earwax may be removed using special instruments, or using water to gently flush out the ear canal. Drops may first be placed in the ear to soften the wax, making it easier to remove.

Don't use an earwax removal kit if your child has a hole in the eardrum (rupture or perforation) or if your child has a possible ear infection (an earache, usually with a cold, sometimes with fever).

When should I call your office?

Call our office if your child has:

- Ear discomfort and reduced hearing that do not clear up after earwax is removed.
- Frequent problems with earwax.
- Severe ear pain, earache with a cold or fever, or fluid draining from the ear—this is usually *not* related to earwax.

Middle Ear Infection (Acute Otitis Media)

Ear infections are very common in infants and young children. Some children have many episodes. Ear infections usually occur along with an upper respiratory infection. Although usually treated with antibiotics, the option of using pain medications for a couple of days in mild cases is reasonable for some children.

What is middle ear infection?

Acute otitis media is inflammation (soreness, redness) of the middle ear (the space behind the eardrum). The inflammation is usually caused by infection with bacteria or sometimes with viruses; it often occurs with a cold. Symptoms may include ear pain, fever, fussiness, and fluid draining from the ear.

Acute otitis media is very common in infants and toddlers, particularly those between the ages of 6 and 20 months. Otitis media can become a frequent or continuing problem for some children.

What does it look like and how is it diagnosed?

- Ear pain is the main symptom. Babies may cry or act fussy. Toddlers and older children can tell you that they have an earache.

- Usually an upper respiratory infection (runny nose, cough, congestion) is present or occurred recently.

- Fever is sometimes present.

- Pus or other fluid may drain from the ear (otorrhea).

- Babies may pull or tug on the ear. However, this isn't always a sign of ear infection—instead it may be a sign of fluid or congestion in the middle ear (otitis media with effusion).

- To make the diagnosis, the doctor will look at the eardrum with an instrument called an otoscope. If infection is present, the drum is usually red and there is fluid or pus behind the drum.

What causes middle ear infection?

- *Acute otitis media* is caused by infection with bacteria. Viruses sometimes play a role.

- *Otitis media with effusion* (serous otitis) occurs when fluid builds up inside the ear, even though no infection is present. Antibiotic treatment is not needed.

What are some possible complications of middle ear infection?

- Frequent doctor's office visits and antibiotic treatment. For some children, acute otitis media becomes a repeated problem. Frequent treatment with antibiotics can encourage the growth of bacteria that are resistant to common antibiotics and therefore are harder to treat.

- Reduced hearing. This is usually temporary. Hearing returns after the fluid is gone from inside the ear. However, hearing loss may be a more lasting problem if your child has repeated infections or if fluid stays in the middle ear for a long time.

- Rupture of the eardrum, with pus draining from the ear. In most cases, the eardrum heals without a problem.

- Persistent ear infection—one that doesn't get better with the usual antibiotic treatment. This may require special antibiotic treatment or drainage.

- Other complications are possible but rare, such as:

  - Infection of the mastoid bone (mastoiditis), which is right behind the ear.

  - Permanent hearing loss, resulting from severe, repeated ear infections or fluid remaining in the ear for a long time.

  - Growth of a cyst within the ear (cholesteatoma).

What puts your child at risk of middle ear infection?

- Colds: Most middle ear infections occur with or soon after a cold.

- Genetic factors: Middle ear disease may "run in families."

- Risk may be higher for boys.

- Risk is high for Native-American children.

- Exposure to tobacco smoke ("passive smoking").

- Using a pacifier may increase the risk.

- Certain medical conditions (for example, cleft palate, Down syndrome) increase the risk.

- The risk is highest for infants and toddlers between 6 and 20 months old.

Can middle ear infection be prevented?

The following steps may reduce your child's risk:

- Breast-feeding.

- Don't smoke or let others smoke around your child.

- If your child has had a lot of trouble with middle ear infections, options may include placing a small tube through the eardrum (see Treatment).

How are middle ear infections treated?

- Antibiotics are often recommended. Treatment usually continues for 10 days but may be less depending on the age of the child and which antibiotic is used.

- To be certain the bacteria causing the infection are eliminated, make sure your child takes all of the prescribed antibiotics. Don't stop treatment just because he or she seems to be feeling better. If your child isn't getting better within 2 to 3 days, call our office.

- If the infection is mild, the doctor may discuss the option of just using pain medication. Many of these milder infections get better just as quickly without antibiotics. Unnecessary use of antibiotics makes it more difficult to treat future infections. If the symptoms get worse or don't get better in a few days, antibiotics will probably be prescribed.

- The doctor may want to re-examine your child after 4 to 6 weeks to see if there is any fluid or congestion behind the eardrum. Even if fluid is present, it usually goes away.

- If infections occur very often or don't get better after a long time, we may recommend a visit to a doctor specializing in ear, nose, and throat diseases (otorhinolaryngologist, or ENT physician). The ENT doctor may perform a procedure to drain fluid from the ear.

- In some situations, the ENT doctor will recommend placing a tube through the eardrum. The tube helps to drain fluid and pus from the ear and to prevent future infections.

- Tubes are usually placed with the patient under anesthesia. The procedure causes little or no pain and the tube often comes out on its own after a few months.

- There are generally few problems with ear tubes. However, sometimes drainage continues despite tube placement, or the tube comes out too early to be helpful. At other times, the tube leaves a hole in the eardrum, which may need to be repaired at a later time.

When should I call your office?

Call our office if:

- Your child's symptoms (ear pain, fever) continue for more than 2 to 3 days after starting treatment.

- Your child's symptoms get better but then return after treatment.

Otitis Media with Effusion

Otitis media with effusion (OME) is a condition in which fluid builds up behind the eardrum in one or both ears. This condition usually occurs with a cold or after a middle ear infection, although it doesn't mean the ear is infected. Otitis media with effusion usually goes away on its own within a few months. If not, the doctor may recommend hearing tests for your child.

What is otitis media with effusion?

Otitis media with effusion (OME) refers to the presence of fluid in the middle ear and inflammation that is not caused by infection. The middle ear space, located behind the ear drum, is where ear infections (acute otitis media) typically occur. Although it is not an ear infection, OME may occur with a cold or after an ear infection.

The inflammation and fluid build-up usually clear up without any treatment, although this may take several weeks. The doctor may want to recheck your child's ear regularly to make sure the fluid clears up. Otitis media with effusion can result in some hearing loss, although it is usually mild. If the hearing problem persists, the doctor may recommend hearing tests.

What does it look like?

- Infants may have no symptoms. You may notice them tugging on or playing with their ears. Unlike ear infections, OME usually causes no pain.

- Older children may feel pressure, fullness, or popping in their ears. Ringing in the ears may also occur.

- Problems with balance may occur but are uncommon.

What causes otitis media with effusion?

Otitis media with effusion usually occurs when the normal drainage system within the ear becomes blocked. The eustachian tube is the connection between the middle ear and the throat. When this tube becomes blocked by swelling, usually from a cold or recent ear infection, fluid cannot drain from the middle ear to the throat. This allows the fluid to build up behind the eardrum.

What are some possible complications of otitis media with effusion?

- The vast majority of children with OME have no problems. The condition gets better on its own.

- Reduced hearing may occur. This is a temporary problem for most children—hearing returns to normal after the fluid is gone from inside the ear. However, hearing loss may be more of a problem if the fluid stays in the ear for a long time. For a small number of children, reduced hearing can lead to problems with speech, language, and other developmental skills if it is not treated.

- Other complications are possible but rare, such as:

  - Growth of a cyst within the ear (cholesteatoma).

  - Damage to some of the structures in the middle ear.

What puts your child at risk of otitis media with effusion?

- Middle ear infections (acute otitis media).

- Colds: Most middle ear infections and OME occur with or soon after a cold.

- Genetic factors: Middle ear disease may "run in families."

- The risk is high for Native-American children.

- Exposure to tobacco smoke (passive smoking).

- Using a pacifier may increase the risk.

- Certain medical conditions (cleft palate, Down syndrome) increase the risk.

- The risk is highest in infants and toddlers between 6 and 20 months.

How is otitis media with effusion diagnosed?

- Most often, the doctor can recognize OME by looking into your child's ear with an otoscope. Children with OME don't have the usual signs of middle ear infection: redness or pus behind the eardrum or bulging of the eardrum.

- Instead, the doctor may see fluid behind the eardrum, or the eardrum does not show the normal movement when the doctor pushes air into the ear canal.

- Medical devices such as a tympanometer or acoustic reflectometer may be used. These instruments use sound waves to tell if there is fluid behind the eardrum.

How is otitis media with effusion treated?

- Most cases of OME clear up without treatment, usually within 3 months. The doctor may want to recheck your child regularly until the fluid is gone.

- Antibiotics, steroids, decongestants, and other medications probably don't help much. Treatment for allergies, if present, might help.

- For some children with OME, hearing loss may be significant and put your child at risk for speech, language, and other problems. If fluid stays in the ears for longer than 3 to 4 months, the doctor may recommend a hearing test.

- Based on the results of hearing tests, other developmental issues, and the parents' feelings about these concerns, the doctor may recommend one of the following treatment approaches:

  - Waiting and watching. Otitis media with effusion usually clears up. Sometimes, it finally goes away on its own during the summer months.

  - Ear tube placement. In some situations, the doctor may recommend placing a tube through the eardrum to help drain fluid from the middle ear. This may be done if your child has more severe hearing loss, if speech or language skills are affected, or if your child is at risk of developmental problems (for example, in very premature infants).

- Ear tubes are usually placed by an ear, nose and throat specialist (otorhinolaryngologist or ENT physician).

- Tubes are usually placed under anesthesia. The procedure causes little or no pain. The tube often comes out on its own after a few months.

- There are generally few problems with ear tubes. However, sometimes fluid continues despite tube placement, or the tube comes out too soon to be helpful. At other times, the tube may leave a hole in the eardrum, which may need to be repaired at a later time.

When should I call your office?

Call our office if:

- Your doctor recommends "watching and waiting." Be sure to keep follow-up appointments.

- Your child has an ear tube. Keep regular follow-up visits with the ENT doctor and with our office. The ENT doctor will provide more details about caring for the ear tube.

- You see fluid draining from the ear after an ear tube is placed. Call the ENT doctor or our office.

Outer Ear Infection (Swimmer's Ear)

> Outer ear infection is an infection of the ear canal, outside the eardrum. This condition is often called "swimmer's ear," although it isn't always related to swimming. Outer ear infections can cause a severe earache. The problem usually clears up quickly with antibiotic eardrops.

What is an outer ear infection?

An outer ear infection is an infection of the skin inside the ear canal with bacteria. Especially in children, this infection commonly occurs when the inside of the ear canal stays wet for a period of time, such as after swimming. That's why it's sometimes called "swimmer's ear"; the medical term is otitis externa. Infection may also result from other causes, such as foreign bodies stuck in the ear. This is not an "inner ear infection" (acute otitis media) which occurs behind the eardrum and is usually accompanied by an upper respiratory infection (a cold).

Outer ear infection can cause a severe earache. Antibiotic eardrops, which are sometimes used to soak a "wick" that is placed in the ear, are an effective treatment.

What does it look like?

- Ear pain, which may be severe.
- The pain is usually worse when you touch or pull on your child's ear.
- Itching in the ear; this may occur before ear pain and/or while the infection is clearing up.
- Swelling and redness of the ear canal.
- Soft, white ear wax or drainage from the ear.
- Lymph glands in the head and neck may be swollen.
- In severe cases, the outer ear may be red and swollen.
- Rarely, inability to move part of the face, dizziness, or hearing loss. These may be signs of a more serious infection—call our office immediately.

What are some possible complications of outer ear infection?

- The infection usually clears up promptly with antibiotic treatment.
- There is a small risk of a more serious infection spreading outside the ear canal. This occurs mainly in children with immune system problems (immune deficiency).

What puts your child at risk of outer ear infection?

- Swimming in lakes, ponds, or swimming pools.
- Anything that causes too much moisture in the ear canal (for example, headphones or hearing aids).
- Being too vigorous about removing earwax.
- Trauma or scratching of the ear canal. Young children may place their fingers or foreign bodies in the ear.
- Previous outer ear infections.

Can outer ear infections be prevented?

- If your child gets a lot of these kinds of ear infections, special ear drops recommended by your doctor placed in both ears immediately may help.
- Avoid sticking anything in your child's ear (including Q-Tips).

How are outer ear infections treated?

- Antibiotic eardrops are an effective treatment for outer ear infections. The drops are placed in the ear a few times per day, usually for 7 to 10 days.
- If the ear canal is badly swollen, it may need to be cleaned out before treatment. The doctor may place a small piece of cotton-like material, called a wick, into your child's ear. Apply antibiotic eardrops to the cotton three times per day, as instructed by the doctor. The swelling should be better after 2 or 3 days, allowing the wick to be removed. Then continue using antibiotic eardrops.
- Keep the ear dry. Your child will have to stop swimming for a while. Keep the ear from getting wet while your child is bathing in the shower or tub.
- Give analgesics (acetaminophen or ibuprofen) if necessary to relieve pain. Pain and swelling should decrease within a few days of starting antibiotic drops.
- Oral antibiotics are rarely needed.

- Occasionally, the ear canal may become infected with a fungus. In this case, other medications will be prescribed.

When should I call your office?

Call our office if:

- Ear pain and swelling aren't getting better after 2 or 3 days of treatment or if they get worse.

- The outer ear is very swollen and red.
- Your child develops an inability to move part of the face, dizziness, or hearing loss. These may be signs of a more serious infection.

Section IX ▪ Emergency

Acute Appendicitis

Appendicitis is a common medical emergency in children. The main symptoms are abdominal pain, vomiting, and fever. If your child has appendicitis, surgery is needed as soon as possible to prevent complications. It can be difficult to be sure that appendicitis is the problem, especially in young children.

What is acute appendicitis?

Appendicitis is inflammation and infection of a pocket of small intestine called the appendix. The opening to the appendix may become blocked off, allowing congestion and infection to develop. The appendix then becomes swollen and inflamed (red and tender). Without surgery, it may burst (rupture). Rupture is a more serious problem that can lead to infection inside your child's abdomen.

The only treatment for appendicitis is an operation to remove the infected appendix (appendectomy). If the doctor thinks that appendicitis is possible, your child may need to go to the hospital for surgery. If the diagnosis is uncertain, tests such as computed tomography (CT scan) may be helpful.

Unfortunately, even with tests, it is sometimes difficult to be sure that your child has appendicitis. Occasionally, surgery is performed but appendicitis is not present.

What does it look like?

Symptoms of appendicitis vary, but the main ones are:

- *Pain in the abdomen.* Pain usually starts around the navel then moves to the lower right side of the abdomen.

- *Nausea and vomiting.* These usually start after pain. Your child may vomit only a little bit or not at all. He or she may have very little appetite.

- *Fever.* Temperature may rise rapidly, usually after the start of pain.

- It is sometimes difficult to tell appendicitis from the "stomach flu," especially in young infants. If you are sure that pain started before other symptoms, this may be a sign of appendicitis.

- Diarrhea may be present.

What are some possible complications of appendicitis?

- If appendicitis is not recognized and treated with surgery, the appendix may rupture. This can lead to a more serious infection inside your child's abdomen. If the appen-

dix is perforated or ruptured, the risk of infection or other complications after surgery is much higher.

- Other complications are possible, especially with a ruptured appendix. All of these complications are treatable:

  - Abscesses (collections of pus) inside the abdomen.

  - Wound infections (infection in the area of skin where the incision was made for surgery).

  - Occasionally, obstruction (blockage) of the intestine.

What puts your child at risk of appendicitis?

- Appendicitis is a frequent problem, affecting about 4 out of 1000 children in the United States.

- The risk is highest in adolescence; appendicitis is rare in infants.

- Some families seem to be at higher risk, and boys may be at higher risk than girls.

Can appendicitis be prevented?

There is no known way to prevent appendicitis. Prompt diagnosis and surgery can avoid a ruptured appendix.

How is appendicitis treated?

- Surgery is the only treatment for appendicitis. Once the doctor diagnoses appendicitis—or even if he or she strongly suspects appendicitis—your child will have surgery as soon as possible.

- The operation for appendicitis is relatively simple. Your child will be under anesthesia (asleep) for the procedure. Medications for pain are given before and after surgery.

- As long as the appendix hasn't perforated or ruptured, complications are uncommon. Recovery is usually quick; your child will probably be able to go home from the hospital within 2 or 3 days.

- If the appendix has perforated and ruptured, additional treatments may be needed before and after surgery. Your child may receive antibiotics through a vein (IV) before surgery and for a while afterward. Recovery after surgery takes longer. Your child will be watched closely for possible complications, especially infections.

When should I call your office?

After surgery, follow the surgeon's instructions for postoperative and follow-up care. Call your surgeon's office or our office if any of the following occur:

- High fever.
- Continued or worsening vomiting.
- Increased pain or swelling of the abdomen.

- Blood in bowel movements.
- Redness around the surgical incision.

Animal and Human Bites

Medical care is often needed for any wounds that breaks your child's skin, including human bites. Antibiotics may be needed to prevent potentially serious infections. Some bite wounds need stitches (sutures), depending on how severe they are and where they are located.

What do you need to know about bite wounds?

Bite wounds are common in children. Children may be bitten by dogs, cats, or other animals. Human bites are also common, especially in preschoolers.

Unless your child's bite is very minor, it should be checked by a medical professional. Antibiotics may be needed to prevent infection with germs from a biting animal's mouth. Stitches may be needed for larger bites or bites located in certain areas, especially on the face. Teaching children some simple safety rules can prevent many animal bites.

What do they look like?

- Dog bites may appear as scrapes (abrasions); puncture wounds, sometimes quite deep; or tears (lacerations). Bites from larger dogs and dogs of more aggressive breeds can be severe.

- Cat and rabbit bites are usually puncture wounds.

- Human bites can be puncture wounds when the upper and lower teeth come together on a body part. Another type of bite wound occurs in fights—the skin of the fist may be cut or torn when it comes in contact with the other person's teeth.

- Rodent (rats and gerbils) bites may also occur.

What are some possible complications of bite wounds?

- *Infection* is the most common complication, whether the bite is caused by an animal or human. The germs causing infection differ, depending on the type of animal. Other important factors include the time since the bite, the depth of the bite, and whether there is any foreign matter in the wound.

- Although they are rare, there is a risk of certain serious infections such as tetanus and rabies. Rabies vaccine may be needed after bites by wild animals, especially rodents, or by stray dogs.

- *Scarring* or other healing-related complications may also occur. Medical evaluation is required to see if stitches are needed to close the wound.

What puts your child at risk of bite wounds?

- Dog bites are most common in boys between the ages of 6 and 11. Most bites occur near home and involve a dog the child knows.

- Dogs are more likely to bite when a child is bothering them. This is especially true for mother dogs who are trying to protect their pups. However, some dogs may bite even when they are not being bothered.

- Serious dog bites are more likely to occur with certain breeds, for example, rottweilers and pit bulls.

- Cat bites occur more commonly in girls and usually involve a cat the child knows.

- Human bites are most commonly seen in preschool and early school-age children.

- Older children may suffer bite wounds when fighting.

Can bite wounds be prevented?

Teach children some simple rules for safety around animals:

- Don't disturb animals that are sleeping or eating.

- Don't go near animals you don't know.

- Don't disturb mother dogs caring for their pups.

- If a dog starts chasing you, don't run.

- Let dogs see and sniff you before touching them.

Parents should not bring animals that may bite into the home. Avoid exotic pets and aggressive dog breeds.

How are bite wounds treated?

- Any animal or human bite that breaks the skin requires medical attention. If your child is bitten, call our office or go to the emergency room.

- The doctor will examine the bite and ask about how it happened. Provide as much information as possible on the type of animal and the circumstances surrounding the bite.

- *Prevention of infection*:

  - The doctor will need to know whether your child has had a tetanus vaccination within the last 5 to 10 years. If not, a tetanus shot will be needed.

  - In human bites, it is important to know whether the child/person who bit your child is infected with hepatitis B virus or human immunodeficiency virus (HIV). If so, medications may be given to your child to prevent these infections.

- In dog or cat bites, it is important to know whether the animal has received rabies vaccine or if the animal was acting abnormally. Your child may need rabies shots if recommended by the local health department. Rabies shots may also be needed for bites from an unknown or wild animal (for example, a raccoon or a bat).

- The bite area should be cleansed and rinsed thoroughly to remove germs. If any skin has been torn, minor surgery may be needed to remove it.

- *Antibiotics*. Antibiotics are generally recommended for:

  - Puncture wounds.

  - Bites in certain areas (face, hands, feet, or genitals).

  - Any bite that is more than just a scrape.

  - Your child may receive antibiotics in oral form or in a shot. If oral antibiotics are given, make sure your child takes the full amount prescribed.

  - The choice of antibiotic depends on the type of biting animal and other factors. Make sure to tell the doctor if your child is allergic to penicillin.

- *Stitches and dressings*:

  - Stitches (sutures) may be recommended to close the wound. Factors affecting the need for stitches include the location of the bite, how long ago it happened, the risk of infection, and the size and depth of the bite.

  - Bites of the face or deep bite wounds may leave unsightly scars. The doctor may recommend a visit to a plastic surgeon or other specialist.

  - A dressing (bandage) will likely be placed on the wound. Follow the doctor's instructions regarding changing the dressing and keeping the wound clean.

  - Get follow-up care within a day or two, or as recommended by the doctor.

When should I call your office?

Call our office if any of the following occurs:

- Severe pain.

- Fever.

- Redness or swelling at or near the area of the bite.

- Pus draining from the bite.

Carbon Monoxide Poisoning

Carbon monoxide is a colorless, odorless gas that is toxic (poisonous) to humans. Carbon monoxide (abbreviated CO) is produced when gasoline, natural gas, or other fuels are burned. At home, faulty furnaces or blocked ventilation systems can quickly lead to deadly levels of CO. Some simple safety tips can help protect your family against CO poisoning.

What is carbon monoxide poisoning?

Carbon monoxide is one of the most common air pollutants because it is produced when nearly any type of fuel is burned. Its chemical abbreviation is CO. When CO is allowed to build up in enclosed spaces—such as in a home, garage, or car—it can quickly reach deadly levels.

Carbon monoxide is generated by cars or other gasoline engines, by gas stoves and furnaces, and by wood or charcoal fires. Carbon monoxide is a silent killer because you can't see it or smell it. Victims may drop off to sleep and never wake up. If your child or others in your family have been exposed to high levels of CO, immediate treatment may be needed. Regular safety inspections and other precautions can prevent accidental CO poisoning.

What does it look like?

Initial symptoms of carbon monoxide poisoning are similar to those of other flu-like illnesses, including:

- Dizziness.
- Fatigue: being tired without a good reason.
- Headache.
- Nausea.

More specific signs of CO poisoning include:

- Absence of other flu-like symptoms, such as fever or sore throat.
- Feeling better once you get fresh air.
- Having other people in the room developing the same symptoms at the same time.

As CO levels rise, more obvious symptoms may appear, such as:

- Worsening headaches.
- Weakness, severe tiredness.
- Vision problems.
- Seizures (uncontrolled body movements).

- Shortness of breath.
- Confusion.
- Victims may also simply fall asleep without experiencing any symptoms. In this situation, people may die without regaining consciousness.

What causes carbon monoxide poisoning?

- Anything that burns carbon fuels produces carbon monoxide gas. Common sources are cars and trucks, gas stoves and furnaces, kerosene-burning heaters and lanterns, wood-burning stoves and fireplaces, and charcoal fires. Methylene chloride, which is used in paint removers and other solvents, can cause CO poisoning if the fumes are inhaled over a long time.
- If CO gas is allowed to collect indoors, toxic levels can build up quickly. This may happen when:
  - A fireplace or chimney flue is blocked.
  - A furnace ventilation system is leaky.
  - A fuel-burning heater or kitchen stove is used for indoor heat.
  - Gasoline-powered engines are run indoors or without proper ventilation.

This is just a partial list—many other situations may lead to accidental CO poisoning!

What are some possible complications of carbon monoxide poisoning?

- Carbon monoxide poisoning can rapidly cause death.
- Survivors may have permanent damage to the brain and nervous system.

What puts your child at risk of carbon monoxide poisoning?

- Any of the situations listed above may rapidly lead to toxic levels of CO.
- Infants and young children can be more rapidly harmed by the toxic effects of CO gas. People with certain heart, lung, and blood diseases are also at higher risk of harm.

Can carbon monoxide poisoning be prevented?

- Make sure stoves, furnaces, water heaters, dryers, and other natural gas-burning appliances are properly installed and ventilated.

- Get regular yearly inspections of your furnace and other home appliances and of your car's exhaust system.

- Never use a kitchen stove for heat. If you must use a fuel-burning space heater indoors, make sure it is properly ventilated. Don't go to sleep while a fuel-burning space heater is operating.

- Never use a charcoal grill, camping stove, or similar devices for cooking indoors. Don't run gas-powered generators or engines indoors.

- Never leave your car's engine running in a garage or other enclosed space. Toxic CO levels can build up even if the garage door is open.

- Install carbon monoxide alarms in your home.

How is carbon monoxide poisoning treated?

If you think there may be a carbon monoxide problem in your home or other enclosed space, *get out! Go outside as quickly as you can.* Because the initial symptoms are vague, CO poisoning may be unrecognized at first. Several people in the same room suddenly feeling ill or woozy or falling asleep may be a warning sign.

Get medical attention as soon as possible. If symptoms are present, call 911 or go to the nearest emergency room.

- In the hospital, treatment will include:

  - Blood tests to determine how severe the CO poisoning is.

  - Oxygen to help eliminate CO from the bloodstream. In severe cases, the patient may be put in an "oxygen room" for administration of very high levels of oxygen (hyperbaric oxygen therapy).

- As the patient recovers, signs of damage to the brain or nervous system may be apparent. Some of these complications are permanent. Others may get better, especially if treatment is started as soon as possible.

- If CO poisoning has occurred as a suicide attempt, psychiatric and other treatment may be needed for the patient.

- After the incident, repair work may be needed to identify and correct the source of the CO (for example, an improperly ventilated furnace).

When should I call your office?

Call our office if any signs of CO poisoning occur.

Dehydration

Dehydration is a common complication of illness in children, especially infants. It can occur any time your child is losing more fluid—through vomiting, diarrhea, or other causes—than he or she is taking in. Dehydration can be a serious problem and always requires prompt treatment.

What is dehydration?

Our bodies must have enough water to function properly, to filter out toxins through the kidneys, and to maintain normal levels of minerals (electrolytes). Dehydration occurs when the body loses fluid more rapidly than it can be replaced. The main ways the body loses water are through urination, evaporation from the skin, and breathing. Vomiting or diarrhea can cause excess fluid losses.

Although dehydration can occur in older children and adults, infants are at highest risk. Pay attention to how much your baby is drinking and urinating any time he or she is ill. Your child should drink enough liquid to replace the fluids lost from the body. *Get medical help immediately any time your child has symptoms of dehydration: not urinating very often, dryness inside the mouth, crying without tears, or sunken eyes.*

What does it look like?

- Dryness inside the mouth, including the tongue.
- Urinating less often. In babies, going 6 hours without wetting the diaper may be a sign of dehydration. (With highly absorbent disposable diapers, this may be hard to judge. It may help to place a cotton ball on the penis or vagina.)
- Crying without tears.
- Sunken eyes or "soft spot" (fontanelle) on the top of the head.
- Extreme tiredness; babies may be irritable instead.
- Confusion or behavior changes.
- Fast heartbeat or breathing (this may also be caused by a high fever).

What causes dehydration?

Dehydration can occur as a complication of any illness in which excess water is lost from the body:

- Diarrhea.
- Vomiting or illnesses that prevent your child from drinking enough fluids.

- High fever causes the body to lose more water; therefore, dehydration can occur more easily.
- Diseases that cause excessive urination, such as diabetes, can also cause dehydration.

What are some possible complications of dehydration?

- Severe dehydration can cause kidney damage.
- Dehydration causes changes in the body's levels of salts (electrolytes), which can lead to seizures or abnormal heart rhythms.
- Dehydration increases the risk of abnormal blood clots.

Can dehydration be prevented?

- Any time your child has a lot of vomiting or diarrhea, keep an eye on the amount of liquids he or she is drinking and how much fluid he or she is losing. Give enough liquids to keep the mouth moist and urination normal.
- Even if it seems as if your child is throwing up all the liquids you give, keep giving them. You may have to give very small amounts of liquids very frequently—a teaspoon every minute or two—to keep up with fluid losses.
- To prevent dehydration, in some children we may recommend it's best to give liquids containing some minerals, such as Pedialyte, Gatorade, or Crystal Light. Kool Aid and juices may make diarrhea worse because of the large amount of sugar they contain.
- For children of all ages (and adults too), make sure they drink enough water on hot days.
- Regular foods should be continued as soon as possible.

How is dehydration treated?

The most important treatment is *fluid replacement* (giving back liquids to make up for what was lost). This is especially true in infants, who can lose body fluids rapidly.

If dehydration is not severe, treatment may be tried in the doctor's office or emergency room with liquids.

- Special solutions such as Pedialyte can be used to replace lost body fluids. These products provide not only water but also sugars, salts, and other chemicals your child's body needs.
- Your child may need large amounts of liquids. The doctor will tell you how much to give; it should be enough to ensure that your child is urinating at least every 6 hours or so, the mouth remains moist, and your child is still

producing tears. The fluids can be given in small amounts frequently—as little as a teaspoon every minute or two.

- Over time, you can gradually give larger amounts of fluid replacement over longer intervals. Your child can eat solid foods too, if tolerated.

- Restarting regular food as soon as possible is important.

If dehyradtion is severe or not enough liquids can be taken by the child to correct or prevent dehydration (because of severe vomiting, large amounts of diarrhea, or refusal to drink), he or she may need intravenous (IV) fluid. Some of these children will have to be hospitalized.

When should I call your office?

If the following symptoms of dehydration appear, seek medical care immediately:

- Dryness inside the mouth, decreased or no tears when crying, fast heartbeat, irritability, or extreme tiredness. In infants, going 6 hours without wetting their diapers may be a sign of dehydration.

- Sunken eyes or soft spot on the top of the infant's head (fontanelle).

Fainting (Syncope)

Syncope is the medical term for fainting. Fainting occurs fairly commonly in children and teens and is usually not serious. In a small percentage of cases, fainting can be caused by heart rhythm problems (abnormal heartbeat) or other uncommon causes. Tests may be needed to determine the origin of the problem.

Fainting during physical activity can be more serious and always requires medical evaluation.

What is fainting?

Fainting is also called "passing out"—the medical term is syncope. People who faint temporarily lose consciousness, often falling down as they do so. The person usually regains consciousness (wakes up) in a minute or two.

Fainting can be scary, but most of the time it doesn't signal any serious disease or health problem. Fainting occurs because not enough blood (oxygen) is getting to the brain. The most common reason involves certain nerves causing the heart to temporarily slow down and pump less blood to the brain. This is called "vasovagal" or "neurocardiogenic" syncope.

In children and teens, fainting often occurs after standing around on a warm day. It can also be related to pain, fear, even straining when going to the bathroom. Most children who faint need no treatment. If fainting is a more frequent problem and not caused by any medical conditions such as problems with heart rhythm, treatments are available.

What does it look like?

- Your child suddenly collapses, losing consciousness.

- He or she may have various symptoms before passing out, such as:

  - Dizziness (lightheadedness)

  - Fast breathing (hyperventilation)

  - Flushing: feeling warm, sweating

  - Vision changes

  - Nausea

- Many other symptoms are possible.

- Sometimes after fainting, muscle twitching occurs. This can make it difficult to tell simple fainting from a seizure (involuntary, uncontrollable muscle movements).

- Your child regains consciousness a minute or two after fainting. He or she should be alert and aware of what's going on. (If not, a seizure may be more likely to have occurred.)

What causes fainting?

- The most common cause of simple fainting in children is "vasovagal" syncope, sometimes called "neurocardiogenic" syncope.

  - An abnormal response of the parasympathetic nervous system (which controls automatic activities such as heartbeat) results in a drop in blood pressure and heart rate. This reduces blood flow to the brain, causing unconsciousness. Blood flow returns to normal when your child falls or lies down.

  - This type of fainting is uncommon before ages 6 to 10 years.

- Fainting can be a sign of low blood sugar in people with diabetes (sometimes even in those without diabetes).

- Rarely, fainting in children can result from some potentially serious heart conditions, including heart rythym problems called *arrythmias*. With arrythmias, the heart beats too fast or, less often, too slowly. This sometimes doesn't allow enough blood to be pumped to the brain and causes fainting. The child may feel his or her heart beating very fast.

- Fainting during exercise always requires medical evaluation!

Can fainting be prevented?

- If the cause is simple fainting (vasovagal syncope), try to make sure that your child avoids factors that seem to trigger fainting spells, for example, not having enough to eat or drink or being emotionally upset. Your child should be aware of the early warning signs of fainting (feeling dizzy, sweating) and sit down immediately.

- If a specific cause of fainting is identified (such as heart disease), treatment given by your doctor will seek to prevent fainting and other complications.

How is the cause of fainting diagnosed?

- Most of the time, your doctor can diagnose simple fainting without any special tests. A test called an electrocardiogram (ECG) may be done to be sure there are no heart rhythm problems.

- If your child has had frequent episodes of fainting, we may recommend a visit to a heart specialist (cardiologist). The cardiologist may perform a simple test called a "tilt-table test."

- This test is just what it sounds like; your child is strapped onto a table, which is then tilted up and down. He or she is monitored closely during the procedure. The response will help to determine whether your child's fainting spells are vasovagal syncope.

● If your child has fainted during exercise or activity, more extensive testing is needed.

How is fainting treated?

In general, you should call your doctor after a fainting spell. If your child has simple fainting and the circumstances surrounding the event seem pretty clear (for example, standing for a long time on a hot day), call the doctor and report the incident.

● If your child has repeated episodes of simple fainting, treatment may be recommended. Several different treatments may be helpful, including increasing salt intake and taking heart medications, such as "beta-blockers."

● If your child has some form of heart disease that is contributing to fainting spells, treatment is obviously needed. Evaluation and treatment by a cardiologist will be recommended.

When should I call your office?

Although fainting spells are usually not a sign of serious disease, it's a good idea to get medical evaluation if your child faints.

● In general, you should call or see the doctor the first time your child faints. The doctor will advise you what to do if fainting occurs again.

● If your child is being evaluated for fainting and the episode appears different than usual, call our office or go to the emergency room. For example:

  ● If your child loses control over urination or bowel movements.

  ● If your child is unconscious for more than a minute or two, or if he or she is confused after waking up.

If your child faints during activity or exercise, call our office or go to the emergency room.

Febrile Seizures (Seizure with Fever)

> Seizures occurring with fever are usually harmless. However, it is important to be sure that a serious infection, like meningitis, is not causing the seizure. Always notify our office when your child has had a seizure, with or without fever.

What are febrile seizures?

There are two kinds of febrile seizures: *simple febrile seizures* and *complicated febrile seizures*. Both can happen in children between the ages of 6 months and 5 years.

Simple febrile seizures are the most common type of seizure in children. They don't last long and usually do not hurt the child. A complicated febrile seizure is one that lasts longer than 15 minutes, involves shaking of just one side of the child's body, or occurs again within 24 hours.

A complicated febrile seizure may mean that your child has a greater chance of developing epilepsy later (although the chance remains small). It may also mean your child is more likely to have a severe infection, like meningitis. Meningitis is an infection of the covering of the brain and can be very serious or fatal if not treated.

What do they look like?

- Your child will have a fever, with or without other symptoms such as a runny nose.

- You may see sudden, rapid, repeated shaking of both arms and legs. Your child's eyes may be rolled back in his or her head.

- A simple febrile seizure is usually brief, lasting only seconds to minutes (less than 15 minutes).

- Following the seizure, your child may be sleepy for a short time.

What should you do if your child has a febrile seizure?

- Place your child on his or her side to prevent choking on food or vomit.

- Give no medications or anything by mouth during the seizure to avoid the risk of choking.

- Call our office to notify us of your child's seizure. At that time, we will let you know whether your child needs to be seen in the office or hospital.

- Don't panic! Remember, most febrile seizures are brief and are not harmful to the child.

If the seizure has not stopped within a few minutes, call an ambulance or seek other medical attention immediately.

What causes febrile seizures?

Febrile seizures occur when the body temperature goes up quickly (fever), as happens early in an illness. The fever is most commonly caused by a viral infection.

What puts your child at risk of febrile seizures?

- If another child in your immediate family has had febrile seizures, your child is at greater risk.

- If your child has had a febrile seizure in the past, he or she is more likely to have seizures with future illnesses.

- Children younger than 12 months at the time of their first seizure have a 50% chance of having another febrile seizure with a later illness.

- Children older than 12 months at the time of their first seizure have a 30% chance of having another febrile seizure with a later illness.

Can febrile seizures be prevented?

- There is no proof that giving drugs to control fever, such as acetaminophen (Tylenol) or ibuprofen (Advil, Motrin), helps to prevent seizures. However, it is certainly reasonable to give your child one of these drugs to prevent a rapid rise in body temperature that might cause a seizure. For children who are under 2 years old, call our office to ask about the correct dosage.

- Daily use of drugs (anticonvulsants) used to control seizures is generally not recommended *for simple febrile seizures.*

What are some possible complications of febrile seizures?

- The seizure itself, if brief, does no harm to the child.

- It is important to be sure that the cause is not a serious infection like meningitis. Complicated febrile seizures that last more than 15 minutes or involve only one side of the child's body may be associated with a greater chance of a severe infection or the development of epilepsy in the future (although the chance remains small).

What follow-up care is needed?

- Febrile seizures usually go away without treatment; however, it is always important to notify our office when your child has had a seizure.

- We may want to run tests to find out whether your child has an infection and determine its cause. The doctor may perform a test called a lumbar puncture, or "spinal tap," to be sure your child does not have meningitis. This test is done by placing a needle between the bones of your child's spine and removing a small amount of fluid (called cerebrospinal fluid). Your child will receive anesthetics so that he or she will not feel the needle. Be assured that this test is safe and will not hurt your child.

When should I call your office?

Call our office any time your child has a seizure, whether or not there is a fever and whether or not your child has had a febrile seizure before.

Foreign Bodies (Swallowed Objects)

Infants and toddlers may swallow small objects, such as coins or toys. These foreign objects may become stuck in the esophagus (swallowing tube) and may at first cause symptoms such as choking, gagging, or difficulty breathing. If needed, a procedure can be performed to remove the object from your child's esophagus.

What do you need to know about swallowed objects?

Infants and toddlers put all kinds of things in their mouths. Most of the time they are swallowed and pass through the digestive tract without a problem. If an object becomes stuck in your child's throat or esophagus (the swallowing tube that leads from the throat to the stomach), it may cause choking, gagging, or difficulty breathing. Even if your child has no symptoms, medical evaluation may be needed.

An x-ray film may be done to see where the object has become stuck. Depending on the situation, the doctor may recommend waiting for a while to see if the object passes into the stomach. If needed, an instrument called an *endoscope* may be used to look into your child's throat and aid in removing the foreign object.

What types of symptoms occur?

- Your child may suddenly start choking, gagging, or coughing.
- Other symptoms may follow, including:
  - Drooling.
  - Painful swallowing or inability to swallow. Your child may refuse to eat or drink.
  - Vomiting.
  - Pain in the neck, throat, or chest.
- **!** Breathing problems may develop if the object is blocking your child's breathing tube (trachea). If your child has noisy breathing or shortness of breath or if his or her skin is turning blue, *call 911* or another emergency number.
- Your child may have no symptoms. However, if you saw your child swallow an object, it's a good idea to get med-ical help, even if he or she doesn't seem to be having any problems.

What are some possible complications of swallowed objects?

Damage to the tissues of your child's esophagus may occur. This risk depends on the object swallowed and where it gets stuck. Swallowed "button" batteries, such as watch batteries, are a special concern.

What puts your child at risk of swallowed objects?

- Infants and toddlers between 6 months and 3 years old are most likely to swallow foreign bodies.
- Children who are mentally retarded or have psychiatric problems are also more likely to swallow objects.

How can you prevent swallowed objects?

With children under age 3, keep all objects that are small enough to go into the mouth—coins, small toys, etc.—out of reach! Make sure food is cut up small enough for your child to swallow easily.

How are swallowed objects treated?

- Treatment for swallowed objects depends on several factors: what the object was, where it became stuck, and what symptoms it is causing.
- X-rays may be performed to make sure that your child swallowed the object and where it is located. Some objects just don't show up on x-rays and so endoscopy will have to be done.
- *Certain objects must be removed immediately,* especially sharp objects and "button" batteries (like watch batteries). Objects causing breathing problems also need to be removed immediately. **!**
- If the swallowed object is something harmless (such as a coin) and it is not causing any problems, the doctor may

recommend waiting as long as 24 hours to see if it passes into the stomach. If so, the object will pass all the way through your child's digestive system. This avoids the need for any treatment.

- If endoscopy is necessary:

  - An endoscope is a long, flexible tube that is placed down your child's throat and into the esophagus. Through the endoscope, the doctor can see, grasp, and safely remove the swallowed object.

  - Your child will be given an anesthetic or sedative—he or she won't be awake or feel much during the procedure. Another tube will probably be placed to protect the airway.

  - The endoscopy procedure is very safe. As soon as the anesthetic or sedative wears off, your child should be back to normal.

- Depending on your child's situation, other simple procedures may be tried to remove the object. The focus will be on removing the object as quickly and safely as possible.

- After returning home, check to make sure that all objects small enough to go into your child's mouth have been picked up and put out of reach!

When should I call your office?

Call our office if your child develops any new symptoms after removal of a foreign object:

- Choking, gagging, or difficulty swallowing.

- Swelling or tenderness in and around the neck.

If your child has noisy breathing or shortness of breath or if his or her skin is turning blue, call 911 or another emergency number.

Frostbite

Frostbite is a risk when the weather is cold. Serious damage can develop quickly on any area of the skin, such as the ears, fingers, or toes. Get medical care immediately whenever a firm, white area with stinging or aching develops on skin that has been exposed to cold temperatures.

What is frostbite?

Frostbite occurs when the skin is exposed to below-freezing temperatures. If it's cold enough, frostbite can develop in a very short time—within minutes of exposure. To prevent frostbite, make sure your child's skin is covered when the weather is very cold and limit time spent outdoors.

A stinging or aching feeling in the skin is an important warning sign of frostbite. If the area becomes numb, serious permanent damage may occur. The most serious complication is gangrene (death of the tissue), which may require amputation (surgical removal) of the affected part. Prompt medical care is essential to maximize recovery from frostbite.

What does it look like?

- At first, the exposed area may become hard and pale. This initial stage is sometimes called *frostnip*. At this point, warming the affected area may prevent further damage. The affected skin may blister or peel over the next few days.

- Aching or stinging develops in the exposed area. Numbness develops gradually. If exposure to cold continues, the area eventually becomes hard, white, and without feeling.

- When the area is rewarmed, it may become blotchy, itchy, swollen, and red. Pain may develop during the rewarming process and can be quite severe.

- Frostbite is most likely to occur on the fingers, toes, nose, and ears, but it can occur on any area of exposed skin.

- Some other problems related to cold exposure may occur:

  - *Hypothermia (low body temperature).* As body temperature drops, the person becomes extremely tired and uncoordinated. Immediate rewarming is essential. Take the child to the emergency room or another medical facility immediately.

  - *Chilblains (pernio).* These are blisters or ulcers caused by exposure to cold. They occur in many of the same areas affected by frostbite.

What causes frostbite?

Frostbite occurs when the fluids inside body tissues freeze. How bad the freezing is and how long it is present determine the severity of tissue damage.

What are some possible complications of frostbite?

Gangrene is the most serious complication. The tissue of the affected body part dies and becomes infected. Without treatment, the infection will spread. Immediate treatment is needed, including surgery to remove (amputate) the infected part. Toes are most commonly affected.

What puts your child at risk of frostbite?

- Being out in cold weather without adequate protective clothing. On very cold days with a high wind-chill factor, exposed skin areas can become frostbitten within minutes.

- Drinking alcohol or smoking.

- Any medical condition that impairs blood flow, including diabetes.

Can frostbite be prevented?

- Make sure your child is dressed properly for cold weather. Have him or her wear layers of warm clothing, as well as gloves, socks, insulated boots, and a hat.

- On cold days, don't let young children play outside for too long. Have them come inside for a break and to warm up. On very cold days, keep children inside if possible.

- If your child is participating in skiing and winter sports, provide plenty of food and liquids. Putting a layer of petroleum jelly (Vaseline) on your child's nose and ears provides some protection against frostbite.

- Make sure your children know the warning signs of frostbite: cold or numbing of body parts, especially the nose, ears, fingers, and toes.

How is frostbite treated?

Before you get to the doctor:

- *Don't* rub the frostbitten area or rub it with snow! This may cause further skin damage.

- *Do* try to rewarm the area by putting it next to warm skin if possible (for example, in the armpit). However, *don't* let the area freeze again, as thawing and refreezing may cause worse damage.

- *Don't* walk on frostbitten feet unless it's absolutely necessary to reach shelter.

- *Do* watch for signs of hypothermia (extreme tiredness, confusion). Don't let the person rest or lie down; keep moving until you reach shelter.

- *Do* seek shelter and medical care as soon as possible. If medical care is not immediately available, place the affected area of the body in a warm (*not hot*) bath. Exposure to high temperatures may damage the numbed skin.

❗ *If normal skin color and sensation do not return after rewarming, it is essential to get the person to the hospital as soon as possible.*

At the hospital:

- Rewarming steps will be carried out, such as a warm water bath or warming blankets.

- Medications may be given to improve blood flow.

- During rewarming, the area may become red and extremely painful. Medications can be given for pain.

- The frostbitten area will be examined. Surgery may be needed to remove severely damaged areas (blisters, broken skin).

- It may take a while to assess the extent of the frostbite damage. If frostbite is not too severe, complete recovery may be possible. Very careful wound care is essential, including frequent dressing changes and close attention to keeping the area clean.

- If permanent tissue death occurs, the area will have to be amputated to prevent or treat gangrene. The area of the amputation will be kept as small as possible while ensuring that all dead tissue is removed.

When should I call your office?

During or after rewarming, call our office if any of the following occur:

- The presence of a hard, numb area.

- Severe pain or burning in the frostbitten area.

- Fever, "feeling ill," or other new symptoms.

- Fluid draining from sores in the frostbitten area.

- A color change in the frostbitten skin.

Head Trauma (Minor)

Most head injuries in children are not serious. Confusion, unsteadiness, and headache usually mean a concussion is present, and your child should see the doctor. Medical attention is also needed if your child has lost consciousness, even for a short time. Imaging tests may be needed to make sure there is no bleeding inside the skull.

What is head trauma?

Children and teens may suffer head injuries in many ways, especially bicycle and motor vehicle accidents. Sports, especially football, are another common cause of head trauma. Medical evaluation is needed for all but the most mild "closed" head injuries, that is, injuries in which nothing penetrated the head or skull.

The main concern is whether your child has suffered swelling or bleeding in or around the brain. Concussions are mild brain injuries producing no damage that can be detected by the usual imaging tests. If your child loses consciousness for even a short time or has any behavior change after a head injury, get medical care as soon as possible.

What does it look like?

Symptoms of head injury depend on how severe the injury was but may include:

- Unconsciousness. If your child loses consciousness even for a minute or two, seek medical care immediately.
- Concussion. The following symptoms are temporary:
  - Behavior changes: drowsiness, confusion, grogginess.
  - Headache.
  - Nausea or vomiting.
  - Dizziness or loss of balance.
  - Memory loss, "temporary amnesia."
- Certain symptoms may signal more severe head injury:
  - A long period of unconsciousness (more than a minute or two).
  - Severe headache.
  - Confusion lasting for a long time.
  - Vomiting lasting for a long time.
  - Changes in the size of the pupils (the black part of the eye), or pupils unequal in size.
  - Seizure (involuntary movements).

- In infants or younger children, irritability (fussiness) may be the only sign of significant brain injury.
- Even if there are no symptoms, it's worthwhile to call the doctor after your child has a hard fall or a blow to the head.

What are some common causes of head trauma?

- Car or motorcycle accidents.
- Bicycle accidents.
- Falls, such as an infant from a changing table.
- Sports, especially football.
- Child abuse.

What are some possible complications of head trauma?

- Brain swelling, which can sometimes be severe enough to cause death.
- Bleeding and clots in the head. The most common type of bleeding is subdural hematoma, which is blood between the tissue lining the brain and the brain itself. If it is severe, subdural hematoma can be very dangerous. Surgery is needed to drain the bleeding.
- Concussions can cause difficulties concentrating, memory loss, or mood changes. It may take a while for your child to return to normal. These changes usually get better, but mild abnormalities may persist if the concussion was severe enough. Repeated concussions are more likely to cause permanent brain injury.

What puts your child at risk of head trauma?

- Riding in a car without a seatbelt.
- Riding on a bicycle without a helmet.
- Playing football and other contact sports.
- Drinking alcohol or using drugs.

How are minor head injuries diagnosed and treated?

- The doctor will ask some questions about the incident and examine your child, including a careful physical examination to evaluate the nervous system (neurologic examination).
- *Brain imaging.* The doctor may recommend special imaging studies to assess the effects of the injury on your child's brain. This is likely to be done if:

- Your child is not acting normally (is confused, groggy, nauseous, etc.) for more than just a short time.

- The physical examination was abnormal.

- Your child has persistent vomiting or severe headache.

- The usual test is an x-ray procedure called computed tomography, or CT scan. The scan will show whether there is any bleeding or blood clot that may pose a danger to the brain.

- *Skull x-rays.* X-rays of the skull may be performed if the doctor thinks there may be a skull fracture.

- *Observation in the hospital.* If treatable problems are found but the doctors are concerned about the injury or the way your child is acting, he or she will be hospitalized overnight for careful observation to see if further treatment is needed.

- *Home monitoring.* In some cases, the child may be sent home for monitoring. You will be asked to watch him or her closely for the first 24 hours.

- *Follow-up.* Children with significant head trauma may need special developmental tests to detect small effects on the brain. These tests are often performed by a specialist called a neuropsychologist.

- *Serious or severe head trauma* resulting in bleeding or swelling of the brain requires treatment by a neurosurgeon (a surgeon who specializes in problems involving the brain) in an intensive care unit (ICU).

When should I call your office?

While monitoring your child at home after being seen and evaluated, call our office if any of the following occurs:

- For any head injury that causes unconsciousness, grogginess or confusion, vomiting, or severe headache.

- Any time your child has a hard injury to the head, even if there are no symptoms.

- Worsening or severe headache.

- Weakness, dizziness.

- Vomiting.

- Difficulty waking.

- Different-sized pupils, or pupils that don't change much in response to light.

- Seizures (involuntary body movements).

- Confusion or irritability; won't stop crying.

Heat-Related Illnesses

> Heat-related illnesses are common and potentially serious problems. They result from too much physical activity when the weather is hot and humid; children are at higher risk. When it's very hot out, it may be necessary to take frequent rest breaks or cancel sports activities.
>
> Get medical help immediately if your child has a very high body temperature and is experiencing confusion.

What are heat-related illnesses?

The milder forms of heat-related illness include heat cramps and heat exhaustion. Most cases of heat-related illness in children and teens occur during sports. When heat-related symptoms develop, it's essential to stop sports or other activities and rest out of the sun. Taking appropriate action can prevent dangerous heatstroke.

Heatstroke is a severe but much less common form of heat illness caused by excessive physical activity on hot, humid days. The body loses its normal ability to regulate temperature and becomes overheated. Heatstroke can cause death in young athletes.

What do they look like?

Mild heat illness: Symptoms occur when your child is very physically active on hot, humid days. Being in direct sun increases the risk of heat illness.

Initial symptoms may or may not occur before heat exhaustion or heatstroke:

- Cramps, especially of the calf and hamstring (back of the thigh) muscles.
- Breathing very fast (hyperventilation) may occur with swelling, tingling, or spasms (jerking movements) of the hands and feet.

Heat exhaustion:

- Headache.
- Nausea and vomiting.
- Dizziness, especially when standing up.
- Weakness.
- Pale, clammy skin.
- Fainting. If your child faints in the heat, immediate medical attention is needed.

Heatstroke is the most serious form of heat-related illness. Get medical help immediately if the following symptoms occur:

- Confusion or other changes in thinking or behavior—possible unconsciousness ("passing out").
- Profuse sweating.

What causes heat-related illnesses?

- Heat-related illnesses occur when your child's body cannot get rid of all the heat generated by intense exercise. The body loses its normal ability to regulate temperature and becomes overheated.
- In children, heat injury most often occurs during sports competition or practice. Although it happens on very hot days, high humidity can make the problem worse.

What are some possible complications of heat-related illnesses?

- Children with milder forms of heat injury usually recover completely. However, it is essential to stop activity and lower body temperature to keep the child from developing heatstroke.
- Heatstroke is a dangerous condition requiring immediate medical attention. Without effective steps to lower body temperature, heatstroke can be fatal.

What puts your child at risk of heat-related illnesses?

- Being very active on hot, humid days. Heat injury usually occurs during outdoor activities in direct sunlight. However, it can also occur in gyms or other indoor locations.
- Not drinking enough liquids on hot days.
- The risk may be higher in child or teen athletes who are obese, not physically fit, and not used to high temperatures. Certain medical conditions and drugs may also increase the risk of heat injury.
- Heat injury often occurs during summer football practice, especially in pads and helmets.

Can heat-related illnesses be prevented?

Heat-related illnesses, including heatstroke, are always preventable!

- If children are exercising on hot days, make sure they take frequent breaks for rest (out of the sun) and water.
- If it is very hot and humid, cancel the activity. Depending on the humidity level, it's a good idea not to do outdoor physical activities when the air temperature is 95°F (35°C) or higher.

● With repeated short exposures, your child will be better able to tolerate physical activity in high heat/humidity.

● *Make sure children drink frequently!* Give liquids before and every 20 minutes during exercise. Cold water is the best choice.

● Schedule practices and games in the early morning or late afternoon. Avoid practicing in full equipment on hot days.

Stop activity and take appropriate steps if early symptoms of heat injury develop!

How are heat-related illnesses treated?

The goal of treatment is to prevent heatstroke. Symptoms of mild heat injury usually improve with rest and other simple measures

● *Heat cramps.* Give your child liquids (water or sports drinks, like Gatorade). Gently stretch the affected muscle(s).

● *Swelling.* Swelling decreases when your child gets used to the heat.

● *Hyperventilation.* Have the child breathe more slowly or breathe into a paper bag.

● *Heat exhaustion* requires more active efforts at cooling:

● Get your child to a cooler location. Use fans to cool the body, if available.

● Remove excess clothing.

● Place ice on the groin and armpit areas.

● Give liquids.

● *Heat stroke is a medical emergency!* If your child cannot drink, becomes confused, or develops any behavior change or reduced consciousness, call 911 or another emergency number. Aggressive cooling and fluid replacement are needed.

When should I call your office?

● For children with milder symptoms of heat-related illness, get the child out of the heat and give fluids. Call your doctor for advice if the symptoms don't improve promptly.

● If the following symptoms develop, go to the emergency room or call 911:

● Fainting or passing out.

● Confusion or behavioral changes.

Lead Poisoning

Lead poisoning can cause brain damage. It is still an important problem in preschoolers, especially those living in older buildings. Peeling paint is the most common source of lead poisoning. Children with high levels of lead in their blood may need treatment. In addition, investigation may be needed to find out where the lead is coming from.

What is lead poisoning?

Lead is a toxic metal that is widely used in many products. Lead poisoning from paint was once a widespread problem. In the United States, paint made since 1978 does not contain lead, but many children are still exposed to lead-containing paint in older buildings. Lead poisoning most often results from "hand-to-mouth" activity by infants and toddlers or from eating paint chips.

Lead poisoning can cause permanent brain damage in children (and adults). This problem is now less common because of the elimination of lead from paint, gasoline, and other sources and because doctors perform screening tests for lead in young children. If your child has high blood lead levels, action is needed to:

- Treat your child, if the lead level is high enough.
- Find the source of the lead.
- Remove the child from the source.
- Correct the lead contamination problem.

What does it look like?

- Lead poisoning can affect the brain, resulting in reduced intelligence and behavior changes. Although this still occurs, effective prevention and screening efforts have made it a lot less common in the United States.

- Today, most children with lead poisoning have their condition detected by screening tests. In general, most children should undergo blood testing for lead at least once between ages 1 and 2. Blood testing for lead will also be performed if your doctor has any reason to suspect your child might be exposed to old paint or other sources of lead.

- If blood tests show higher than accepted levels of lead, the health department or other agency will need to check the home or other possible sources of lead. The child may have to be removed from the home until the lead contamination is corrected. The goal is to detect elevated lead levels before any permanent damage occurs.

- High levels of lead poisoning causing acute symptoms are now uncommon. However, the following symptoms are possible:

- Abdominal pain.
- Constipation.
- Decreased appetite.
- Anemia (low levels of red blood cells or hemoglobin).
- Headaches, seizures, and coma.

Where does the lead come from?

- Most lead poisoning results from exposure to old lead paint. The most common cause is hand-to-mouth activity; lead dust gets on your child's hands, and from there into his or her mouth. Children may also eat chips of peeled lead paint.

- Much less often, lead exposure comes from old water pipes in the home or ceramic bowls with a lead glaze from which food is eaten. Poisoning can also result from industrial sources.

What are some possible complications of lead poisoning?

- When it is severe, lead poisoning can interfere with brain growth and development.

- Children with less severe exposure to lead may be at increased risk of other problems, including:
  - Reduced intelligence and school performance.
  - Behavior problems, such as hyperactivity.

What puts your child at risk of lead poisoning?

- Preschool age.

- Living in older buildings, particularly in houses built before the 1950s, but in any building in which cracked or peeling paint is present. Children living in recently renovated buildings may also be at risk.

- If one child in your family has had lead poisoning, other children may be affected as well.

Can lead poisoning be prevented?

Screening and early detection are the best ways to prevent lead poisoning. Follow your doctor's recommendations for blood testing.

How is lead poisoning treated?

- *Early detection.* In the United States, 99% of children with lead poisoning are identified by screening tests. At age 1 or 2, the doctor may order a test to measure the level of lead in your child's blood. This is most likely to be done if there is some reason to suspect your child may be exposed to lead—for example, if you live in an older home with peeling paint or if your child is a recent immigrant from a country without environmental lead controls.

- *Blood lead level.* If the screening test shows a higher than normal blood lead level, further tests may be done to confirm the result. About 10% of American children have elevated blood lead levels. However, unless your child has had a very high exposure to lead, his or her blood lead level will be far below the level causing serious or immediate health problems.

- *Identifying and removing lead.* If your child has elevated blood lead levels, the first step is to find out where the lead is coming from. Old, peeling paint is the most common source. Your child has not necessarily been eating paint chips; instead, the lead may be coming from dust in your home. Sometimes the lead comes from an occupational source—for example, the clothes of a parent exposed to lead at work or from a factory in the neighborhood.

  - Removing lead from old buildings can be a difficult job. If not done correctly, such attempts may make the problem worse. The local health department may play a role in identifying and eliminating lead exposure.

  - If a source of lead is found in your home, a contractor with special knowledge and experience will be needed to do lead clean-up (abatement).

- *Changing your child's behavior.* Efforts are needed to reduce the "hand-to-mouth" activity that causes lead poisoning in infants and toddlers. Washing your child's hands frequently may help to reduce the amount of lead getting into his or her system.

- *Diet changes.* Adequate amounts of vitamin C, calcium, and iron may help to prevent higher levels of lead in the body.

- *Removing lead from your child's body* is difficult, because the lead is absorbed into bone and other tissues. If your child's blood lead level reaches a certain point, drugs are used to help remove the lead. This is called *chelation therapy.* If your child has milder lead exposure, his or her blood lead levels will eventually return to normal without chelation therapy as long as the source is removed.

- *Follow-up.* Your child should receive regular medical follow-up checks to be sure his or her blood lead levels are going down. Close attention will be paid to your child's developmental skills and behavior, depending on how high his or her blood levels were.

When should I call your office?

Call your doctor's office if you have any questions about: blood lead testing or concerns about possible exposure to lead by your child.

Nosebleeds

Nosebleeds may result from many different causes. Most nosebleeds stop on their own in a few minutes; it may help to have your child sit quietly with his or her head tilted forward and gently squeeze the nostrils. If nosebleeds do not stop or if they occur frequently, call our office.

What are nosebleeds?

Nearly all kids get a "bloody nose" once in a while. Nosebleeds are very frequent in preschool-aged children; they are less common after puberty. There are a number of possible causes, including excessive nose picking, dry air, allergies, and injuries. Nosebleeds rarely signal a serious medical problem.

Most childhood nosebleeds come from the septum—the hard tissue between the nostrils. Nosebleeds nearly always stop after a few minutes. If your child has a nosebleed that simply won't stop or if he or she has a lot of nosebleeds, get medical help.

What do they look like?

- Blood coming from one or both nostrils.
- Blood flow is usually slow but steady. Occasionally, there is a lot of blood running freely from the nose.
- Much less often, vomiting of blood or blood in a bowel movement may be the first sign that your child has had a nosebleed. (This may occur if a nosebleed happens at night and your child swallows the blood.)

What causes nosebleeds?

- Abnormal or excessive nose picking. All children (and adults!) pick their nose at times. However, very frequent or forceful nose picking can cause nosebleeds.
- Injuries, for example, falling or getting hit in the nose.
- Foreign bodies; younger children may place objects in their noses.
- Dry air may irritate the sensitive lining of the nose (especially in winter).
- Certain diseases involving the nose and upper airway: infections (including colds), sinusitis, allergies, or polyps.
- Rarely, nosebleeds are caused by blood vessel abnormalities, bleeding problems, or other diseases.

What are some possible complications of nosebleeds?

- Usually none.
- Very rarely, severe or repeated nosebleeds may cause a lot of blood loss, resulting in anemia (low levels of red blood cells or hemoglobin).

What puts your child at risk of nosebleeds?

- Conditions leading to irritation of the lining of the nose such as allergies or colds.
- Blood disorders that lead to easy bleeding, for example, hemophilia.

Can nosebleeds be prevented?

- Teach children to keep objects out of their noses.
- In the wintertime, use a humidifier to avoid dry air indoors.
- If instructed by the doctor, use saline (saltwater) nose drops or put a thin layer of petroleum jelly (Vaseline) on the septum (the hard tissue between the nostrils).

How are nosebleeds treated?

At home:

- Most nosebleeds stop on their own in a few minutes. The following steps may be helpful:
  - Put gentle pressure on the nostrils. It may help to hold a cold washcloth to the nose.
  - Have your child sit quietly. Keep the head tilted forward; this helps keep blood from trickling back into the throat.
  - If the nosebleed doesn't stop within several minutes, try a nasal spray such as Afrin or Neo-Synephrine.
  - If there is a lot of blood coming from your child's nose, or if the nosebleed doesn't stop within 5 to 10 minutes, it's a good idea to seek medical help.

At the doctor's office or emergency room:

- The doctor may place a small gauze pack inside the nostril to control the bleeding.
- Once the bleeding is under control, the doctor may try to locate the blood vessel that is causing the bleeding. A medication called silver nitrate can be placed to seal off the bleeding vessel. This must be done carefully to avoid injuring the delicate tissues inside the nose.

- *If nosebleeds are severe or frequent,* further examination and tests may be needed to find out what's causing them. This may include:

  - A visit to an ear, nose and throat (ENT) doctor (also called an otorhinolaryngologist).

  - Tests to be sure your child doesn't have a bleeding disorder.

When should I call your office?

Call our office if your child has any of the following:

- Nosebleeds that are very frequent (at least once a month) or take a long time to stop (more than 5 to 10 minutes).

- A lot of blood coming from the nose, or if the nosebleed simply won't stop.

- Blood in vomit or bowel movements. (Bowel movements may look tarry and black, not red.)

- Bruises or easy bleeding, or if you or others in your family have a bleeding disorder.

Poisoning

Poisoning is a common and often serious emergency in children. Poisoning most often occurs when toddlers and preschoolers find poisons in the home and eat or drink them. If you have an infant or toddler, you need to "poison-proof" your home and make a plan for what to do if poisoning occurs.

What types of poisoning occur in children?

The average home contains many products that could cause poisoning in a young child. Many common medications can be harmful when taken in large doses. Infants and toddlers are at risk of poisoning because they love to explore their environment and will put almost anything in their mouths.

- *If you have an infant or toddler, it is essential to "poison-proof" your home so that your child cannot find and eat or drink anything harmful. All potential poisons must be locked up!*

Some common and dangerous household poisons include medicines, cleaning and chemical products, and auto antifreeze.

- *Always get medical advice before attempting any treatment for poisoning!* For some types of poisons—especially caustic substances such as drain openers—you should *not* induce vomiting. If your child eats, drinks, or inhales something that may be poisonous, call 911 or another emergency number.

What does it look like?

- Poisoning symptoms depend on what type of poison your child has taken. Often, there are no symptoms—the parent just discovers that a child has drunk or eaten a possible poisonous substance.
- Possible symptoms include:
  - Nausea and vomiting.
  - Very fast or very slow breathing.
  - Confusion, behavior changes.
  - Changes in the pupils (the black part of the eye); they become dilated (large) or constricted (small).
  - Extreme sleepiness or unconsciousness.
  - Burns around the mouth.
  - Coughing or choking.

What puts your child at risk of poisoning?

- *Crawling infants and toddlers are at highest risk!* Most poisonings occur in children under age 5.
- Poisoning is much less common at ages 6 and older. Teenagers may poison themselves in suicide attempts or while attempting to get "high."
- *Not poison-proofing your home!* Ninety percent of poisonings in children occur at home.

How can poisoning be prevented?

- Poison-proof your home by putting away all medicines, household cleaners, and other possible poisons. All of these products should be locked up or put away where your child cannot see or find them. (Remember, toddlers love to climb!)
- Teach your child never to put anything but food or drink into his or her mouth. Never tell your child that medicine is "candy."
- Buy medicines with childproof caps. (Remember, grandparents may have medicine bottles without safety caps.) Keep medicines in their original containers.
- *Have a plan in case poisoning occurs!*
- Get medical help as soon as possible. Call our office or the Poison Help Line (1-800-222-1222).
- Don't make your child vomit, *unless* you are told to do so by a doctor or the poison control center. Some poisons may cause more damage if your child vomits.

What are some possible complications of poisoning?

The harmful effects of poisoning depend on what type of substance your child has taken, along with other factors such as how much was taken, when it was taken, and your child's age and size. Some poisons and common medications taken in large amounts can cause serious complications are:

- *Acetaminophen* (brand name: Tylenol, among others). Widely used as a "safer" alternative to aspirin but may cause severe liver damage.
- *Aspirin.* May also cause abnormalities of body salts (electrolytes) or blood clotting. (Use of aspirin is generally not recommended in children because it may lead to Reye's syndrome, a disease involving brain swelling and liver damage.)
- *Antidepressants.* Can affect the nervous system causing drowsiness, coma, and seizures. They can also cause heart and breathing problems.

- *Clonidine.* Sometimes used for attention deficit–hyperactivity disorder (ADHD) treatment. Dangerous poisoning can occur at relatively low doses, causing breathing problems and coma.

- *Corrosive products* (for example, drain openers, bleach, or any kind of acid). Can seriously damage the esophagus (swallowing tube), skin, or eyes. Do not induce vomiting!

- *Antifreeze* (ethylene glycol). A common cause of poisoning because it tastes sweet. Causes organ failure if not treated, including seizures, kidney failure, and coma.

- *Insecticides* (organophosphates or carbamates). Can cause nervous system damage.

- *Hydrocarbons* (such as refrigerants). Can cause lung damage if inhaled.

- *Plants.* Many house plants and wild plants are potentially toxic.

How is poisoning treated?

If you think your child may have been poisoned, get medical help immediately. Call your regional poison control center (1-800-222-1222), or call 911. Don't wait for symptoms to occur. Be prepared to provide as much information as possible about the substance your child was exposed to.

- For swallowed poisons, do not give syrup of ipecac or anything else to induce vomiting unless instructed to do so by the poison control center or a doctor.

- For inhaled poisons, get the child to fresh air as soon as possible.

- If poison has gotten on the skin or in the eyes, rinse with lots of fresh water for several minutes.

Home treatment: Your child may be managed at home, depending on the dangers of whatever he or she was exposed to. For example, although some kinds of medicines are very dangerous, others are unlikely to cause serious poisoning. If your child is managed at home, you'll be given specific instructions on when to seek emergency medical care.

- If your child develops new or unexpected symptoms, get medical advice immediately.

Hospital treatment: If your child has been exposed to a dangerous poison or has overdosed on certain medicines, he or she will need to go to the hospital. There he or she may undergo various types of treatment, including:

- Activated charcoal may be given to absorb the poison from your child's stomach. This may be given as a "slurry" drink or placed in your child's stomach through a nasogastric (NG) tube. This is a small tube placed down the nose and into the stomach.

- The NG tube may be used to remove the poison from your child's stomach. This is called gastric lavage, or stomach pumping.

- Treatments to help eliminate the poison. For certain poisons, a treatment called dialysis may be used to filter the poison from the blood.

- Blood tests. Blood and urine tests may be performed to measure the amount of poison in your child's body and how it is affecting the organs and blood salt (electrolyte) levels.

- Supportive care. Other treatments may be needed to support your child while the poison is eliminated. If breathing is severely affected, your child may need to be connected to a machine to help with breathing (mechanical ventilation).

- If the poisoning was part of a suicide attempt, psychiatric care may be needed.

When should I call your office?

Call the regional poison control center (1-800-222-1222) any time you think your child may have drunk or swallowed any type of poison.

Seizures Without Fever (Nonfebrile Seizures)

When a child has a seizure without a high fever or other known cause, medical evaluation is needed. Nonfebrile (without fever) seizures are sometimes a sign of epilepsy, a treatable disease involving repeated seizures. However, many other causes are possible. You should always call our office when your child has had a seizure, with or without fever.

What are seizures?

Seizures are involuntary, uncontrollable muscle movements and/or behavior changes. Many kinds of seizures can occur in children. The most common type, *febrile seizures,* result from a high fever. When seizures occur, medical evaluation is needed to identify the cause.

Less than one third of seizures in children are caused by epilepsy, a disease in which repeated seizures are triggered from within the brain. Epilepsy is defined as repeated seizures not caused by other medical conditions (such as fever, infection, or head injury). Many children who have a seizure without fever or other known cause never experience another seizure.

What do they look like?

Several types of seizures are possible:

- Your child may experience sudden, rapid, repeated shaking of the arms and legs on one or both sides of the body. His or her eyes may be rolled back in the head. When the whole body is involved, it may be called a "grand mal" or "generalized (tonic-clonic) seizure."

- Your child's entire body may become very tense or very relaxed. Sometimes there is no movement at all—your child simply becomes unresponsive during the seizure.

- Parts of the body, such as an arm or leg, may shake or become stiff. Even holding onto the part doesn't make it stop shaking.

- Seizures usually last for only a few minutes but can last longer.

- Your child may have other symptoms, such as numbness or pain in a specific area, may make involuntary noises, and may lose control over urination or bowel movements.

- Your child may be conscious or unconscious during the seizure. Afterward, he or she may be very sleepy.

What causes seizures?

- There are many possible causes. For some children with seizures, the cause is unknown.

- Some causes of seizures other than epilepsy include the following:
  - Fever or infections.
  - Head injuries.
  - Toxic substances, including medication side effects and drug abuse.
  - Abnormal heart rhythms.
  - Low blood sugar (hypoglycemia).

- Other events may look like seizures but really aren't, such as breath-holding spells, fainting, chills and shivering, and many others. Rarely, events similar to seizures may be a symptom of a mental health problem. (These are called "pseudoseizures," but are not true seizures.)

What are some possible complications of seizures?

- The seizure itself, if brief, does no harm to the child.

- Your child may be injured during seizures, especially if they are violent.

- Although it is rare, brain injury may occur if a seizure is very prolonged.

What puts your child at risk for seizures?

- Any of the causes listed above, such as head injuries or low blood sugar.

- If you or anyone else in your family has had epilepsy or other seizure disorders, your child may be at higher risk.

- If your child has had one seizure, he or she is at risk of having additional seizures. However, less than half of children with one seizure without fever go on to experience a second seizure.

Can seizures be prevented?

- Anticonvulsant drugs may be used to control seizures for epilepsy and other seizure disorders.

How are seizures treated?

If your child has a seizure at home:

- Place your child on his or her side to prevent choking on food or vomit.

- Do not give any medications or anything by mouth during the seizure to avoid the risk of choking.

- ❗ It is always important to call our office when your child has had a seizure.

Diagnosis:

- At the doctor's office or hospital, provide as much information as possible on the seizure as well as any factors that you think might have contributed to it.

- Depending on the history and type of seizure, certain tests can help to determine the cause of seizures:

  - If your child has had a head injury, special types of x-rays (called CT or MRI scans) may be done to see if there is any damage to the brain.

  - Blood or urine tests may be done.

  - If your child has fever or other symptoms of infection of the brain (such as meningitis), a test called lumbar puncture, or "spinal tap," may be performed. The test is safe and is generally not very painful. A spinal tap is more likely to be performed if your child has a seizure with fever. The doctor may perform a test called a lumbar puncture, or "spinal tap," to be sure your child does not have meningitis. This test is done by placing a needle between the bones of your child's spine and removing a small amount of fluid (called cerebrospinal fluid). Your child will receive anesthetics so that he or she will not feel the needle.

- An electroencephalogram (EEG) may be performed. This is a painless test that measures patterns of electrical activity in your child's brain (brain waves). The results may help in identifying the cause of your child's seizure and in predicting the risk of future seizures.

- We may recommend a visit to a specialist in brain and nervous system diseases (a neurologist). This specialist has the expertise to diagnose the cause of your child's seizure and recommend the most appropriate treatment, if any.

If this is your child's first seizure, we will not likely recommend any treatment at first. This is especially likely if there were no other unusual features and if no specific medical problem is suspected. Even if no specific cause is identified, many children with an initial seizure never have another seizure.

If your child has repeated seizures, further evaluation and treatment will be recommended. Detailed evaluation of your child's seizures will guide the choice of treatment.

- Treatment will likely include anticonvulsant drugs. These medications have many possible side effects. Your child will need careful follow-up. Other treatments may be recommended as well.

- If a specific cause is identified, treatment may help to control the risk of future seizures.

📞 When should I call your office?

- Call our office any time your child has a seizure—whether or not there is a fever and whether or not your child has had a seizure before.

- If the seizure has not stopped within a few minutes, call an ambulance or seek other medical attention immediately. ❗

Skin Wounds (Lacerations, Punctures, and Abrasions)

Cuts, punctures, and other skin wounds should be cleansed to prevent infection. Certain types of wounds require a visit to a doctor, including deep wounds, wounds in which the edges won't stay together, or wounds containing visible dirt. Some wounds require a tetanus "booster" shot, especially puncture wounds and unclean wounds.

What are skin wounds?

A wound is any type of injury that causes a break in the skin:

- *Lacerations (cuts or incisions).* Wounds caused by something sharp, such as a knife or broken glass. Cuts may cause a lot of bleeding.

- *Punctures.* Wounds caused by a pointed object stuck deep into the skin, such as a nail. If the puncture wound is deep and difficult to clean or if the object was contaminated, there is an increased risk of infection.

- *Abrasions (scrapes).* Wounds caused by rubbing against something rough, such as a sidewalk. Abrasions are often contaminated by dirt or grit.

What kinds of wounds require a doctor's visit?

Children with the following types of wounds should be taken to the doctor's office or emergency room:

- Deep or large wounds, especially:
  - Deep puncture wounds.
  - Wounds in which the edges won't stay together.
  - Wounds with deeper layers (fat or muscle) visible inside.
- Wounds with jagged edges.
- Wounds that don't stop bleeding after a few minutes or that spurt blood.
- Lacerations or puncture wounds with visible contamination, such as dirt or grit.
- Wounds that are very painful.
- Wounds on the face, unless they are very minor.

What are some possible complications of skin wounds?

- Wounds may interfere with the function of the injured part (such as bending a finger or leg).

- If wounds don't heal properly, they may leave scars.

- Wounds may become infected, usually with bacteria. Without proper care, even minor wounds may lead to serious infections.

- One particularly serious infection is *tetanus* (sometimes called lockjaw). Tetanus vaccine prevents this complication. Your child may need a booster shot if his or her tetanus vaccinations are not up-to-date.

What puts your child at risk of skin wounds?

- Obviously, children get a lot of cuts and scrapes. Most are minor and heal without problems.

- Provide age-appropriate supervision when children play. Make sure that play areas such as backyards are free of hazards that could cause injuries.

How are wounds treated?

Minor wounds can be treated at home:

- Wash your hands with soap and water before cleaning the wound.

- Wash the area gently with soap and water, then rinse with lots of clean water. All dirt, sand, and debris need to be removed.

- To stop bleeding, put gentle pressure on the wound.

- Putting a thin layer of antibiotic ointment on the wound may help reduce pain and promote healing. However, to prevent infection, cleaning the wound is more important than using an antibiotic.

- After applying antibiotic ointment, place a bandage over the wound. This will help it heal more quickly.

- When a scab forms, be sure your child leaves it alone. Scabs serve the same purpose as bandages, sealing the wound off from germs. Picking at scabs increases the risk of infection.

Other wounds should be evaluated and treated by a health professional, including large wounds, wounds with jagged edges, deep puncture wounds, "dirty" wounds, and certain other types.

Don't wait to see the doctor! Cleanse the wound immediately, as described for minor wounds.

- At the emergency room or doctor's office, the wound will be carefully cleansed. This is especially important for abrasions or other wounds with visible dirt and for deep puncture wounds.

- *Tetanus prevention.* If your child's tetanus vaccinations are not up-to-date, he or she may need a tetanus booster shot. Unless you are positive your child has had a tetanus shot in the past 5 years and has had a total of three shots, a tetanus shot is needed after any wound involving a contaminated source.

- Even if your child's tetanus shots are up-to-date, vaccination is recommended after certain types of wounds that are at high risk of tetanus contamination, such as:

  - Animal bites.

  - Crush or puncture wounds.

  - "Dirty" wounds contaminated by soil, saliva, or feces. Immediate and thorough cleaning of such "dirty" wounds is essential to reduce the risk of tetanus as well as other infections. Home cleaning is a good start, but cleaning by a doctor or other health care professional is recommended for skin wounds that are deep or appear contaminated. Seek medical care immediately if your child has a "dirty" wound with obvious contamination.

- *Stitches (sutures).* If the wound is large or deep or if the edges do not line up properly, the doctor may decide to place stitches, also known as sutures. This is done to promote proper healing while reducing the chances of scarring.

  - An anesthetic will be used so that your child will not feel pain when stitches are placed.

  - Your doctor will provide you with instructions for taking care of the stitches. Keep the area clean and covered, or as directed by your doctor.

  - Certain cuts may be treated with tissue adhesives (glues) instead of sutures.

When should I call your office?

Call our office if your child has a wound and you are not sure whether medical attention is needed or if the wound shows any of the following signs of not healing properly:

- Wound edges are coming apart.

- Signs of infection (redness, soreness, tenderness, fever).

- For new or old wounds, call our office if your child is experiencing a lot of pain or is having difficulty moving the injured part.

Section X ▪ Endocrine Disorders

Breast Enlargement in Boys (Gynecomastia)

Enlargement of the breasts, sometimes called gynecomastia, is relatively common in boys. It can be an embarrassing problem during adolescence, when boys may be self-conscious about their bodies. Most cases are caused by normal hormones produced during puberty, although other causes are possible. Usually the breasts return to normal size without any special treatment.

What is gynecomastia?

Enlargement of the breast in boys or men is called gynecomastia. A number of different diseases can cause the male breast to grow larger. This can also be caused by exposure to the hormone estrogen or certain drugs.

Most often, however, breast enlargement is a temporary response to hormonal changes occurring around puberty. In most cases, the breasts eventually return to normal size. This is called physiologic pubertal gynecomastia, and no treatment is needed. Treatment is possible, however, if gynecomastia is causing severe emotional distress.

Boys who are overweight or obese may appear to have enlarged breasts. However, this is not the same as gynecomastia but is caused by excessive body fat. For these boys, losing weight is the best way to reduce breast size.

What does it look like?

- One or both breasts become enlarged and sometimes tender. Breast tissue may develop at different rates or different times.

- The enlargement appears as an area of firm breast tissue located under the nipple. It is not the same as the soft, fatty tissue that can make the breasts seem enlarged in boys who are overweight or obese.

- The breasts may be tender; this is usually temporary.

- In most cases, the breasts gradually return to normal. This may take a few months or may take as long as up to 2 years.

What causes gynecomastia?

- Pubertal gynecomastia. Most often, breast enlargement is caused by hormone changes in your son's body around puberty. As many as two thirds of boys have at least mild breast enlargement and/or tenderness sometime during early to middle puberty.

- Many other causes are possible but much less common:

- Exposure to the hormone estrogen.

- Exposure to other drugs, including certain antacids, diuretics ("water pills"), and heart medications.

- Drug abuse, including marijuana and heroin.

- Certain genetic diseases (such as Klinefelter's syndrome).

- Various gland and hormonal diseases, including tumors of the adrenal glands or testicles and hyperthyroidism (overproduction of hormones by the thyroid gland).

What are some possible complications of gynecomastia?

- Usually none. In most cases, the condition clears up on its own.

- For some boys, breast enlargement is an embarrassing problem. Treatment is available if needed.

How is gynecomastia treated?

- Usually, boys with breast enlargement around the time of puberty require no treatment. The condition is normal and temporary.

- In most cases, breast enlargement goes away on its own within a few months. However, in some children it may take up to 2 years for the problem to go away completely.

- For boys who are overweight or obese, apparent breast enlargement is usually related to fatty tissue, not to hormone-related enlargement. Weight loss through diet and exercise is the best way to reduce breast size.

- Some boys with gynecomastia are very embarrassed about this problem. If your son is experiencing serious emotional issues related to breast enlargement, we may recommend seeing a counselor.

- Because the enlarged breasts generally return to normal or become significantly smaller, surgery is rarely recommended.

- If the cause is estrogen exposure or drug use, the breasts should return to normal once exposure to these substances is eliminated.

- If the cause is a genetic or hormonal disorder, we will recommend a visit to an appropriate specialist.

When should I call your office?

After evaluation for gynecomastia, the doctor may want to re-examine your son every 6 months, just to be sure no other problems are present. Between visits, call our office if:

- Breast size continues to increase.

- You have any concerns about your child's possible drug abuse or accidental drug exposure, for example, smoking marijuana or exposure to even small amounts of estrogen.

- Your son is experiencing severe embarrassment or emotional distress that is interfering with other areas of his life.

Breast Enlargement in Infants (Premature Thelarche)

> Premature thelarche is a condition in which the breasts of baby girls begin to enlarge. It is usually a temporary, harmless condition. Breast enlargement in infants and young girls is sometimes the first sign of early (precocious) puberty, but this is uncommon.

What is premature thelarche?

Premature thelarche is enlargement of the breasts in infant girls. Most often, breast enlargement is the only abnormality. It is occasionally the first sign of early (precocious) puberty. This is more likely if the breasts become enlarged after ages 2 to 3.

Usually there is no apparent cause of early breast enlargement, although it can result from exposure to medications or to sources of the hormone estrogen. The breasts may remain enlarged for as long as a few years but eventually go down in size before your daughter starts puberty.

What does it look like?

- Your daughter's breasts start getting bigger.

- One or both breasts may be enlarged. They may go up and down in size.

- Breast enlargement usually occurs before age 2. Occasionally, a baby girl is born with enlarged breasts.

- There are no other signs of puberty, for example, growth of pubic hair (hair around the genitals) or rapid body growth.

- Medical tests, if performed, show no other signs of approaching puberty.

- Breasts eventually stop growing and may become reduced in size. It may take a few years before the breasts completely return to normal. Girls go on to have a normal puberty.

What causes premature thelarche?

- Usually, no specific cause is identified.

- Premature breast enlargement can be caused by exposure to the hormone estrogen, for example, a child eating the mother's birth control pills.

What are some possible complications of premature thelarche?

- Usually none. The condition often goes away on its own, although this may take a few years.

- Infrequently, premature thelarche is the first sign of early (precocious) puberty. This is most likely when the breasts start to enlarge after ages 2 to 3, accompanied by other signs of puberty such as an enlarged clitoris or development of pubic hair. Treatment may be needed to halt the process of early maturation.

What puts your child at risk of premature thelarche?

There are no known risk factors.

Can premature thelarche be prevented?

There is no way to prevent this condition.

How is premature thelarche treated?

- Usually, no treatment is needed. Your daughter's breasts will eventually go down in size or stop enlarging.

- Your doctor will examine your child for any other signs of puberty. Medical tests are usually not needed. If the doctor has any reason to suspect an abnormality, various tests may be performed as well, such as measuring hormone levels, x-rays to assess bone growth, or ultrasound scans of the uterus and ovaries.

- The doctor will continue to monitor your daughter to make sure there are no other signs of early puberty.

- If there is any reason to suspect a medical cause of early puberty, we will probably recommend a visit to an endocrinologist (a doctor specializing in the treatment of gland and hormone diseases). This specialist can perform tests and recommend treatments designed to interrupt the process of puberty, if necessary.

When should I call your office?

Between visits, call our office if your daughter develops any of the following:

- Further enlargement and development of the breasts.

- Repeat enlargement of the breasts after they have gone down in size.

- Any other signs of early puberty, such as hair around the genital area and under the arms or very rapid bodily growth.

Diabetes Mellitus, Type 1

Type 1 diabetes mellitus is a chronic disease in which the body makes no or only low levels of the hormone insulin. This results in higher than normal levels of sugar, or glucose, in the blood. Diabetes can cause serious complications. However, with good medical care and education, your child with diabetes can lead a healthy, active life.

What is type 1 diabetes mellitus?

Children with type 1 diabetes cannot make enough insulin, which the body needs in order to use glucose (blood sugar) for energy. Lack of insulin allows blood sugar to rise high enough that it comes out in urine. Glucose in urine brings water along with it, so urination becomes frequent and the body loses water. This makes it easier for your child to become dehydrated.

Without insulin, the body uses fats for energy, which results in the body's becoming more acidic. This "acidosis" is not healthy and can cause certain symptoms. Your child will need insulin injections to replace the missing insulin.

Type 1 diabetes is a lifelong problem that requires close attention to medications, diet, and activity. Living with diabetes is difficult for children, especially during the teen years. However, learning to control diabetes allows your child to live a relatively normal life. Type 1 diabetes mellitus was formerly called "insulin-dependent" or "juvenile" diabetes.

What does it look like?

- Type 1 diabetes usually develops in previously healthy children. It can start at any age but most often occurs in children between the ages of 7 and 15.

- Typical symptoms of diabetes may develop gradually over time or all of a sudden:

  - Tiredness, lack of energy.

  - Frequent thirst; drinking a lot of water.

  - Frequent urination and sometimes wetting the bed.

  - Weight loss, despite eating a lot.

  - In girls, yeast infections of the vagina.

- *Hypoglycemia* is a complication of treatment with insulin, occurring when the blood sugar level drops too low. It is very important to identify hypoglycemia. In infants and young children, it can affect intellectual development. Symptoms include:

  - Shakiness.

  - Sweating.

- Fussiness in infants.

- Behavior changes, such as drowsiness.

- In severe cases, confusion, coma, and seizures.

It can be difficult to recognize hypoglycemia in infants and young children. That's one reason why blood sugar levels are allowed to be higher in this age group than in older children.

- *Ketoacidosis.* If insulin levels become very low and blood glucose levels very high, your child may develop a condition called *diabetic ketoacidosis.* Inability to use glucose leads to production of acids in the body. Symptoms of diabetic ketoacidosis include:

  - Abdominal pain.

  - Nausea and vomiting.

  - Weakness or dizziness.

  - Confusion.

As ketoacidosis becomes worse, your child becomes more dehydrated. He or she may pass out and have trouble breathing. *This is an emergency!*

What causes type 1 diabetes?

- In type 1 diabetes, the body's own immune system destroys special cells in the pancreas. These cells, called beta cells, make the body's insulin. After the beta cells are destroyed, your child's body can no longer make enough insulin. The reason why the immune system destroys beta cells is unknown.

- A combination of factors may affect the risk of diabetes. These include genetic and environmental factors, such as infections or chemicals. Sometimes type 1 diabetes occurs when the pancreas is infected with a virus.

What puts your child at risk of type 1 diabetes?

- If you or any family members have diabetes, your child may be at higher risk.

- Certain racial/ethnic groups are at higher risk of diabetes, for example, people from Northern Europe.

- Another type of diabetes, type 2, is more frequent in overweight or obese children.

What are the possible complications of type 1 diabetes?

Type 1 diabetes can cause many types of complications. Learning to manage your child's blood glucose levels can reduce the long-term risk of these complications. Complications of diabetes include:

● Damage to the retina of the eye.

● Damage to the kidneys.

● Increased risk of diseases involving the blood vessels, including heart disease and stroke.

(!) Patients with diabetes are at risk of life-threatening complications:

● *Ketoacidosis,* as previously described.

● *Hypoglycemia,* caused by very low blood glucose levels.

● It is very important to know how to recognize and treat these complications. See later, under "Treatment of diabetic emergencies."

How is type 1 diabetes treated?

If your child has type 1 diabetes, we may recommend a visit to an endocrinologist (an expert in treating hormone-related diseases, including diabetes). Treatments for type 1 diabetes include:

● *Insulin shots.* Treatment for type 1 diabetes focuses on replacing the insulin that the body cannot produce on its own. This is done by giving insulin injections (shots) on a regular schedule:

  ● You'll be taught to give your child insulin injections. Older children will learn to give themselves insulin shots.

  ● The type, dose, and timing of insulin shots depend on your child's blood glucose levels. For example, your child may need to take three or four shots of insulin per day. Shots are usually given before meals and at bedtime.

  ● An insulin pump is a good choice for some diabetic patients, especially teens. A battery-powered pump is placed under the skin to provide a continuous supply of insulin.

  ● Your child's insulin treatment will be adjusted according to his or her blood glucose levels or other factors.

  ● Additional changes may be needed in certain situations, for example, when your child gets sick or during periods of high stress.

● *Blood glucose monitoring.* You (or your child) will be taught to measure his or her blood glucose level several times a day. Recording the results will help to make sure diabetes is under the best possible control. Modern test devices have made blood glucose monitoring easier than ever.

● *Education.* You and your child will receive training in how to use insulin, how to monitor blood glucose levels, how to recognize danger signs of low or high glucose levels, and how to prepare appropriate meals for a person with diabetes.

(!) *Treatment of diabetic emergencies.* Learning how to recognize and treat hypoglycemia and ketoacidosis is an essential part of your child's diabetes care:

● *Hypoglycemia* occurs when blood sugar levels drop too low:

  ● If symptoms are mild, the first step is to check your child's blood sugar level. If symptoms are more severe (for example, if your child is becoming drowsy), start treatment immediately and check blood sugar levels later.

  ● Give your child something sweet, for example, juice or candy.

  ● Give your child a shot of glucagon. You will be supplied with and taught how to use this emergency medication. It is used when the blood sugar level needs to be raised immediately.

● *Ketoacidosis* occurs when your child's blood sugar rises to a high level, meaning not enough insulin is present and so *acids* are produced.

  ● Call your endocrinologist or call our office—get medical help immediately! (!)

  ● Give insulin as instructed by the doctor.

  ● Give as much fluid as possible to manage dehydration.

● It can be very difficult to remember all of the information you need to manage your child's diabetes, especially at first! With time, however, you and your child can learn what you need to know to keep diabetes under control. This allows your child to live as normal a life as possible while reducing the risk of serious complications.

Psychological issues. Having a child diagnosed with type 1 diabetes is a traumatic event for your family. Parents may feel anxious and guilty. Your diabetic child may feel rebellious, especially during the teenage years. Counseling may help your family to deal with difficult feelings and family conflicts.

(📱) When should I call your office?

Call your endocrinologist, or call our office, if any of the following occurs:

● Your child develops any of the symptoms of diabetes mellitus (fatigue, frequent thirst or hunger, excessive urination).

● You and your child are having difficulty performing diabetes self-management or keeping blood glucose levels under control.

● Your child develops symptoms of ketoacidosis (abdominal pain, nausea and vomiting, weakness or dizziness, and confusion). *This is an emergency!* (!)

● Your child has frequent episodes of hypoglycemia or develops moderate/severe hypoglycemia (confusion, weakness, sweating, paleness, unconsciousness, or seizures). *This is an emergency!*

Where can I get more information?

- American Diabetes Association: *www.diabetes.org* or 1-800-DIABETES (1-800-342-2383).

- National Diabetes Information Clearinghouse: *www.diabetes.niddk.nih.gov*or 1-800-860-8747.

Diabetes Mellitus, Type 2

Type 2 diabetes mellitus is a chronic disease in which the body becomes resistant to the effects of the hormone insulin. This results in higher than normal levels of blood sugar (glucose). Once rare in children, type 2 diabetes has become relatively common in obese children and teens. Any type of diabetes can cause serious complications. However, with good medical care and education, your child with diabetes can lead a healthy, active life.

What is type 2 diabetes mellitus?

Children with type 2 diabetes become resistant to the effects of insulin (the insulin isn't working as well as it should), which the body needs to use glucose (blood sugar) for energy. This leads to abnormally high glucose levels in the blood. Unlike children with type 1 diabetes, many with type 2 will not need insulin to control their blood sugar.

Type 2 diabetes is a serious medical problem that requires close attention to your child's medications, diet, and activity. Living with diabetes is difficult for children, especially during the teen years. However, learning to control diabetes allows your child to live a relatively normal life. Type 2 diabetes mellitus was formerly called "non–insulin-dependent" or "adult-onset" diabetes.

What does it look like?

Type 2 diabetes usually develops in obese children, most commonly during the teen years.

- Your child may have no symptoms of diabetes. Type 2 diabetes may be detected initially because of elevated blood sugar levels on a routine laboratory test.

- Your child may have symptoms, such as tiredness or rapid weight gain.

- You may notice dark areas along skin creases, especially the armpits and neck (called acanthosis nigricans).

- Other symptoms are more common in children with type 1 diabetes (in which the body cannot make enough insulin) but may also occur in type 2 diabetes:
  - Frequent thirst—drinking a lot of water.
  - Frequent urination—sometimes bedwetting.
  - Frequent infections—girls may have yeast infections of the vagina.

- *Hypoglycemia* is a complication of treatment with insulin or with medications used to treat type 2 diabetes, occurring when the blood sugar level drops too low. It is very important to identify hypoglycemia. Symptoms include:

- Shakiness.

- Sweating.

- Behavior changes, such as drowsiness.

- In more severe cases, confusion, coma, and seizures may occur.

- *Ketoacidosis.* This condition occurs much less commonly with type 2 diabetes than with type 1. If insulin levels become very low and blood glucose levels very high, your child may develop a condition called *diabetic ketoacidosis.* The inability to use glucose leads to production of acids in the body. Symptoms of diabetic ketoacidosis include:

- Abdominal pain.

- Nausea and vomiting.

- Weakness or dizziness.

- Confusion.

As ketoacidosis becomes worse, your child becomes more dehydrated. He or she may pass out and have trouble breathing. *This is an emergency!*

What causes type 2 diabetes?

Type 2 diabetes occurs when the muscles and other body tissues become resistant to the effects of insulin. The level of glucose in the blood becomes abnormally high. Eventually, the body has problems making its own insulin.

What puts your child at risk of type 2 diabetes?

- Obesity and lack of exercise are the main risk factors for type 2 diabetes. Habits that increase your child's risk of obesity—such as eating too much, eating the wrong kinds of foods, and not getting enough exercise—also increase the risk of type 2 diabetes.

- Certain racial/ethnic groups seem to be at higher risk for type 2 diabetes, including African Americans, Mexican Americans, and Native Americans.

- If you or others in your family have had type 2 diabetes, your child may be at higher risk.

Can type 2 diabetes be prevented?

In many cases, yes. Nearly all children with type 2 diabetes are obese and get little exercise. If your child is obese or overweight, a weight-loss program, including diet changes and exercise, will reduce his or her chances of developing diabetes.

What are the possible complications of type 2 diabetes?

Type 2 diabetes can cause many different types of complications. Learning to manage your child's blood glucose levels can reduce the long-term risk of these complications:

- Damage to the retina of the eye.

- Damage to the kidneys.

- Increased risk of diseases involving the blood vessels, including heart disease and stroke.

- *Hypoglycemia* and *ketoacidosis,* described under "What does it look like."

How is type 2 diabetes treated?

- *Weight control, diet, and exercise* are essential first steps in the treatment of type 2 diabetes. Losing weight and increasing physical activity can greatly reduce the impact of the disease. We may recommend visits with a dietician, diabetes educator, or other professional to help your child (and family) learn healthier diet and exercise habits. We may also recommend a visit to an endocrinologist (an expert in treating hormone-related diseases) including diabetes.

- *Medications.* A number of different oral medications can help to reduce your child's blood glucose level. Some children with type 2 diabetes require insulin injections (shots), temporarily or permanently. The type, dose, and timing of medications, including insulin shots, depend on your child's blood glucose levels.

- *Blood glucose monitoring.* You or your child will be taught to measure his or her blood glucose level several times a day. Recording the results will help to make sure that your child's diabetes is under the best possible control. Modern test devices have made blood glucose monitoring easier than ever.

- *Education.* You and your child will receive training on how to use insulin if needed, how to monitor blood glucose levels, how to recognize danger signs of low or high glucose levels, and how to prepare appropriate meals for a person with diabetes.

- *Treatment of diabetic emergencies.* Learning how to recognize and treat hypoglycemia and ketoacidosis is an essential part of your child's diabetes care:

  - *Hypoglycemia* occurs when blood sugar levels drop too low:

    - If symptoms are mild, the first step is to check your child's blood sugar level. If symptoms are more severe (for example, if your child is becoming drowsy), start treatment immediately and check blood sugar levels later.

    - Give your child something sweet, for example, juice or candy.

    - Give your child a shot of glucagon. You will be supplied with and taught how to use this emergency medication. It is used when the blood sugar level needs to be raised immediately.

  - *Ketoacidosis* occurs when your child's blood sugar level is high, meaning not enough insulin is present and so *acids* are produced. Ketoacidosis occurs very in frequently in type 2 diabetes.

    - Call your endocrinologist or call our office. Seek medical help immediately.

    - Give insulin as instructed by the doctor.

    - Give as much fluid as possible to manage dehydration.

It can be very difficult to remember all of the information you need to manage your child's diabetes, especially at first! With time, however, you and your child can learn what you need to know to keep diabetes under control. This allows your child to live as normal a life as possible, while reducing the risk of serious complications.

Psychological issues. Having a child diagnosed with type 2 diabetes is a traumatic event for your family. Parents may feel anxious and guilty. Your diabetic child may feel rebellious, especially during the teenage years. Counseling may help your family to deal with difficult feelings and family conflicts.

When should I call your office?

Call your endocrinologist, or call our office, if any of the following occurs:

- Your child develops any of the symptoms of diabetes mellitus (fatigue, frequent thirst or hunger, excessive urination).

- You and your child are having difficulty performing diabetes self-management or keeping blood glucose levels under control.

- Your child has frequent episodes of hypoglycemia or develops moderate/severe hypoglycemia (confusion, weakness, sweating, paleness, unconsciousness, or seizures). *This is an emergency!*

- Your child develops symptoms of ketoacidosis (abdominal pain, nausea and vomiting, weakness or dizziness, and confusion). *This is an emergency!*

Where can I get more information?

- American Diabetes Association: *www.diabetes.org* or 1-800-DIABETES (1-800-342-2383).

- National Diabetes Information Clearinghouse: *www. diabetes.niddk.nih.gov* or 1-800-860-8747.

Puberty: Normal, Early, and Late Development

Puberty is the time when your child goes through many types of changes: physical, sexual, intellectual, emotional, and social. Certain diseases can cause puberty to occur early ("precocious" puberty) or late ("delayed" puberty). In healthy children, the timing of puberty varies widely. Monitoring your child's development is a key part of your child's medical care during the middle childhood to early teen years.

What is normal puberty?

Puberty is the period of life during which boys and girls start undergoing the bodily changes that will make them men and women. These changes are caused by increased levels of sex hormones. They include growth of pubic and underarm hair, enlargement of the testicles in boys, and development of the breasts in girls. Children also go through many intellectual, emotional, and social changes during puberty.

Puberty generally occurs between the ages of 10 and 12— a little sooner in girls and a little later in boys. Actually, the hormone changes that eventually lead to puberty begin much earlier in childhood.

Parents are sometimes concerned that their child is going through puberty too early or too late. It's true that there are some medical causes of precocious (too early) or delayed (too late) puberty. However, these are uncommon. Chances are your child is going through puberty at the time that's right for him or her. Your child's doctor will check your child's physical development at each visit.

What does it look like?

- *Sexual development.* Your child's sex organs will begin to grow and mature into their adult form:

  - In girls, breast buds and pubic hair can start to develop anywhere between ages 8 and 13. Menstrual periods start a little later, usually between 9 and 16 years.

  - In boys, the testicles begin to enlarge by about 10 years of age; the process may begin as early as 9 years. Pubic hair may start to develop around this time or a little later. Many boys develop slight enlargement of the breasts, but this usually goes away with time.

  - Both boys and girls become more interested in sex and relationships. Masturbation and sexual fantasies are common and normal. Boys often have their first ejaculation while asleep ("wet dream") and may worry that it's abnormal.

- *Physical development.* Both boys and girls begin to grow rapidly. Girls start growing faster in the early part of puberty, while boys grow faster in the later part. The peak "growth spurt" usually occurs 2 or 3 years later in boys than in girls. In addition, boys generally continue growing for 2 to 3 years after girls have stopped.

  - Growth may occur unevenly, giving your child a "gawky" appearance. Other changes may make your child feel awkward as well, such as sudden changes or "cracking" of the voice and acne (the result of hormone changes).

- *Intellectual and social changes.* Puberty has a major impact in practically every area of your child's development, including intellectual ability, self-esteem, and relationships. It is normal for young teens to be self-conscious about their appearance and to feel that everyone else is noticing them.

What causes early or late puberty?

- Parents and children are sometimes concerned that they are going through puberty too early or too late. The timing of puberty varies widely.

- Several medical conditions can cause puberty to occur early or late. All, in one way or another, have to do with the production or effects of hormones. Most of these conditions are uncommon.

- *Early (precocious) puberty.* There are many possible causes of early puberty. Early puberty is much more common in girls than boys. In 90% of girls with precocious puberty, no specific cause is detected. Whether the cause is known or not, specific hormone-blocking drugs can be used to treat precocious puberty if it is severe enough.

  - Usually no specific cause ("idiopathic").

  - Certain tumors of the ovaries, adrenal glands, or brain.

  - Rare syndromes or genetic diseases.

  - Certain medications.

- *Late (delayed) puberty.* Delayed puberty may occur in children with certain growth disorders. Other possible causes include:

  - Hard physical training (in girls).

  - Chronic diseases (such as cystic fibrosis or sickle cell disease).

  - Certain syndromes and genetic diseases (such as Turner's syndrome in girls).

What are some possible complications of early or late puberty?

- Even when no specific cause is detected, treatment is available for most children with early or late puberty if needed. Complications are uncommon.

- If not detected and treated early enough, late puberty may lead to reduced final height.

- Some children experience psychological effects related to early or late puberty. Visits to a psychologist can be helpful.

How are early and late puberty treated?

- Your child's doctor will monitor his or her physical development at each medical visit. Although parents are often concerned about the timing of their child's puberty, problems that need treatment are uncommon. Your child may simply be reaching puberty a little ahead of or behind other children of the same age.

- Even if early or delayed puberty is not medically abnormal, it may be a source of embarrassment to your child. It may help your child to know that puberty and adolescence are awkward periods for nearly everyone and that he or she is just a little ahead of or behind other kids of the same age.

- If there is any reason to suspect a medical cause of early or delayed puberty, we will probably recommend a visit to an endocrinologist (a doctor specializing in the treatment of gland and hormone diseases). This specialist can perform tests and recommend treatments designed to slow (or less commonly, speed up) the process of puberty. Treatment usually consists of hormone-blocking drugs (for early puberty) or hormones (for delayed puberty).

- If a tumor or other specific cause is identified, treating that problem will likely help. However, serious medical problems are unlikely.

When should I call your office?

Call our office if:

- You and your child have questions about the normal changes of puberty.

- Worries about early or delayed puberty are making your child anxious.

- Your child seems to be developing typical changes of puberty (for example, breast buds, pubic and underarm hair) at an early age:

  - Before age 8 for girls.

  - Before age 9 for boys.

- Your child's growth and maturation seem far behind those of other children of the same age.

Short Stature (Below Normal Height) ■

You may be concerned if your child is shorter than others of his or her age. Most likely, your child is genetically short or is growing at a slower rate than "normal." Less often, short stature results from poor health or nutrition or from certain uncommon diseases.

What is short stature?

Short stature simply means that your child is below "normal" height for his or her age. He or she may be shorter than his or her classmates. This may lead to teasing or problems with self-esteem. Your child's actual height in inches is not as important as whether he or she is gaining in height and weight at a normal rate.

What causes short stature?

- *Familial short stature.* Some children are simply shorter than others because it's "in the genes"—if the parents are short, the child is likely to be short as well.

- *Constitutional growth delay.* Some children start out growing more slowly than others but don't seem to have any disease or other abnormality responsible for slow growth. Most of these "late bloomers" eventually catch up in height to other children their age.

- *Hormone deficiencies or abnormalities.* Less commonly, short stature results from problems with *growth hormone* and other hormones such as *thyroid hormone* produced by the pituitary gland.

- *Chronic diseases or illnesses.* This refers to a disease or health problems that are present for a long period of time, such as cystic fibrosis or sickle cell disease.

- *Certain genetic (inherited) diseases or conditions.*

- *Malnutrition.* This refers to not getting enough food and calories over a long period of time. There are many causes of this, including neglect, chronic disease, or poverty. A child's weight is affected first, then height.

What does it look like?

The appearance of a child with short stature depends on the cause.

- If your child has familial short stature or growth delay, he or she will otherwise be normal.

- Children with certain genetic conditions may have other abnormalities in appearance or on physical examination.

- Malnourished children will appear very thin.

What puts your child at risk of short stature?

- Genetics: Short parents often have short children.

How is the cause of short stature diagnosed?

- If your child is growing slowly but otherwise appears healthy, no further tests may be needed. If the parents or other family members are short or were "late bloomers," the same may be true for your child.

- If your child has stopped growing normally, further tests may be recommended to see if the cause is a disease or other abnormality. These may include:

  - X-rays (radiographs).

  - Blood tests to measure levels of growth hormone and other hormones produced by the pituitary gland.

  - Genetic testing for causes of an underactive pituitary gland.

  - Tests to diagnose other diseases that can cause slow growth, if needed.

How is short stature treated?

Treatment for short stature depends on the cause:

- If your child seems to have constitutional growth delay, his or her growth will be checked over time. If your child's growth "catches up," then no treatment is needed. If not, tests for other possible causes of slow growth may be performed.

- For hormone problems such as *growth hormone deficiency* or *low thyroid*, treatment can be given to replenish the low levels. This usually requires seeing an endocrinologist (a specialist in treating hormonal diseases) for further tests and treatment.

- If other diseases are present, your child's growth may improve after those diseases are treated. Growth hormone treatment may help in some children.

- Some children without any hormone deficiencies or health problems are simply are very short. Growth hormone therapy may increase their adult height but there may be side effects and risks. If you are very concerned about how tall your child will be, we can refer you to an endocrinologist.

 When should I call your office?

Call our office if:

- Your child is growing slowly or stops growing normally.

Thyroid Disorders (Hypothyroidism, Hyperthyroidism)

The thyroid is a gland in the neck that produces several essential hormones. Problems can occur when thyroid hormone levels are too low (hypothyroidism) or too high (hyperthyroidism). Hypothyroidism can be present at birth and can cause growth and developmental disorders if not detected and treated. Thyroid problems can also develop later in childhood and adolescence, especially in girls, causing a number of problems.

What are thyroid disorders?

There are many types of thyroid disorders. In children, the most common are *hypothyroid* disorders, meaning that thyroid hormone levels are too low. The most serious disease in this category is *congenital hypothyroidism*. Babies who are born with inadequate thyroid activity can develop serious growth and mental deficiencies if not treated within the first few months of life. Fortunately, congenital hypothyroidsm is usually detected by routine screening tests performed at birth. Treatment to replace thyroid hormone prevents most complications.

Older children may have *acquired hypothyroidism*, which means the problem with low thyroid hormones occurred some time after birth. The most common cause is lymphocytic (Hashimoto's) thyroiditis, which is caused by antibodies made by the body that attack the thyroid gland. This is an *autoimmune* disease that occurs when the body's own immune system attacks itself. Hypothyroidism can cause delayed growth, decreased energy, constipation, and other symptoms. It is treatable with thyroid hormone replacement.

In *hyperthyroid* disorders, thyroid hormone levels are too high. The most common type is *Graves' disease*, which occurs most often in teenage girls (and in women). It is also caused by the person's immune system affecting the thyroid gland. Treatment consists of thyroid-blocking drugs.

What do they look like?

- Babies with *congenital hypothyroidism* appear normal at birth. However, without treatment they gradually develop delayed growth and development, including mental retardation. The problem is usually detected at birth by routine screening tests. If the diagnosis is missed, early symptoms may include feeding problems, sluggish behavior, sleepiness, and constipation.
- For children with *acquired hypothyroidism,* the main sign is slower than normal growth. However, you may notice other symptoms first, including puffy swelling of the skin, constipation, always feeling cold, low energy, and sleepiness. Signs of puberty may occur early in younger children or be delayed in older children. A goiter, swelling of the thyroid gland in the neck, is often present.
- *Hyperthyroidism,* including Graves' disease, is most common in girls between the ages of 11 and 15. Initial symptoms may include hyperactivity, extreme mood swings, and reduced attention, causing problems at school. A goiter and bulging of the eyes (exophthalmos) also may be present. Your child may seem to eat a lot but never gain weight. Many other symptoms are possible, including excessive sweating, fast heartbeat, and muscle weakness.

What puts your child at risk of thyroid disorders?

- Thyroid disorders are more common in girls than in boys.
- A family history of thyroid or autoimmune disorders, including type 1 diabetes.
- Hypothyroidism may occur more often in children with certain genetic disorders such as Down syndrome, Turner's syndrome, or Klinefelter's syndrome.

How are thyroid disorders treated?

Once they have been detected, thyroid disorders can be treated. Hypothyroid disorders are treated by replacing the low levels of the thyroid hormone thyroxine. Hyperthyroid disorders in children are most often treated by giving drugs to block thyroid hormones. For expert diagnosis and treatment, your doctor will probably recommend a visit to an endocrinologist (a specialist in treating hormone diseases).

- *Congenital hypothyroidism.* Your child will need immediate treatment with thyroxine. Careful monitoring is essential to make sure your child is getting the correct dose of thyroxine. In the first few years of life, tests are needed to determine whether your child's thyroid gland has started functioning or whether hypothyroidism is a permanent problem. Your child should receive close medical follow-up to ensure that his or her growth and mental and physical development continue to stay on track.
- *Acquired hypothyroidism.* Tests are performed to identify the cause of your child's low thyroid activity. Treatment with thyroxine is given to make up for the missing thyroid hormone levels. Close follow-up is needed to make sure your child is receiving the correct thyroxine dose.
- *Hyperthyroid disorders.* The usual treatment for Graves' disease in children is medications that block thyroid hormones.

- These drugs have a number of possible side effects. Careful medical follow-up is needed.

- Treatment may have to continue for several years. There is a chance that hyperthyroid disease will recur after the end of treatment. In that case, your child will have to go back on antithyroid medications.

● In some cases, surgery may be recommended to remove most of the thyroid gland. This is generally a safe procedure. However, there is a risk that surgery may lead to the opposite problem, that is, thyroid function may become too low (hypothyroidism).

● Another possible alternative is radioiodine treatment: medications are used instead of surgery to eliminate overactive thyroid tissue. Again, there is a risk of hypo-

thyroidism. Surgery and radioiodine treatment are used more often in adults than in children.

When should I call your office?

Thyroid disorders are complex diseases that require careful follow-up, often by a specialist. Call your endocrinologist or our office if any of the symptoms of thyroid disease return after treatment:

- Hyperthyroidism: shakiness, fast heart rate.

- Hypothyroidism: low energy, sleepiness, weight gain, constipation.

Section XI ▪ The Eye

Blocked Tear Duct

Many babies are born with blocked tear ducts. You may notice tears overflowing down your child's cheeks, or thicker material draining from the eye. Infections may occur in and around the blocked tear duct. A simple, nonsurgical treatment usually solves the problem.

What is blocked tear duct?

The tear ducts are tiny openings in the corner of the eye that let tears flow out of the eye. As many as 6% of babies are born with blocked tear ducts. Because tears can't flow normally, they build up and overflow out of the eye. Tears help keep the eyes free of bacteria and debris, so blocked tear ducts can lead to infections in and around the lacrimal glands (tear glands) and ducts. Inflammation (redness, irritation) of the area around the eye can also occur.

In many babies, blocked tear ducts eventually open up on their own, with no need for treatment. We may recommend frequent, gentle massage of the area to help the duct open up sooner. If the blockage doesn't clear by about age 12 months or if your child has frequent infections, a simple procedure can be done to unblock the tear duct.

What does it look like?

- You may see excessive tears coming from your child's eyes, even when he or she isn't crying. You may not notice the problem until your child is a few weeks old.

- You may notice thicker material, consisting of mucus or even pus, coming from your child's eyes—this may be a sign of minor infection.

- If the blockage is only partial, you may see overflow only when the eye is producing a lot of tears; for example, when your child is exposed to cold, wind, or sunlight. If the blockage is more complete, tears may leak out of your child's eye constantly.

- Tears and other discharge may make the skin around the eye red and irritated. This may be a sign of mild infection. If the infection gets more severe, the area around the inner corner of the eye may become swollen and tender. Other symptoms of more severe infection include fever and fussiness.

What causes blocked tear ducts?

Many infants are born with blocked tear ducts. They can also occur in older children (and adults), occasionally after an eye infection.

What are some possible complications of blocked tear ducts?

Blocked tear ducts increase the risk of infection. However, ost of these infections are mild and easily treated.

What puts your child at risk of blocked tear ducts?

- In babies, blocked tear ducts are a common problem that is usually not preventable.

How are blocked tear ducts treated?

- We may recommend frequent, gentle *massage* to unblock the tear ducts. Gently massage the area around the blocked duct two or three times per day, as instructed by your doctor. Make sure to wash your hands before touching the area around your baby's eyes. After you're done, wash the area with warm water. Don't use soap because it could irritate the eyes.

- If the blockage doesn't clear up by age 12 months or if frequent infections are a problem, we may recommend a visit to an eye specialist (ophthalmologist). He or she may perform a simple procedure called *probing*.

  - The doctor gently inserts a tiny tube (called a catheter) into the blocked duct. This almost always opens up the blockage.

  - Babies are usually given anesthesia so that they will be asleep during the probing procedure. In older children, it can be done without anesthesia.

- If the eye is infected, your child will need antibiotic eyedrops. Treatment usually continues for 5 to 7 days, depending on how quickly the infection clears. For more severe infections, oral antibiotics may be recommended.

When should I call your office?

Call our office if:

- Your child still has symptoms of blocked tear ducts (overflowing tears) by age 12 months.

- Your child has thicker material (mucus or pus) draining from the eye.

- The area around the eye becomes red, tender, or swollen. *These may be signs of more serious infection—call our office immediately.*

Conjunctivitis (Pinkeye)

Conjunctivitis, often called pinkeye, is a common, easily spread infection. It usually goes away on its own, but treatment can be helpful. Conjunctivitis in newborns can be more serious, requiring medical attention.

What is conjunctivitis?

Conjunctivitis (pinkeye) means inflammation (redness, soreness) of the white part of the eye and the inside of the eyelid. Pinkeye is caused by bacteria or viruses, which can easily spread to others.

In newborns, conjunctivitis can be caused by bacteria or viruses transmitted during birth. These infections can be more serious and require medical attention.

What does it look like?

- The white part of one or both eyes is pink or red.

- There is a gritty or "scratchy" feeling in the eye, with little or no pain.

- Eyelids may be swollen but not red or tender.

- Eyes may be mildly sensitive to bright light.

- There may be a clear, green, or yellow discharge from the eye. While your child is sleeping, a crust may develop on his or her eyelashes, causing the eyelids to stick together.

What causes conjunctivitis?

- Infection with bacteria or viruses. Sometimes this happens when your child has a cold or sore throat.

- Other things can irritate the eye, such as allergies or dust. These are sometimes confused with pinkeye.

What are the possible complications?

- Children with conjunctivitis may also develop middle-ear infections (otitis media).

What puts your child at risk of conjunctivitis?

- The bacteria or viruses that cause pinkeye can spread quickly among children. This commonly happens at school or in day care, especially in young children.

Can conjunctivitis be prevented?

- To avoid spreading the infection, children with pinkeye may not be permitted to go to school or day care.

- Having your child wash his or her hands frequently may help avoid spreading the infection.

How is conjunctivitis treated?

Pinkeye is caused by bacteria in about half of cases and by viruses in the other half. It can be difficult to tell the two causes apart.

- *If the cause is a virus,* antibiotics won't help. The infection usually goes away on its own in a few days.

- *If the cause is bacteria,* the infection may go away more quickly with the use of antibiotic eye drops. Drops are usually given four times per day for about a week.

- Your child will usually be allowed to go back to school or day care in a day or two.

- Warm or cold water soaks may help the eyes feel better. Use lukewarm water to remove crusty material that builds up on the eyelids.

- Older children and teens should avoid using eye makeup or wearing contact lenses until the eye looks and feels better.

When should I call your office?

If your child is being treated for conjunctivitis, call our office if he or she develops

- Fever.

- Increased pain.

- Increased sensitivity to light.

- A change in vision.

Also call if conjunctivitis doesn't get better in 1 week.

Conjunctivitis in newborns may be more serious. If your baby develops redness or fluid draining from the eyes anytime before 1 month old, call our office.

Corneal Abrasions

Eye injuries are common in children, especially boys. Scratches (abrasions) of the cornea and foreign bodies in the eye are among the most common injuries. They are usually not serious but may still require medical care. Some important steps can reduce your child's risk of serious eye injuries.

What are corneal abrasions?

The cornea is the clear layer of the eye that covers the iris (colored part of the eye) and pupil. It works to help direct light into the eye. Scratches of the cornea are a very common injury.

Corneal abrasions can be caused by a scratch from a fingernail, tree branch, or other object. They may occur when very small foreign bodies, such as sand or grit, get into the eye. Corneal scratches often occur when your child rubs his or her eyes after a foreign body makes its way into the eye. If at all possible, keep your child from rubbing the eyes to avoid further damage.

If your child has a foreign body in the eye that cannot be removed easily, seek medical attention. Corneal abrasions are generally minor but can be very painful. They are treated with antibiotic eyedrops and usually heal quickly.

Children are also at risk of other, more serious eye injuries. Common causes include playing sports, using fireworks, and exposure to projectiles such as sticks and stones. BB gun injuries and chemical burns can cause particularly serious damage to the eye.

If your child has any penetrating injury or chemical injury of the eye, get medical help immediately.

What do they look like?

- Foreign bodies and corneal abrasions usually cause sudden, sometimes intense eye pain.
- Tears may flow.
- Eyes are sensitive to light. Your child may refuse to open the injured eye to let you look at it.
- Your child may experience decreased vision.
- You may or may not see any foreign object in the eye.
- You probably won't see any scratch or abrasion. The injuries usually aren't visible without using a special dye and examining light.

What are some possible complications of corneal abrasions?

- Usually none. Minor corneal scratches generally heal within a few days. However, it's important to get treatment to prevent the cornea from becoming infected.
- If there is a foreign body that is not removed, it may cause further damage.

Can eye injuries be prevented?

Certain activities commonly lead to eye injuries:

- Make sure your child is very cautious around BB guns and fireworks.
- Make sure your child wears appropriate eye protection during sports (such as racquetball).
- Safety goggles should be worn during any activity that could lead to small objects flying into the eye, for example, mowing the lawn, using power tools.

How are corneal abrasions diagnosed and treated?

- The doctor can use a special green dye and blue light to detect corneal scratches that can't otherwise be seen. These may be used along with an instrument called an ophthalmoscope, which provides light and magnification. Special equipment may be needed to detect foreign bodies in the eye.
- For corneal abrasions, antibiotic drops or ointment will be prescribed. Place these medicines in the eye a few times a day until the scratch has healed—usually by 24 to 48 hours. We probably won't recommend placing a patch over the eye as it doesn't help the injury heal any faster.
- Give your child acetaminophen or ibuprofen for pain. Anesthetic eyedrops are usually not recommended because they may delay healing or increase the risk of further injury.
- If there is a foreign object in the eye, the doctor will attempt to remove it. If there is any problem finding or removing the foreign object or any sign of penetrating injury, we will probably recommend a visit to the eye doctor (ophthalmologist).

When should I call your office?

- Corneal abrasions should heal within a few days. If your child is still having eye pain or other symptoms (tearing, light sensitivity, feeling of "something in the eye") after 48 hours, call our office.

- If your child has other types of eye injuries—such as cuts or tears of the eyelid, any kind of penetrating injury or burn, blood in the eye, or hard trauma to the area around the eye (such as occurs in playing sports, a fight, or auto accident)—seek immediate medical attention.

Glaucoma

Glaucoma is a serious eye disease caused by increased pressure inside the eye. Some babies are born with glaucoma. Prompt diagnosis and treatment are needed to save the child's vision. In other infants or in older children, glaucoma may result from injuries or other eye diseases.

What is glaucoma?

Glaucoma refers to several types of eye diseases in which the pressure inside the eyeball is higher than normal. This causes damage to the optic nerve, which is essential for vision. The optic nerve damage may lead to blindness.

Glaucoma is relatively rare in children, but it can occur. Most infants and toddlers with glaucoma have the congenital form of the disease: they are born with an abnormality that doesn't allow normal drainage of fluid from the eyeball. Glaucoma can also result from other eye defects or diseases or from trauma.

Glaucoma requires expert treatment to protect your child's vision. Unfortunately, glaucoma can be difficult to recognize in children. Treatment often includes surgery.

What does it look like?

The typical symptoms of glaucoma in infants are tearing, sensitivity to light, and hard blinking. Other symptoms may include:

- "Bloodshot" eyes—redness of the white part of the eye.

- Big irises (the colored part of the eye).

- Clouding of the cornea (the normally clear part of the eye that covers the iris and pupil). This makes the irises appear cloudy.

- Enlarged eyes. This may be more noticeable if just one eye has glaucoma.

- Vision problems; these can be difficult to recognize in infants.

What causes glaucoma?

- In most infants with glaucoma, the disease is caused by an abnormality of the drainage system of the inner eye.

- Glaucoma in infants may also occur as part of more complex eye problems and congenital (present from birth) diseases.

- Later in childhood, glaucoma may result from eye injuries, including bleeding inside the eye (not on the white part of the eye). It can also be a complication of other diseases.

What are some possible complications of glaucoma?

Vision loss is the main complication. The goal of treatment is to preserve your child's vision as much as possible.

What puts your child at risk of glaucoma?

- Certain genetic diseases.

- Other eye diseases, eye surgery, and severe eye injuries.

Can glaucoma be prevented?

- Most of the time, there is no way to prevent childhood glaucoma. If you or others in your family have genetic diseases associated with glaucoma, genetic counseling may help you to understand this risk.

- Make sure your child wears protective eyewear when playing certain sports (for example, racquetball) or during other activities that could result in objects flying into the eye.

How is glaucoma diagnosed?

- Glaucoma is suspected if you or your doctor notices the typical symptoms in your child: light bothering the eyes, blinking, redness and tearing.

- If glaucoma is suspected, we will recommend a visit to an eye specialist (ophthalmologist). The ophthalmologist will perform a test called tonometry to measure pressure inside the eyeball. The test is painless, but an anesthetic may be placed into the eye to numb it.

- Determining the exact cause and type of your child's glaucoma is essential to deciding on the best treatment.

How is glaucoma treated?

- Treatment for glaucoma varies, depending on the cause. At all times, the goal of treatment is to reduce the pressure within your child's eye to as close to normal as possible! This prevents further loss of vision.

- Surgery is usually needed for children with glaucoma. One of several different procedures may be recommended, either to allow fluid to drain from the eyes or to reduce the amount of fluid produced. Some children require repeated eye surgeries as they grow.

- Other treatments may be needed as well, including special glasses and medications. The eye doctor will monitor your child's vision closely to achieve the best possible results.

When should I call your office?

Children being treated for glaucoma should have regular follow-up visits to the eye doctor. Call your eye doctor if there is any change in your child's vision.

Strabismus

Strabismus is a condition in which the eyes are not lined up (aligned) normally. The eyes point in different directions: either inward ("crossed eyes") or outward ("walleye"). Treatment usually consists of eye patching or special glasses to train the eyes to work together. Visits to an eye doctor (ophthalmologist) are needed to diagnose and treat this condition. Your child also may need eye surgery.

What is strabismus?

Strabismus, sometimes called "lazy eye," is a common vision problem in children. One eye is not aligned with the other, so they don't move together properly. The eyes may point inward (crossed eyes, or esotropia) or outward (walleye, or exotropia). Strabismus doesn't always cause obvious vision problems, but treatment is needed to protect vision in the weaker eye.

A visit to an eye doctor (ophthalmologist) is needed to determine the type of strabismus and the best treatment. Most often, treatment consists of an eye patch or special glasses to help train the weaker eye to work normally. Some children with strabismus need surgery.

What does it look like?

- Your child's eyes do not line up or move together properly. This may be noticeable all the time or only when your child looks in one direction.

- The affected eye may turn inward (cross-eyed) or outward (walleyed). In some children, the eyes have difficulty moving up and down together, rather than side to side.

- Your child may or may not have vision problems, such as double vision. Vision is usually quite a bit weaker in one eye. This may cause problems with depth perception and judging distances, which require accurate vision in both eyes.

- Occasional turning in or turning out of one eye is normal in babies during the first 3 to 4 months.

What causes strabismus?

- For various reasons, your child has an imbalance in the muscles that move the eyes or in their ability to focus. Eventually, the brain "learns" to ignore the vision in the weaker eye. If this happens, the vision in that eye will grow weaker and weaker over time (called *amblyopia).*

- Most often, the cause of strabismus is unknown. If the problem is discovered at birth or before 6 months of age, it may be called "congenital" or "infantile" strabismus.

- Less often, strabismus is caused by specific injuries or diseases affecting the eye muscles or the nerves that move them.

What are some possible complications of strabismus?

- Permanent loss of vision in the weaker eye. Prompt diagnosis and treatment will preserve your child's vision as much as possible.

- Certain types of strabismus are difficult to eliminate completely. Your child may require long-term treatment, or the problem may return after treatment.

What puts your child at risk of strabismus?

- If you or others in your family have had strabismus, your child may be at higher risk.

- Certain genetic diseases, including Down's syndrome.

- Certain types of brain or nerve injuries, including cerebral palsy.

- Certain eye diseases, including retinopathy of prematurity; or tumors, including retinoblastoma.

Can strabismus be prevented?

There is usually no way to prevent strabismus. Early treatment gives your child the best chance for normal vision.

How is strabismus diagnosed?

Proper treatment of strabismus requires tests and evaluation to determine what type of strabismus your child has. An eye doctor (ophthalmologist) will coordinate your child's care. The tests are not painful. The doctor will likely have to put drops in your child's eyes to perform a complete examination.

There are several types of strabismus:

- *Pseudostrabismus.* Some infants whose eyes don't seem to work together properly don't really have strabismus at all. This pseudostrabismus ("false" strabismus) is a misleading appearance that will eventually go away as your baby's face continues to grow and develop. However, it's important to remember that your child could still develop true strabismus later in life. If the cross-eyed appearance doesn't go away within a few months, your child should be checked again.

- *Esotropia (crossed eyes).* Your child may be born with crossed eyes but more often the problem becomes apparent during the first 6 months. This is called "congenital" or "infantile" esotropia. Other children develop crossed eyes a little later on, usually around age 2 or 3. This is called "accommodative" esotropia.

- *Exotropia (walleye).* Walleye (eyes pointing in opposite directions) may be noticeable all the time or just some of the time. It may be more noticeable when your child is tired or sick, or when he or she is focusing on something at a distance. The problem may not develop until your child is 4 to 6 years old.

- *Paralytic strabismus and other special types.* Some children with strabismus have damage to the nerves that move the eye muscles. Your child may be born with these problems (congenital), or they may result from some injury or illness developing later on. Children with these types of problems are more likely to need eye muscle surgery.

How is strabismus treated?

- Depending on the cause of strabismus, treatment may consist of using patches, glasses, and/or eye muscle surgery.

- For congenital esotropia, patching of the good eye is often done to improve the function of the bad eye. Surgery to correct the problem is done after patching. Surgery may be needed if glasses or patching don't work, or if your child still has some leftover strabismus after this treatment.

- The exact treatment depends on the ophthalmologist's evaluation. The earlier you notice the problem with eye alignment, the earlier treatment can begin and the better the chance of good results.

When should I call your office?

Most children with strabismus make regular visits to their ophthalmologist. Call your ophthalmologist if your child's strabismus symptoms don't improve with treatment or if they return after treatment.

Stye (Hordeolum)

> A stye is an infection causing a red, swollen bump on the eyelid. It occurs when the glands under the skin of the eyelid become infected. Treatment, possibly including antibiotics, is important to prevent the infection from spreading.

What is a stye?

A stye is an infection of the glands under the skin of the eyelid, at the base of the eyelashes. The medical term is "hordeolum." Styes can be quite irritating, and there is a risk that the infection will spread.

Treatment usually consists of frequent soaks with a warm washcloth. Your doctor may recommend an antibiotic ointment as well. If the stye doesn't go away within a few days, or if it seems to be getting worse, call our office.

What does it look like?

- A red, tender, swollen bump on the edge of the eyelid. You may be able to see the infected gland on the eyelid or it may be under the skin.

- The infection may quickly become quite large and painful.

- The eyes are teary. Your child may feel like there's something in the eye.

What causes a stye?

One or more glands under the skin of the eyelid become infected, most often with "staph" bacteria.

What are some possible complications of a stye?

The infection may enlarge and spread. This can lead to a more serious infection of the skin of the eyelid and surrounding area (cellulitis).

What puts your child at risk of a stye?

- Anything that irritates the eye, including frequent rubbing, eye makeup, or contact lenses, may increase the risk of infection. However, most styes occur without such risk factors.

- Other infections of the eyelid (such as blepharitis) may increase the risk of styes.

Can styes be prevented?

Good hygiene, including regular washing of the face and hands, may reduce the risk of styes.

How are styes treated?

- *Warm soaks.* Soak a washcloth in warm water and place it over the eye. Keep the warm washcloth on the eye for 10 minutes or so, a few times per day. This will reduce pain and help the stye to heal faster.

- *Antibiotics.* Your doctor may recommend an antibiotic ointment, especially if the stye is large or painful. Follow the doctor's instructions for using this medication.

- *Keep the area clean.* Discourage your child from touching or squeezing the area. The stye will eventually clear up on its own. Your child should stop wearing eye makeup and contact lenses until the stye has healed.

- *Surgery.* If needed, a minor surgical procedure can be done to drain the stye.

When should I call your office?

Call our office if:

- The stye does not clear up within a week or so.

- The stye seems to be getting worse; that is, the area of redness and tenderness gets larger.

- Your child has eye pain or any change in vision.

Section XII ▪ Gastrointestinal Disorders

Anal Fissure

An anal fissure is a small tear of the tissues around your child's anus (the opening where bowel movements come out). Usually, the tear occurs when your child passes a hard bowel movement that causes too much stretching of the delicate tissues in this area. Treatment includes medications to soften your child's bowel movements. It may take a while for the fissure to heal completely.

What is anal fissure?

Anal fissures are a fairly common problem in infants. They are tears that occur when the delicate tissues around the anus are stretched too far when your child passes a hard bowel movement (BM). Injury from hard wiping around the anus may also cause tears.

Your baby may cry when having BMs, and you may see some bright red blood on the BM. Constipation can either cause or result from anal fissures.

Treatment includes keeping the area as clean as possible, applying a lubricant, and giving a stool softener to prevent hard BMs. Normally, anal fissures heal without any problem. It's important to break the cycle of constipation and anal fissures: if BMs hurt because of the injured tissue, your child may try to hold them in, which will make the problem work.

What does it look like?

- Pain during bowel movements. Your child may strain or cry when passing BMs.

- You may see bright red blood on the surface of your child's BM (or on diaper wipes or toilet paper).

- The fissure usually looks like a small tear in the tissues around the anus. It may be difficult to see because of the normal folds of skin in this area.

- Your child may have constipation: hard BMs being passed less often than normal. Constipation may occur before or after anal fissure.

What causes anal fissure?

- Passing hard BMs is the most common cause of anal fissures. If your child has been constipated, this is probably what caused the fissure. However, sometimes constipation is the result, rather than the cause, of an anal fissure.

- Whichever happens first, constipation and anal fissures can set up a vicious circle: BMs hurt, so your child tries to avoid having them. This makes the BMs hard, which may make the anal fissure worse.

- The area around the anus may also be injured during diaper changes, for example, from wiping too hard or accidental scratches from long fingernails.

What are some possible complications?

- Usually none. Anal fissures nearly always heal with simple treatments. Complete healing may take several days, or even weeks.

- Some anal fissures don't heal as promptly as they should. This problem is most often related to continued constipation. Chronic fissures may require minor surgery, but this is rare.

- A small skin "tag" may develop around the fissure. This is caused by skin irritation and is considered harmless.

Can anal fissures be prevented?

- Avoiding constipation may reduce the risk of anal fissures.

- Wipe your child's bottom gently during diaper changes.

How are anal fissures treated?

- The most important factor is to try to avoid hard BMs and constipation. If your child continues to have hard BMs, it will be difficult for the fissure to heal.

- We may recommend a medication called a stool softener (such as Metamucil). Use these medications as recommended by your doctor. Your may have to adjust the dose, depending on how your child responds. Too much stool softener can cause diarrhea (loose, watery BMs).

- For babies who haven't started solid foods:

  - Add corn syrup (Karo syrup) to your baby's formula: 1 teaspoon per 4-ounce bottle, a few times a day.

  - It may also help to give your baby juice, especially prune juice. However, since juices don't have a lot of nutritional value for babies, don't give too much.

  - Your doctor may recommend other oral solutions.

- For older children, add more fiber to the diet: give plenty of fresh fruits and vegetables and bran cereals.

- Spread a small amount of lubricant, such as petroleum jelly (Vaseline), on the anal area to help protect it.

- Make sure your child gets plenty of water and other liquids.

- If any other cause of constipation is present, your doctor may recommend additional treatments.

- Keep the area as clean as possible. Be gentle when cleaning.
- Encourage older children to use the toilet frequently, as needed. Holding in BMs will only make the problem worse.

When should I call your office?

Call our office if:

- Your child is having continued constipation and hard BMs, despite the use of stool softeners and other treatments.
- Your child is having continued pain and/or bleeding during BMs.

Celiac Disease (Sprue)

Children with celiac disease have damage to the intestines, which may cause diarrhea and other symptoms. The damage is caused by exposure to gluten, contained in wheat and other grains. Treatment consists of carefully avoiding all gluten in your child's diet, which can be difficult to do. To avoid continued symptoms and possible complications, your child must follow a gluten-free diet throughout his or her life.

What is celiac disease?

Celiac disease is damage to the small intestine, often causing diarrhea, fussiness, and slow weight gain and growth. It is caused by exposure to gluten, a protein found in wheat, rye, and barley, which is present in many bread and cereal products. Celiac disease most often occurs several months after solid foods are first introduced into your baby's diet. It is sometimes called "sprue."

If the doctor suspects your child has celiac disease, he or she will probably recommend a visit to a specialist in stomach and intestinal diseases (a gastroenterologist). This doctor may perform special procedures and tests to make sure the diagnosis is correct. A special gluten-free diet will eliminate most symptoms and complications of celiac disease.

What does it look like?

- Symptoms most often develop a while after your child starts on solid foods, usually around ages 6 months to 2 years. However, celiac disease can be present for quite a while before it is recognized.

- Symptoms of celiac disease vary. Your child may have some or all of the following symptoms:

  - Diarrhea; sometimes vomiting.

  - Poor growth; your child may be underweight or short for age.

  - Irritable behavior.

  - Decreased appetite.

  - Bulging (distended) belly, despite being skinny and underweight.

- Many other symptoms are possible. Other patients have gluten intolerance and intestinal damage without the typical symptoms of celiac disease.

What causes celiac disease?

- People with celiac disease are "gluten-intolerant." When they eat cereal or foods containing gluten, this causes damage to a part of the small intestine. The intestinal damage takes a while to occur—it doesn't happen the first time your child eats wheat or other grains.

- It's not certain why some people develop celiac disease. A genetic component (inheritance) may play a role, along with factors in your child's diet and environment. Some people have the typical intestinal damage of celiac disease but never develop symptoms.

What are some possible complications of celiac disease?

- Slow weight gain and growth; height may be lower than normal. In older children, onset of puberty may be delayed.

- Anemia: low levels of hemoglobin, which lets blood cells carry oxygen.

- "Celiac crisis": sudden severe diarrhea, weight loss, and other symptoms.

- Other problems may occur in adulthood, including weak bones and increased risk of certain types of cancer. Following a gluten-free diet lowers the risk of these complications.

What puts your child at risk for celiac disease?

- Celiac disease appears to be most common in people of Northern European descent. However, it does occur in other races and ethnic groups.

- Genetic factors affect the risk of developing celiac disease. If you or others in your family have celiac disease, your child may be at increased risk.

- The risk of developing gluten intolerance and celiac disease is higher in children with certain other diseases, including diabetes, rheumatoid arthritis, thyroid disease, Addison's disease, and Down's syndrome.

Can celiac disease be prevented?

- Since it is genetically determined, there is no practical way to prevent celiac disease.

How is it diagnosed and treated?

- Special tests may be needed to make the diagnosis of celiac disease, including measurement of specific antibodies. A referral to a gastroenterologist (a specialist in diseases of the intestine) is often made.

- To be certain of the diagnosis, the doctor may recommend a procedure called endoscopy. A special instrument like a telescope is used to examine the inside of your child's intestine and to take a sample of tissue (called a biopsy).

- There is no cure for celiac disease. The main treatment is a *gluten-free diet*. You must carefully eliminate all bread and cereal grains from your child's diet, including wheat, rye, and barley.

- *Foods to avoid* include breads, cakes, cookies, and other baked goods. Also, many types of processed foods include thickeners and other grain products. Parents of children with celiac disease must become experts in reading labels to determine which products contain gluten.

- *Foods that are allowed* include any food that doesn't contain gluten, such as fruits and vegetables (including potatoes, beans, and corn), meats, dairy products, and rice. Some cereals are made without wheat, and special gluten-free products are increasingly available.

- Most children with celiac disease do fine on a gluten-free diet. Diarrhea and other symptoms may start to improve within a week or so. If your child has been very ill, improvement may take a little longer.

- Your doctor may recommend iron and vitamin supplements. Additional medications, such as pancreatic enzymes,may be used as well.

- Some children have trouble following a gluten-free diet. This is a special problem in the teen years, when children are more independent and want to eat the foods their friends enjoy (for example, pizza). You may need to remind your child that gluten intolerance is a lifelong problem, even when he or she isn't having any symptoms. Staying on the diet not only reduces your child's risk of complications but will also help him or her look and feel better.

When should I call your office?

Call our office if:

- You need help developing a gluten-free diet for your child.

- Your child has continued diarrhea and other symptoms, despite a gluten-free diet.

If your child has symptoms of celiac crisis (severe diarrhea, rapid weight loss), call our office immediately. This is a potential emergency, requiring immediate treatment.

Colic

Newborns with colic have long-lasting periods of crying and fussing. The cause of colic is unknown; several factors probably contribute. Babies usually outgrow colic by 3 months of age. In the meantime, we can recommend a few simple measures that may be helpful.

What is colic?

Colic is prolonged periods of crying for no apparent reason in an otherwise normal, healthy newborn. Doctors most often define colic as crying for 3 or more hours per day, at least 3 days per week, for at least 3 weeks. Whether or not your baby fits this definition, you may need advice on how to deal with his or her crying.

Doctors don't know exactly what causes colic or why it's a problem for certain babies. A number of factors are probably involved. Taking steps to ensure proper burping and to reduce stress and overstimulation may help to reduce crying. Nearly all infants "outgrow" colic by age 3 to 4 months.

What does it look like?

- Periods of crying and fussing that last a long time. Compared with "usual" infant behavior, the crying is louder and more intense, and the baby is more difficult to comfort.

- Crying usually occurs around the same time each day—often in the evening.

- Your baby's face may be red and flushed or sometimes pale around the lips.

- Your baby's belly may seem swollen and tense. He or she may pull the legs up over the belly.

- It may seem like nothing you can do helps stop the crying. Your baby may simply continue crying until he or she falls asleep from exhaustion. Sometimes, the crying finally stops when your baby passes gas or has a bowel movement.

What causes colic?

- Several factors are probably involved, but no clear cause has been identified. Colic does not *necessarily* mean that your baby is having abdominal pain. In some cases, colic seems to be related to a combination of the baby's temperament and the parents' responses.

- For a small number of infants, colic may be related to formula intolerance, swallowing excess air, or gastroesophageal reflux disease (GERD).

What are some possible complications of colic?

- None. Colic attacks rarely continue past 3 or 4 months of age.

- Obviously, having a screaming baby can be very stressful for parents.

What puts your child at risk of colic?

- Colic usually occurs only in infants between birth and 3 months old.

- There is no way to predict which babies will develop colic. Being overstressed or overtired seems to contribute to the symptoms.

How is colic treated?

- The first step is to understand the nature of the problem. In many cases, colic seems to reflect the baby's temperament and the parents' responses. Healthy babies cry for lots of reasons; crying doesn't necessarily mean that they are in pain.

- Improve feeding techniques:

  - Make sure to burp your baby after each feeding; hold him or her upright until you hear air coming out of the stomach. Patting the baby gently on the back may help.

  - Feed your baby in a quiet, calm environment. Feed around the same time every night.

  - Avoid overstimulation, especially around feeding time. Try soothing techniques, such as rocking or quiet music.

- Try not to get too upset yourself! High stress and emotion in the parents sometimes seem to contribute to colic attacks. It's difficult, but try to keep your emotions under control. If you really need a break, there's no harm in leaving your baby in his or her crib for a few minutes or with another caretaker.

- If the crying doesn't get better, your doctor may recommend a change in formula. (A small percentage of babies with formula intolerance may have symptoms similar to those of colic.) Remember that the condition is not serious. Babies almost always outgrow it by age 3 months.

- During colic attacks, try different techniques to see what works best for your baby. For example, try holding him or her upright. You may also try placing the baby on his or her belly across your lap, or on a hot-water bottle or heating pad. *Make sure the heating pad is warm, not hot!*

- Gas-reducing drugs (for example, simethicone) or other medications may not help, but your doctor may recommend trying them. Other medications or herbs may be tried as well. However, these are often avoided because of the risk of side effects.

When should I call your office?

Call our office if:

- Colic attacks are very severe or last a very long time.

- Crying is accompanied by other symptoms, such as vomiting, diarrhea, swollen or tender abdomen, or fever.

- Your baby continues having colic attacks after age 3 to 4 months.

Constipation

There are a number of possible causes of constipation in infants and children. Whatever the cause, once it has started, constipation can be a continuing problem. Your doctor can evaluate your child to be sure there is no medical reason for constipation and can recommend the most appropriate treatment.

What is constipation?

Constipation is difficult, uncomfortable, or infrequent bowel movements (BMs). Having BMs less than once daily can be perfectly normal, as long as they aren't too hard and aren't causing any discomfort. However, constipation is present if BMs are hard, difficult or painful to pass, or very infrequent.

Although there are many possible causes of constipation, it does not usually result from any medical condition. Making some simple changes in your child's diet (for example, more water, more fiber) can help a lot. The main risk is that constipation will become a continuing problem. Occasionally constipation signals a medical problem in need of treatment.

What does it look like?

- Infrequent, hard BMs that are difficult or uncomfortable to pass. Younger children especially may try to hold back and avoid having BMs as long as possible, which will make the problem worse.

- Straining or pain when having BMs. Sometimes bleeding occurs; you may see blood on the outside of the stool or on the toilet paper.

- Your child may have pain and/or swelling of the abdomen. Even after having a BM, your child may still feel like he or she has to go to the bathroom.

- Leakage of watery stool from the rectum. This is called *encopresis*. Although it may look like diarrhea, it is actually caused by stool leaking around the hard BM. This activity is not voluntary; your child is probably not even aware when it is happening.

What causes constipation?

- Most children with constipation have "functional constipation." This means that there is no medical reason for the constipation. It often begins with a painful BM or a stressful situation when having a BM. It may also be related to diet, especially not drinking enough liquids or not eating enough high-fiber foods.

- Other causes are possible:

- Medications: for example, some drugs used for mental health disorders or pain.

- Certain medical conditions, such as hypothyroidism (low thyroid hormone activity).

- Spinal nerve problems.

- Hirschsprung's disease (absence of normal nerves in the large intestine).

What are some possible complications of constipation?

- The main complication is that constipation will become an ongoing or chronic problem. If passing BMs is difficult or uncomfortable, your child may try to avoid them. This can make the problem worse.

- Other possible problems include:

- Chronic abdominal pain ("stomach aches"), often accompanied by reduced appetite.

- Hemorrhoids (painful outpouches of veins in and around the anal region), although these are very uncommon in a child.

- *Encopresis.* Uncontrolled soiling. Your child soils his or her underwear without even knowing it's happening. This occurs because the rectum has become so dilated (swollen) that your child cannot even sense when watery stool is leaking around harder BM.

What puts your child at risk of constipation?

Some factors increase the risk of functional constipation:

- Stressful experiences or pain while having BMs.

- Not enough liquids or fiber in the diet.

- High stress.

- Various medical causes and diseases (such as hypothyroidism or Hirschsprung's disease).

- Certain congenital conditions (such as Down's syndrome or cystic fibrosis).

Can constipation be prevented?

- Don't make toilet training a stressful situation. If you have questions about your approach to toilet training, ask your doctor.

- Make sure your child gets a balanced, high-fiber diet, including lots of fresh fruits and vegetables and whole grains. It's also important for your child to drink enough water and other fluids.

How is constipation treated?

Correcting bowel habits.

- Most of the time, constipation in children is related to problems with bathroom habits, problems with diet, or both.

- To start correcting bowel habits, have your child sit on the toilet for 5 minutes after meals and after coming home from school. Keep track of how often BMs occur; this will help in determining how often and when your child needs to move his or her bowels.

- If constipation has been present for a while, fecal (BM) material may become impacted (stuck) in your child's rectum. The doctor may recommend or perform an enema (placing water through a tube in your child's rectum) to dislodge the stool.

Medications.

- Your doctor may recommend laxatives to relieve constipation.

- There are different kinds of laxatives. Some work by softening the stool, while others work by stimulating the bowel to produce BMs.

- In infants less than 1 year old, corn syrup (Karo syrup) may be mixed with formula. Try 1 teaspoon of corn syrup mixed in one or two bottles of formula per day; more may be needed. Other medications are available.

- For older infants and children, there are many options, including:
  - Mineral oil (usually mixed with milk).
  - Milk of Magnesia.
  - Metamucil.

- Your doctor may recommend a different medication, possibly a prescription drug.

- The goal of treatment with laxatives is to adjust the dose until the stools are soft, without producing diarrhea. Keep your child using laxatives for at least a few months, until healthy bowel habits are established and your child no longer worries about pain during BMs.

Diet changes.

- Your doctor may recommend some changes in your child's diet. If your child has only mild constipation, diet changes alone may be helpful.

  - Increase the amount of fiber in your child's diet. Feed your child lots of fresh fruits and vegetables and whole-grain breads and cereals; avoid white bread and processed foods. Large amounts of milk and cheese may contribute to constipation.

  - Make sure your child gets plenty of water and other liquids.

Constipation is usually the only abnormality present. It often clears up with a change in bathroom habits and diet changes. Sometimes, however, it can be a symptom of other medical problems. This is most likely if constipation occurs with other symptoms, such as weight loss or slow growth. If your child has other symptoms in addition to constipation, be sure to let the doctor know about them.

ⓘ When should I call your office?

Call our office if:

- Your child continues to have difficult, infrequent BMs, despite recommended treatment.

- Your child has other symptoms, such as weight loss or slow growth.

Gastroesophageal Reflux Disease

Gastroesophageal reflux occurs when the contents of the stomach, including stomach acid, move upward ("reflux") into the esophagus (swallowing tube). In infants, reflux is a fairly common problem ("spitting up") that usually clears up with time. Gastroesophageal reflux becomes a disease (GERD) when it occurs enough to cause heartburn, respiratory symptoms, and other problems. Over time, GERD can cause damage to the esophagus and other complications.

What is gastroesophageal reflux disease?

Gastroesophageal reflux disease (GERD) occurs when the stomach contents, including stomach acid, regularly move backward: up from the stomach and into the esophagus. The stomach has a special lining that normally protects it from the harmful effects of acid. The esophagus does not; therefore, when acid gets into the esophagus it can cause irritation, pain, and tissue damage. GERD can also cause respiratory (breathing-related) problems, including making asthma worse.

Treatment includes avoiding certain foods and taking medications to reduce stomach acid. Surgery is rarely needed. In infants, some reflux ("spitting up") is normal. However, treatment is needed if your baby is having reflux that is causing other symptoms or interfering with gaining weight.

What does it look like?

- In babies, you may see milk or formula coming out of the mouths. Older children may complain of a sour taste in their mouths.

- Infants with GERD may be fussy. Your baby may cry, arch his or her back, or refuse feedings. He or she may vomit frequently and gain weight slowly.

- Young children may complain of stomachaches. Older children and teens may have typical "heartburn."

- Symptoms occur commonly after meals. In older kids and teens, symptoms may get better after taking antacids (for example, Tums).

- If GERD becomes severe, it may cause problems with eating and swallowing.

- If stomach acid gets into the throat and airway, it may lead to other symptoms, including:

- In infants: gagging, choking, episodes of apnea (temporary interruption of breathing).

- Hoarse, scratchy voice.

- Coughing, throat-clearing.

- If your child has asthma, GERD may make it worse.

What are some possible complications of GERD?

- GERD can cause feeding problems and slow weight gain in infants (although this is uncommon).

- Frequent reflux of stomach acid can cause damage to the teeth (erosion).

- GERD may cause or contribute to breathing-related symptoms, including laryngitis (hoarseness); throat, sinus, and ear infections; and sleep apnea (temporary interruptions of breathing during sleep).

- GERD seems to be common in children with asthma and may even worsen asthma. GERD in children with asthma or other respiratory diseases may require long-term treatment.

- Other long-term complications are possible, but rare in children:

  - Acid can damage the lower esophagus, causing scarring and narrowing (strictures).

  - If GERD continues into adulthood, it may increase the risk of cancer of the esophagus.

What puts your child at risk of GERD?

- GERD is a common and increasingly recognized condition. It may run in families.

- In teens (and adults), being obese, overeating, and using alcohol and tobacco may all contribute to GERD.

How is GERD diagnosed?

- It can be difficult to recognize GERD, especially in infants and younger children. Older children and teens are more likely to have the typical pattern of heartburn after eating.

- If the doctor suspects your child has GERD, he or she may recommend tests, such as:

- *X-rays.* An "upper GI series," using a material called barium that shows up on x-rays. This test can show any abnormalities of the stomach and esophagus.

- *pH Probe.* A tube may be placed into the esophagus to test for stomach acid.

- *Endoscopy.* A flexible instrument like a telescope is used to examine the esophagus and stomach directly.

- At other times, the doctor will simply recommend trying acid-reducing drugs. If the medications reduce your child's heartburn or other symptoms, then GERD is probably present.

How is GERD treated?

Medications are the main treatment for GERD:

- Several types of acid-reducing drugs are available. Examples include Tagamet (generic name: cimetidine) and Prilosec (generic name: omeprazole). These medications work by reducing acid production by the stomach.

- Antacid drugs (for example, Tums) can reduce heartburn symptoms. However, they have to be given very frequently and may cause side effects.

- Drug treatment may have to continue for a while, especially if your child is having asthma or other airway-related symptoms. If heartburn or other symptoms improve, the doctor may try stopping medication for a while to see if the problem has cleared up.

Other treatments:

- For infants:

  - For some infants with GERD, the doctor may recommend thickening the formula.

- Elevating the head of the bed does not appear to help much in infants. Feeding the baby in a seated position (for example, in a car seat) is also not helpful and may actually increase reflux.

- Laying the baby on his or her stomach to sleep may help reflux but is not recommended because of the risk of sudden infant death syndrome (SIDS).

- For older children and teens:

  - Avoid giving your child acid-producing foods, such as caffeine and chocolate. Teens with GERD should avoid alcohol and smoking.

  - Since many reflux episodes occur at night, it may help to raise the head of your child's bed. Place the legs of the bed on 6-inch wood blocks.

- We may recommend a visit to a doctor specializing in stomach and intestinal diseases (a gastroenterologist) if the diagnosis is uncertain, if treatment doesn't help, or if your child has complications related to GERD.

When should I call your office?

Call our office if symptoms of GERD continue or return, especially if your child has:

- Frequent vomiting: in infants, vomiting with weight loss, slow growth, or fussiness.

- Heartburn, chest pain, or stomach pain.

- Painful swallowing or difficulty swallowing.

- Choking, gagging, or apnea (temporary interruptions of breathing during sleep).

Inflammatory Bowel Disease

> Inflammatory bowel disease is chronic inflammation of the intestines, causing attacks of symptoms such as diarrhea, abdominal pain, and cramping. The two main types of inflammatory bowel disease are Crohn's disease and ulcerative colitis. The exact cause is unknown. Inflammatory bowel disease is not curable, but helpful treatments are available.

What is inflammatory bowel disease?

Inflammatory bowel disease (IBD) is a group of digestive diseases causing inflammation (irritation, tenderness) of the intestinal system. These diseases are fairly common in children, most often in teens, but they can occur at younger ages. IBD causes unpredictable attacks of disease, with symptoms including diarrhea, abdominal pain and cramping, and bleeding from the intestines.

The two main types of IBD are:

- *Ulcerative colitis.* Inflammation is found only in the lowest parts of the intestinal tract: the colon (large intestine) and rectum. The main symptoms are bloody bowel movements and diarrhea. Symptoms may continue for a prolonged period or may come and go in unpredictable attacks.

- *Crohn's disease.* Sometimes called "regional enteritis," Crohn's disease is inflammation anywhere in the intestinal tract, including the large and small intestines and the anus. The exact symptoms depend on where the inflammation is found.

Symptoms unrelated to the digestive system may occur, including fever, slow growth, and arthritis. These are more common with Crohn's disease but may also occur in ulcerative colitis. Unfortunately, there is no cure for IBD. However, treatments are available to reduce symptoms, prevent complications, and reduce the number of attacks.

What does it look like?

Symptoms of inflammatory bowel disease vary. They most commonly begin after age 15 but can occur in younger children. Common symptoms and problems include:

Ulcerative colitis:

- Blood in bowel movements.
- Diarrhea, but some patients have constipation instead.
- Feeling like you have to have a bowel movement very frequently or urgently.

- Symptoms may develop gradually or suddenly.
- Symptoms last a long time without improving, often more than 2 weeks.
- Weight loss or slow growth.
- Arthritis, although this is more common in Crohn's disease.

Crohn's disease:

- Symptoms depend on what parts of the intestinal system are involved.
- Patient may have bloody diarrhea, as in ulcerative colitis.
- Stomach pains and cramping.
- Symptoms outside the intestinal system are more common, including fever, tiredness, "feeling sick."
  - Slow growth may be the first sign.
  - Ulcers (open sores) in the mouth.
  - Arthritis (swollen, painful joints).
  - Kidney stones/gallbladder stones.
- Other symptoms are possible.

What causes IBD?

- The causes of IBD are unclear. Both genetic and environmental factors are probably involved. Abnormal immune system responses lead to inflammation in the intestinal system.
- IBD is *not* caused by emotional stress. However, stress does seem to affect how often attacks of IBD symptoms occur.

What are some possible complications of IBD?

There are many possible complications of IBD. Getting regular medical care and following a healthy lifestyle can reduce your child's risk of complications.

- Constant inflammation and irritation can lead to complications affecting the intestines:
  - People with IBD, especially ulcerative colitis, are at increased long-term risk of colon cancer. This risk doesn't develop until the disease has been present for many years.
  - People with Crohn's disease are at risk for strictures (scarring, narrowing), fissures (open sores), or fistulas (abnormal connections between the intestines and other structures, such as the skin, anus, or vagina). These complications may require additional treatment or surgery.

- Other problems outside the intestines may occur, including anemia, vitamin deficiencies, weight loss/growth problems, and many others. These problems are sometimes the initial symptoms of IBD, or they may develop later.

- In adulthood, other complications may develop, including arthritis, bone loss, eye problems, and kidney and liver disease.

What puts your child at risk of IBD?

- If you or someone else in your family has IBD, your child may be at higher risk.

- In the United States, the risk is higher for whites and African Americans, lower for Hispanics and Asians.

- Ulcerative colitis is slightly more common in males; Crohn's disease is slightly more common in females.

Can IBD be prevented?

- There is no known way to prevent IBD.

- Good treatment, including medical follow-up and diet changes, can reduce the risk of complications.

How is IBD treated?

- Unfortunately, there is no cure for IBD. Effective treatments can improve symptoms, reduce the number of attacks, and reduce the risk of complications.

- We will recommend a visit to a specialist in stomach and intestinal diseases (a gastroenterologist). This specialist has the expertise to diagnose your child's IBD and recommend the most effective treatments.

- *Diagnosis.* Various tests may be needed, including tests to determine whether your child has ulcerative colitis, Crohn's disease, or some other intestinal problem. Tests may include blood tests, endoscopy (using a special instrument like a telescope to examine the inside of the intestinal system), and x-rays.

- *Medications* are an important part of treatment for IBD. The drugs and doses chosen depend on how ill your child is. Common medications include:

  - Sulfasalazine. A drug that can reduce inflammation of the colon (large intestine). It may also help to prevent repeat attacks. However, aspirin allergy can cause problems for patients using this drug.

  - Steroids. Steroid drugs such as prednisone are very effective in reducing inflammation. They have various side effects, including interference with growth, the development of cataracts, and others. Your doctor will try to keep your child's steroid dose as low as possible.

  - Immunosuppressant drugs (for example, azathioprine) may be helpful. These medications help the person's own immune system from doing damage.

  - Antibiotics seem helpful in some people with IBD. They may work by killing bacteria in the intestines that contribute to inflammation.

- *Surgery* is avoided if possible. However, it is sometimes needed if IBD has caused irreparable damage to part of the intestine.

- *Diet.* Because IBD can interfere with absorption by the intestines, it's important to make sure your child gets adequate nutrition.

- *Emotional support* can help your child and family live with IBD. Visits with a social worker or family counselor or participating in an IBD support group can be helpful.

When should I call your office?

Call your gastroenterologist or our office if any of the following occurs:

- Fever.
- Severe abdominal pain.
- Vomiting.
- Blood in bowel movements.

Inguinal Hernia

Inguinal hernia occurs when a part of the intestine slips through an opening in the muscle separating the abdomen from the groin (genital area). The intestine feels like a lump or bump. The lump may be felt in the scrotum in boys or the vaginal area in girls. Inguinal hernias are more common in premature infants, especially boys. Prompt surgery is needed to repair the hernia and prevent complications.

What is an inguinal hernia?

Inguinal hernia is a relatively common problem in infants. Part of the intestine slips though the abdominal muscle wall, causing a noticeable lump. In girls, the hernia may include one of the ovaries. The lump may be noticeable only some of the time, such as when your child cries or coughs.

Hernias are usually not emergency situations, but surgery is needed to prevent complications. The operation is a simple one, with quick recovery and no further problems.

What does it look like?

- A bulge or lump in the groin area. The bulge may be located anywhere in the area between the legs, including inside the scrotum (the sac containing the testicles) in boys or around the vagina in girls.

- The bulge may be most noticeable when your child cries, coughs, or strains when passing a bowel movement.

- When your child relaxes, the bulge may disappear. Sometimes it disappears if you push it gently upward.

- The hernia is often present within the first 6 months of life but may not be noticed until later on.

- Some serious complications can develop and may be present when the hernia is first noticed:

  - The bulge may appear suddenly, causing pain and crying, sometimes accompanied by a bulging belly and vomiting. This may mean that the hernia has become trapped ("incarcerated") or choked ("strangulated").

  - An incarcerated hernia can no longer move back into its normal position. Unlike in adults, this problem can develop quickly in children.

  - In a "strangulated" hernia, the blood supply to the hernia may be reduced or cut off completely. The lump becomes more swollen and tender. Your child may vomit, and the intestine may become obstructed (blocked). Immediate surgery is needed to prevent permanent damage to the trapped portion of intestine. If this happens, there is also a risk of serious infection.

What causes an inguinal hernia?

- Most inguinal hernias in children are present at birth. They occur when a small opening between the abdomen and groin fails to close normally during prenatal development. The herniated intestine slips through this opening.

- Other causes are possible, including muscle strains that allow part of the intestine to slip through. However, this is rare in children.

What are some possible complications of an inguinal hernia?

- The main complications are incarceration and strangulation: the herniated portion of the intestine may become trapped in its abnormal position and its blood supply may be cut off. A strangulated hernia is a medical emergency.

- An incarcerated hernia may cause further damage to surrounding structures, especially the reproductive organs.

What puts your child at risk of inguinal hernia?

- Premature infants are at highest risk, especially very premature infants. However, up to 5% of full-term infants have congenital inguinal hernias.

- Inguinal hernias are much more common in boys than in girls.

- If you or someone else in your family has had an inguinal hernia, your child may be at increased risk.

- Inguinal hernias are more common in infants with specific birth defects or diseases, including:

  - Other congenital problems of the urinary/reproductive organs.

  - Any condition with abnormal fluid or pressure within the abdomen.

  - Chronic lung diseases.

  - Connective tissue diseases (such as Marfan's syndrome).

How is an inguinal hernia treated?

- *Surgery* is almost always needed for children with inguinal hernias. The hernia does not get better on its own. The goals of surgery are to move the herniated intestine back into its normal position and to close the abnormal opening that allowed the hernia to occur.

- Surgery should be done as soon as possible to reduce the risks of incarcerated or strangulated hernia. Performing surgery before the hernia becomes incarcerated greatly lowers the risk of complications.

- If the hernia is incarcerated (trapped), the doctor may gently try to move it back into normal position before surgery. This may allow the operation to be delayed for a few days.

- If the hernia is strangulated (blood supply is cut off), surgery is needed.

- Hernia repair is one of the most common operations performed in children. It is fast and safe, with a low complication rate. Most children can go home the same day. Others may stay in the hospital overnight (especially premature infants).

- During the operation, the surgeon will check to make sure that the hernia hasn't caused any damage to the reproductive organs, including the testicles in boys and the ovaries and uterus in girls. If any other abnormalities are present, they can usually be repaired during the same operation.

- Children usually recover very quickly after hernia operations. Follow the surgeon's instructions for activity permitted and pain medication.

When should I call your office?

The surgeon will probably want to recheck your child within a few weeks. In the meantime, call the surgeon's office or our office if your child develops pain or swelling in the groin area.

If your child develops symptoms of acute illness—such as severe pain, fever, vomiting, bulging belly, or bloody bowel movements—get medical help immediately.

Intestinal Obstruction

There are many possible causes of intestinal obstruction (or blockage) in children. The intestine becomes blocked off, partially or completely, interfering with normal bowel movements. Intestinal obstruction is sometimes present at birth. In other cases, it develops later as a result of illness, injury, or a malformation of the intestines. Prompt treatment is needed to restore the function of the intestines and prevent complications.

What is intestinal obstruction?

Intestinal obstruction is blockage somewhere along the intestinal tract (small or large intestine). Infants may be born with intestinal obstruction. This can result from malformations (abnormal development) of the intestines or from conditions that interfere with the intestine's normal emptying ability.

The intestines may be blocked completely or partially. Partial obstructions may be less easily recognized. Intestinal obstruction requires prompt treatment to prevent complications, including permanent damage to the intestines. If the blockage cannot be removed in any other way, surgery must be performed as soon as possible.

What does it look like?

The symptoms of intestinal obstruction vary a lot, depending on the cause. Some symptoms are present at birth or shortly afterwards, whereas others develop later on. Some of the main symptoms are:

- Vomiting, especially of yellowish-green material (bile).
- Episodes of sudden, intense crying caused by abdominal cramps. Vomiting is common but may not be the first symptom (for example, intussusception).
- Belly sticking out (distended abdomen).
- Lack of the normal first bowel movement (meconium) after birth. In some conditions, the meconium stool passes, but normal bowel movements don't start after that (for example, Hirschsprung's disease).

Intestinal obstruction can lead to serious complications, including infections and shock. For some causes of intestinal obstruction, or if serious damage to part of the intestine (gangrene) has occurred, surgery must be performed as soon as possible.

What causes intestinal obstruction?

There are many possible causes:

- *In newborns and infants,* blockage may result from:
  - Various malformations of the intestines, which means the intestines didn't develop normally.
    - Atresia (lack of normal intestinal passages).
    - Stenosis (narrowing of the intestines).
    - Malrotation (twisting of part of the intestines).
    - Intussusception (part of the intestine gets stuck in another part).
  - Hirschsprung's disease (lack of normal nerve cells in the large intestine).
  - Blockage of the intestines with meconium (which babies normally pass as their first bowel movement after birth). This occurs mainly in infants who have the genetic disease cystic fibrosis.
- *In older infants and children*, blockage may be caused by:
  - Hernias (part of the intestine slipping through a hole in the muscle wall).
  - Foreign bodies: objects that children swallow may block the intestines.
  - Adhesions: scars after surgery that narrow or block the intestines.
  - Paralytic ileus: lack of normal intestinal function after surgery or injury.

What are some possible complications of intestinal obstruction?

Intestinal obstruction can lead to serious complications, including infections, perforations (holes in the intestine), or death of the involved part of the intestine (gangrene). Prompt treatment is needed to relieve the blockage and prevent these complications.

What puts your child at risk of intestinal obstruction?

Risk factors depend on the cause of the obstruction:

- Many types of intestinal malformations are more common in infants with other birth defects or genetic diseases.
- Any type of abdominal surgery increases the risk of adhesions.

How is intestinal obstruction treated?

- Intestinal obstruction must be treated as soon as possible to restore normal intestinal function and reduce the risk of complications.

- If your child has symptoms of obstruction, seek medical care immediately.
- Treatment depends on the cause; surgery may be needed (for example, if your child has an inguinal hernia or a malformation of the intestines).

When should I call your office?

If your child has been treated for intestinal obstruction, call our office if similar symptoms occur again (for example, vomiting of bile, swollen abdomen, lack of bowel movements, abdominal cramps).

Irritable Bowel Syndrome

All children and teens have occasional stomach-aches, diarrhea, or constipation. If these symptoms occur regularly and start to interfere with your child's life, the doctor may make a diagnosis of irritable bowel syndrome. This is a "functional" disorder, which means it has no recognizable cause and no lasting health effects. Although there is no cure for irritable bowel syndrome, treatment can help to reduce symptoms.

What is irritable bowel syndrome?

Irritable bowel syndrome (IBS) is a common chronic disease causing abdominal pain, gassiness and bloating, and constipation or diarrhea. It may also be called "spastic colon."

IBS is a "functional" disorder. This means that the symptoms result from some change in the way the stomach and intestines work rather than any specific physical problem. Your doctor usually will diagnose IBS after examination and tests to make sure there is no other, more serious cause of his or her symptoms.

IBS can be difficult to live with, and there is no specific cure. However, it causes no permanent damage. Symptoms may improve with simple treatments, such as avoiding certain foods and using medications when needed. Although stress doesn't cause IBS, managing stress can help to reduce symptoms.

What does it look like?

- Stomach pain, especially cramps. Pain happens frequently, not just occasionally.

- Bloating.

- Diarrhea or constipation may happen at different times. Abdominal pain may seem to get better after a bowel movement.

- Abdominal pain and constipation/diarrhea interfere with normal activities. Your child may start missing school or social activities or avoid going to places where no bathroom is available.

- The usual symptoms of "stomach flu" are absent, such as fever, vomiting, and dehydration.

- Your child may be anxious or worried, especially if abdominal symptoms have been present for some time. Usually, symptoms must be present for 3 months or longer before the diagnosis of IBS is made.

What are some possible complications of irritable bowel syndrome?

- There are no physical complications.

- Effective treatment can reduce the impact of IBS on your child's school and social life.

What puts your child at risk of IBS?

- Little is known about the risk factors for functional disorders such as IBS. If you or other members of your family have similar bowel problems, your child may be at higher risk.

- Girls and boys are at similar risk. (In adults, IBS is more common in females.)

- Although stress doesn't cause IBS, high stress levels may contribute to symptom flare-ups. Children with IBS have increased rates of anxiety and depression.

Can IBS be prevented?

- There is no practical way to prevent IBS.

- Good treatment, including diet changes and stress reduction, may lessen the impact of IBS on your child's life.

How is IBS treated?

Proper diagnosis is an important first step in recognizing and treating IBS. After initial examination, your doctor may recommend a visit to a specialist in stomach and intestinal disorders (a gastroenterologist) for further evaluation and treatment. Many children with IBS (and their parents) are relieved to find out they do not have a serious physical problem.

There is no specific test for IBS. The diagnosis is based on your child's symptoms and how frequently and regularly they occur.

There is also no specific cure for IBS, but various treatments may be helpful:

- Some simple *diet changes* may help to control IBS symptoms:

  - If there are foods that seem to make your child's symptoms worse, avoid them. Keeping a food diary may help to identify the foods that cause problems.

  - Make sure your child gets plenty of fiber, including fresh fruits and vegetables and whole-grain breads, and plenty of liquids. This helps to avoid both constipation and diarrhea. Your doctor may recommend a fiber supplement, such as Metamucil.

- It may help your child to eat frequent, smaller meals.

- *Stress reduction* can help in living with the symptoms of IBS. Lower stress levels can also help to reduce the frequency and severity of symptoms:

  - Try not to let the symptoms interfere much with your child's life. Simply knowing that the symptoms aren't caused by a serious disease may help to reduce stress.

  - Encourage your child to resume regular school and social activities.

  - Encourage your child to engage in regular exercise and relaxation techniques.

- *Medications* may be helpful but generally should be used only for short periods. Your doctor may recommend certain medications, including:

  - Antispasmodics (drugs to reduce stomach cramps).

  - Medications for diarrhea.

  - Laxatives, especially bulk laxatives that work by adding extra fiber (such as Metamucil). Avoid stimulant laxatives.

  - Antidepressants.

- *Dealing with chronic pain.* Techniques may include relaxation therapy, biofeedback, evaluation by a pain medicine specialist.

- Treatment for anxiety or depression, if present.

- *Medical follow-up* is an important part of treatment for IBS. Your doctor will likely recommend regular visits to check for improvement or any other change in your child's condition.

It sometimes takes a while to determine the best combination of treatments for a patient with IBS. The goal is to minimize your child's symptoms and their impact on his or her life as much as possible.

When should I call your office?

During treatment for IBS, call our office if there is any sudden or significant change in your child's symptoms, especially:

- Black, tarry-looking bowel movements.

- Vomiting.

- Weight loss.

Pancreatitis

Pancreatitis has many possible causes, including injuries, infections, and other diseases. Acute pancreatitis causes abdominal pain, vomiting, and fever. Children with pancreatitis can become very ill quite rapidly and often need hospital treatment. As long as no other serious illness or injury is present, most children with pancreatitis recover in a few days.

What is pancreatitis?

The pancreas is a small organ, located behind the stomach, with several important functions. It makes digestive juices and the hormone insulin, which allows the body to use sugar (glucose) for energy.

When the pancreas becomes infected or inflamed for any reason, the disease is called pancreatitis. Pancreatitis has many causes, any of which can make your child very ill. When pancreatitis occurs in children, it is usually "acute"; this means that the problem develops suddenly.

Many children with acute pancreatitis need hospital treatment to relieve pain and avoid dehydration. Most recover completely. Chronic pancreatitis, with repeated episodes of inflammation, is uncommon in children.

What does it look like?

- Abdominal pain, which can become quite severe within a short time. Back pain may also be present. Pain may be so severe that your child doesn't want to move or be touched.

- Vomiting, which may be frequent or constant.

- Fever.

- Bulging or distended belly.

- Symptoms of dehydration (dry mouth, little or no urine produced, crying without tears) caused by vomiting and lack of fluids.

- In severe cases, shock, severe abdominal pain, and jaundice (yellow color of the skin).

If your child has any of these symptoms, get medical care as soon as possible.

What causes pancreatitis?

There are many possible causes, including:

- Infections, usually caused by viruses. Common viral causes include coxsackievirus and influenza A virus.

- Injury, especially a hard blow to the abdomen (for example, from a car crash or child abuse).

- Stones or other causes of blockage in the pancreas.

- Certain genetic diseases (including cystic fibrosis).

- Drugs and toxic substances, including alcohol, acetaminophen, and many others.

- Pancreatitis can occur as a complication of other diseases, such as diabetes or kidney disease.

What are some possible complications of pancreatitis?

- Dehydration, caused by severe vomiting and lack of fluids.

- Most other complications are related to the severity of the illness or injury causing pancreatitis.

- Rarely, pancreatitis in children becomes severe, causing potentially life-threatening complications such as bleeding or major infection.

- Chronic pancreatitis: repeated episodes of pancreatitis (uncommon in children).

Can pancreatitis be prevented?

- Most causes of pancreatitis in children cannot be prevented.

- Preventing certain injuries, especially by having your child always wear a seatbelt, would prevent many cases of pancreatitis caused by trauma.

How is pancreatitis treated?

- Children with acute pancreatitis can become very ill. They usually need to go to the hospital for tests and treatment.

- Tests include measuring levels of certain enzymes made by the pancreas. X-rays and other imaging studies (ultrasound or computed tomographic [CT] scan) may be performed.

- In the hospital, your child will receive:

  - Medications to control pain.

  - Fluids given through a vein (intravenous [IV]) to treat and prevent dehydration.

  - In severe cases, antibiotics may be given to reduce the risk of infection.

  - Your child may receive specific treatments to address the cause of his or her pancreatitis. For example, if the bile duct in the pancreas has become blocked, a procedure can be performed to unblock it. If your child has suffered blunt trauma, for example, in an automobile accident, treatment for other injuries may be needed.

- Acute pancreatitis usually gets better within 2 to 5 days. Once vomiting has stopped, your child can gradually begin drinking liquids and eating solid foods again. As soon as your child has returned to a normal diet, he or she can continue to recover at home.

- Although it rarely occurs in children, severe pancreatitis can result in shock, which means not enough blood and oxygen are getting to the important organs of the body. Your child's doctors and nurses will monitor his or her condition carefully.

- After recovery, your child will receive follow-up care to detect possible complications. Repeated attacks of pancreatitis (chronic pancreatitis) are possible. However, this is uncommon unless there is some abnormality of the pancreas or other condition such as very high lipid levels (cholesterol and other fats in the blood).

When should I call your office?

While your child is recovering from acute pancreatitis, call our office if any of the following occurs:

- Abdominal pain.

- Vomiting.

- Not eating or drinking.

Peptic Ulcer Disease

> Ulcers of the stomach or duodenum (the upper part of the small intestine) are uncommon in children. They are most often related to major injuries, certain medical conditions, or the use of certain medications. In otherwise healthy children, most ulcers occur when the stomach is infected with a certain type of bacteria. Treatment depends on the cause. Ulcers generally heal after treatment with acid-reducing drugs and other medications.

What is peptic ulcer?

A peptic ulcer is a deep sore that forms in the stomach (gastric ulcer) or the upper part of the small intestine (duodenal ulcer). In children, ulcers are most often a complication of a severe illness or injury, or medications. Ulcers occurring in otherwise healthy children are usually caused by a stomach infection with bacteria called *Helicobacter pylori*. However, this infection is much more common in adults.

Treatment depends on the cause of the ulcer. After a major injury, your child may receive acid-reducers or other drugs to prevent or treat ulcers. If infection with *Helicobacter pylori* is the cause, antibiotics and acid-reducing drugs will be used. Very few children need surgery for peptic ulcer disease.

What does it look like?

- *Abdominal pain* is the main symptom of peptic ulcer disease.
  - Your child may feel pain anywhere in the abdomen, most commonly in the upper abdomen or around the navel (belly button).
  - Pain may get better after your child eats or after he or she takes antacids. (This pattern is more common in older children and adults.)
- Less often, bleeding is the first sign of an ulcer. Your child may vomit blood or may have black, tarry bowel movements (blood in the stool). Even less often, bright red blood may be seen coming from your child's rectum.
- *If signs of bleeding occur, get medical help as soon as possible.*
- In infants, recurrent vomiting and slow weight gain are the most common symptoms of ulcer.
- Injured children with ulcers may not have any symptoms.

What causes peptic ulcer?

- Most children with ulcers have serious disease or illness, such as burn patients in the intensive care unit (ICU).

- Ulcers may also occur in patients taking certain medications, such as ibuprofen. In these situations, the natural barriers that protect the stomach lining are disrupted, allowing stomach acid to injure the inside of the stomach.
- In otherwise healthy children, infection with *Helicobacter pylori* is usually the cause.

What are some possible complications of peptic ulcer?

- Bleeding may occur.
- The ulcer may penetrate the stomach or intestinal wall (called a perforated ulcer), allowing the stomach contents to leak out. This can result in bleeding and/or infection.

What puts your child at risk of peptic ulcer disease?

- Major injuries, such as head trauma or serious burns. Ulcers are a frequent complication in critically ill patients.
- Regular use of aspirin, ibuprofen, and related medications (called non-steroidal–anti-inflammatory drugs), which can irritate the stomach. Acetaminophen (Tylenol) does not cause stomach irritation.
- If you or others in your family have had stomach ulcers, your child may be at higher risk.
- Certain diseases increase the risk of ulcers, including inflammatory bowel disease or various types of gastritis (inflammation of the stomach lining).

Can peptic ulcer disease be prevented?

- In critically ill or injured children, acid-reducing drugs or other medications are commonly given to prevent ulcers.
- If you or others in your family have ulcers related to *Helicobacter pylori* infection, getting effective treatment may prevent the bacteria from spreading to your child.

How is peptic ulcer diagnosed?

- If gastric or duodenal ulcer is suspected, your doctor may recommend a procedure for your child called endoscopy. An instrument like a telescope is placed through the mouth, down into the stomach and duodenum. This allows the doctor to see if there are any ulcers and to take a sample of the tissue (biopsy). This sample can be checked for infection with *Helicobacter pylori* bacteria. Your child is sedated during the endoscopy procedure.
- Some simple tests (such as a breath test, blood test, or stool test) can help to determine whether your child is infected with *Helicobacter pylori*.

How is peptic ulcer treated?

Treatment for peptic ulcer depends on the cause:

- If your child has a critical illness or injury, he or she will receive medications to control stomach acid. This may be done either to prevent or to treat peptic ulcer.

- If your child is taking aspirin, ibuprofen, or other medications that irritate the stomach, those medications should be stopped.

- If your child is infected with *Helicobacter pylori,* antibiotics are needed to kill the bacteria. Acid-reducing medications such as Tagamet (generic name: cimetidine) and Prilosec (generic name: omeprazole) work by reducing acid production by the stomach.

- Older antacid drugs (for example, Maalox) are not as effective as drugs that affect acid secretion and may cause side effects.

- It takes a few weeks for ulcers to heal. Your child will receive medical follow-up visits to confirm healing.

When should I call your office?

During treatment for peptic ulcer, call our office if:

- Your child has any sign of bleeding: vomiting blood, blood in his or her bowel movements (black, tarry stools), or bleeding from the rectum.

- Your child's symptoms of peptic ulcer disease (stomach pain, heartburn) don't seem to be getting better.

- Your child develops new symptoms, such as severe abdominal pain.

Pyloric Stenosis

Pyloric stenosis is a relatively common condition in infants. The bottom portion of the stomach becomes narrowed, blocking the normal passage of food. This can cause forceful vomiting, called projectile vomiting. Surgery is highly successful in curing pyloric stenosis.

What is pyloric stenosis?

Pyloric stenosis occurs when the part of the stomach leading to the small intestine, called the pylorus, becomes narrowed and blocked so that food cannot reach the intestines. The cause is unknown. The main symptom is vomiting, which often comes out in a strong stream.

If the condition goes unrecognized for a long time, inadequate nutrition and growth problems may occur. Although pyloric stenosis is a potentially serious condition, it is curable with surgery.

What does it look like?

- The main symptom is vomiting:

  - Vomiting usually starts after the first few weeks of life—rarely after 5 months.

  - It usually occurs shortly after feeding.

  - Projectile vomiting often occurs: the vomit comes out in a forceful stream.

  - If vomiting has been going on for a long time, the vomit may appear brown (like coffee grounds). *This is a sign of bleeding in the stomach; call our office or go to the emergency room immediately.*

- Because of vomiting, your child may become dehydrated. Symptoms of dehydration include dry mouth, decreased tears, fewer wet diapers.

- If pyloric stenosis is not recognized and treated, your infant may have signs of poor nutrition. He or she may show signs of slow growth and be hungry all the time.

- Your doctor may be able to feel a small, "olive-shaped" bump in your child's abdomen. This is the narrowed part of the pylorus, and it's a key sign that pyloric stenosis is causing your baby's vomiting.

- A small number of infants with pyloric stenosis have other congenital abnormalities or birth defects.

What causes pyloric stenosis?

- An abnormal thickening of the circular muscle (pylorus) around the "outlet" leading from the stomach to the intestine.

- The cause of this abnormal thickening of the pyloric muscle is unknown.

What are some possible complications of pyloric stenosis?

- It prevents your baby from getting enough to eat or drink, causing dehydration. If the condition goes on long enough, problems with nutrition and growth may occur.

- An imbalance of salts (electrolytes) in your child's body may occur. This could lead to further complications if not corrected.

- Complications of the operation performed to treat pyloric stenosis are possible but very uncommon.

What puts your child at risk of pyloric stenosis?

- Pyloric stenosis is a relatively common condition, affecting 2 to 3 out of 1000 infants.

- It is more common in first-born children.

- It is more common in boys than in girls.

- It is most common in families of Northern European origin.

Can pyloric stenosis be prevented?

There is no known way to prevent this condition.

How is pyloric stenosis diagnosed and treated?

- If the doctor suspects pyloric stenosis, he or she may order tests such as ultrasound scans or an "upper GI (gastrointestinal) series." The upper GI series uses a material called barium that shows abnormalities of the stomach and duodenum on x-rays. However, if the doctor can feel the olive-shaped bump (the narrowed part of the pylorus) in your child's abdomen, these tests may be unnecessary.

- Babies with pyloric stenosis need hospital treatment. The first step is intravenous (IV) fluids to treat dehydration and electrolyte imbalances caused by frequent vomiting.

- Your baby needs a relatively simple operation, called a *pylorotomy,* to treat pyloric stenosis. An anesthetic is used to put your child to sleep during the operation.

- The surgeon splits the abnormally enlarged muscles surrounding the pylorus. This allows food to pass normally from your baby's stomach into the small intestine.

- Vomiting may continue for a while as your child is recovering from the operation. However, it gradually disappears as healing occurs.

- There is a low risk of other complications after pylorotomy, such as infection or scarring. Your baby will receive close follow-up care after the operation.

- The surgeon will provide detailed instructions on caring for your infant, including wound care, after the operation.

- Pylorotomy almost always cures pyloric stenosis immediately and permanently. Feeding usually starts within 12 to 24 hours after the operation. Your baby should be eating normally within a few days.

When should I call your office?

After treatment for pyloric stenosis, call our office if any of the following occurs:

- Continued and/or worsened vomiting. (Vomiting may continue for a few days after the operation but should gradually decrease.)

- High fever or pain, swelling, redness, bleeding, or fluid draining from the surgical wound.

- No improvement in feeding and/or weight gain in the weeks after the operation.

Section XIII ▪ Genetics

Down Syndrome (Trisomy 21)

> Down syndrome is a relatively common chromosomal disorder. Most children with Down syndrome have mild to moderate mental impairment. About half have heart defects or other medical problems such as hearing and vision problems. Prenatal testing may be able to recognize Down syndrome before the baby is born. Your doctor can help to arrange for appropriate medical care for your child with Down syndrome, along with services and support for your family.

What is Down syndrome?

Down syndrome is a genetic disease caused by a chromosomal abnormality. The child usually has a certain appearance that is common to children with Down syndrome. These children also have differing degrees of mental deficiency, heart disease, and other problems.

Down syndrome usually results from an extra copy of chromosome 21, although other chromosomal abnormalities are possible. It occurs in about 1 of every 600 to 800 live-born babies.

Your child will have screening tests to look for medical problems associated with Down syndrome. Visits to some medical specialists may be recommended as well. We can help you access appropriate medical care for your child as well as support for your family, including early intervention and special education services.

What kinds of problems occur with Down syndrome?

Physical appearance. Children with Down syndrome have a certain typical appearance:

- Flat, broad head.
- Slanted eyes, pointing upward.
- Small mouth; tongue tends to stick out.
- Short, broad hands with a single crease across the palm. The little finger is short and curves inward. There is a wide space between the first and second toes.
- Poor muscle tone during the newborn period ("floppy").
- As they grow, children with Down syndrome have shorter than average height.

Medical problems. Children with Down syndrome are at increased risk of many different medical problems:

- Heart problems. About half are born with heart defects, most commonly atrial septal defect (ASD). In this condition, a hole is present between two chambers of the heart. As children get older, problems with the heart valves may develop.
- Mental impairment. Most children with Down syndrome have mild to moderate mental retardation. Some have severe mental impairment.
- Hearing loss and ear infections are frequent.
- Vision problems, including cataracts and strabismus.
- Snoring and difficulty breathing during sleep (obstructive sleep apnea [OSA]) occur in about half of children.
- Thyroid problems. Usually low thyroid function (hypothyroidism), but sometimes high thyroid function (hyperthyroidism).
- Infections are more frequent than in the average child.
- Gastrointestinal problems, especially obstruction (blockage) of the small intestine during the newborn period. There is also an increased risk of celiac disease: sensitivity to gluten, a substance present in cereals and breads.
- Obesity.
- Leukemia. Risk is higher than average, although only about 1% of Down syndrome children are affected.
- Instability of the cervical spine (neck). This can affect the spinal nerves, causing weakness and other neurologic symptoms.
- Females with Down syndrome are fertile and able to bear children. Almost all males are infertile.
- People with Down syndrome have a shortened lifespan. They are also at increased risk of early Alzheimer's disease.

What causes Down syndrome?

In over 90% of children with Down syndrome, the disease results from the presence of an extra chromosome. Normally, people have 46 chromosomes—23 from each parent. Most children with Down syndrome have 47 chromosomes, with an extra copy of chromosome 21; that's why this condition is also called "trisomy 21." A small number of children have the right number of chromosomes, but an extra piece of chromosome 21 is attached to one of the other chromosomes. This is called a *translocation,* and affected children have the same problems as those with typical Down syndrome.

In 1% to 2% of children with Down syndrome, some cells contain the normal 46 chromosomes, while others contain 47 chromosomes. This is called *mosaicism.* These children have fewer problems than those with other chromosomal abnormalities.

What increases the risk of Down syndrome?

- Older age of the mother. The rate of Down syndrome pregnancies is increased for mothers over 35.

- Having another family member with Down syndrome.

How is Down syndrome diagnosed?

- After the baby is born, a simple chromosome test can confirm whether or not Down syndrome is present.

- Women over 35 and other pregnant women at high risk of having a Down syndrome child can undergo prenatal (before birth) testing. This may include procedures to obtain samples of the amniotic fluid in the womb (called amniocentesis) or the placenta (called chorionic villus sampling).

- New strategies to detect Down syndrome before birth are now being used. A combination of blood tests and ultrasound scans is performed during the first and second trimesters of pregnancy. The results help to determine if amniocentesis or other additional tests are needed. If not, the mother can avoid the risks of these tests.

- If Down syndrome is diagnosed before birth, the parents face the difficult decision of whether to terminate the pregnancy.

How is Down syndrome managed?

Medical issues. During regular checkups, your child will be screened for various health problems that may occur:

- Thyroid function is checked as part of regular newborn screening tests and rechecked frequently.

- A test called an echocardiogram ("echo"), which uses sound waves to take pictures of your child's heart, will be done to check for heart defects. If any are found, your doctor will recommend a visit to a heart specialist (cardiologist). Some heart defects require surgery.

- By age 6 months, your child should be checked by an eye specialist (ophthalmologist) for eye problems.

- Hearing is checked at birth and rechecked at certain times. We may recommend visits to an ear, nose, and throat specialist (ENT or otorhinolaryngologist) and an audiologist (a professional trained to evaluate hearing problems).

- The ENT specialist can also evaluate and treat snoring and sleep-related breathing problems.

- Screening for celiac disease (gluten intolerance) may be recommended at around age 2 or 3.

Developmental issues. Education is an important aspect of care for Down syndrome:

- *Early intervention* should start as soon as your child's condition is diagnosed. Every state has an early intervention program; our office can put you in touch with resources to get you started. Early intervention experts can assess your child and develop an Individualized Family Support Plan (IFSP) based on your child's development, need for support, and goals for independence.

- *Special education* services are also available in every state (although children with less severe impairment may not qualify for services). You are entitled to expert evaluation of your child. Based on the results, an Individualized Education Program (IEP) can be developed to meet your child's educational needs.

- Speech therapy can be helpful.

- Having a child with Down syndrome is a life-changing event for your family. We can help to put you in touch with community resources to help children with Down syndrome and their families.

When should I call your office?

Your child will receive regular checkups to look for medical problems associated with Down syndrome. Call our office if problems come up between visits or if you have any questions about your child's testing, treatment, or educational intervention.

Where can I get more information about Down syndrome?

A good place to start is the National Down Syndrome Society. On the Internet at *www.ndss.org*, or call 1-800-221-4602.

Fragile X Syndrome

Fragile X syndrome is the most common inherited cause of mental retardation in boys. It is usually caused by a gene abnormality passed on from mother to son. Certain physical abnormalities and behavior problems are also present. There is no cure for fragile X syndrome. Special education and various types of therapy can be helpful for children with fragile X syndrome and their families.

What is fragile X syndrome?

Fragile X syndrome is a relatively common genetic disease causing mental retardation. It is more common and severe in boys, although it can occur in girls. The disease is most often caused by an abnormal gene passed on from mothers to sons. Fragile X syndrome does not result from anything the parents did wrong or anything that happened during pregnancy or childbirth.

Most children with fragile X syndrome have problems with intellectual functioning. Some have relatively mild learning disabilities; others have moderate mental retardation. Some physical abnormalities occur along with certain medical problems. Social and behavior problems are common as well.

There is no cure for fragile X syndrome. However, special education and other services can help to make the most of your child's intellectual abilities and other skills. The benefits are greatest if the condition is recognized and services are started as early as possible. Genetic counseling can help you to understand your risk of passing the disease on to future children.

What kinds of problems occur with fragile X syndrome?

Intelligence/development.

- Children with fragile X syndrome have lower than normal intelligence. Your child may be slow to reach normal language milestones. In less severe cases, the problem may not be detected until your child reaches school age. In girls with the syndrome, intelligence may be closer to normal.

- Language and speech problems, such as difficulty using the right words and problems with pronunciation (such as stuttering).

- Emotional and behavioral difficulties, especially in boys. Your child may be shy and anxious, especially around unfamiliar people and situations. In these circumstances, angry outbursts or temper tantrums may occur.

Sometimes it may be difficult to tell what's making your child upset.

- Children with fragile X syndrome may be diagnosed with other psychiatric or developmental disorders, especially attention deficit–hyperactivity disorder and autism.

Physical abnormalities.

- In infants and young children, appearance is normal. During puberty, your child develops a large face, jaw, and ears. In boys, the testicles may be enlarged (sexual function is normal).

- Loose joints ("double-jointed") are related to an abnormality of the body's connective tissue. This can lead to problems such as joint dislocations or hernias.

Medical problems.

- Heart problems. Later in life, the connective tissue abnormalities may lead to heart problems such as mitral valve prolapse.

- Girls may have premature ovarian failure, causing early menopause. This means the ovaries are no longer producing eggs and therefore pregnancy cannot occur.

Individual symptoms and behaviors vary a lot. Your child may have different symptoms or the problems may be more or less severe.

What causes fragile X syndrome?

- This disease is caused by an abnormality in the fragile X mental metardation 1 (*FMR1*) gene. The *FMR1* gene makes proteins that affect how the brain works.

- The *FMR1* gene mutation is found on the X chromosome. Females have two X chromosomes (XX), while males have an X chromosome and a Y chromosome (XY). Since females have two X's, one of them will be normal; that's why girls are less likely than boys to be affected by fragile X syndrome. Males can only pass the abnormal *FMR1* gene to daughters, not sons. This is because males have to donate a Y chromosome (not an X) to have a male child.

How is fragile X syndrome diagnosed?

- Fragile X syndrome is recognized based on your child's symptoms, a physical examination, and information on your family history. Once the diagnosis is suspected, it can be confirmed by a special chromosome test.

- Genetic counseling can help you to understand the risks of having another child with fragile X syndrome.

How is fragile X syndrome managed?

Many of the problems associated with fragile X syndrome can be improved with treatment. It is especially important to seek help with behavioral or emotional disorders, which can be stressful for your family.

- Education is probably the most important aspect of care:
  - *Early intervention* should start as soon as your child's condition is diagnosed. Every state has an early intervention program; our office can put you in touch with resources to get you started. Early intervention experts can assess your child and develop an Individualized Family Support Plan (IFSP) based on your child's development, need for support, and goals for independence.
  - *Special education* services are also available in every state (although children with less severe impairment may not qualify for services). You are entitled to expert evaluation of your child. Based on the results, an Individualized Education Program (IEP) can be developed to meet your child's educational needs.
- Several professionals may play a role in your child's care. For example:
  - A speech/language pathologist can help with stuttering or other language difficulties.
  - An occupational therapist may help in identifying the best adaptations to your child's needs.
  - A behavioral therapist may help in dealing with emotional and behavioral problems.
  - Other types of services can be helpful. Family counseling may help to deal with the emotional or social problems associated with having a special needs child.

When should I call your office?

Call our office if you have any questions about your child's testing, treatment, or educational intervention.

Where can I get more information about fragile X syndrome?

- Contact the National Fragile X Foundation on the Internet at *www.fragilex.org*, or call 1-800-688-8765.
- The National Institute of Child Health and Human Development (NICHD) offers an informative booklet on "Families and Fragile X Syndrome." It is available on the Internet at *www.nichd.nih.gov/publications/pubs/fragileX/*, or call 1-800-370-2943.

Genetic Counseling

> Genetic counseling may be recommended in many situations, for example, pregnancy in a woman over age 35, a family history of inherited disease, or diagnosis of a genetic disease in a child. Counseling is done by experts in the nature of genetic disorders, the risks of passing these disorders to future children, and caring for affected children. The information provided in genetic counseling can help you make important decisions about your child's and family's health.

What is genetic counseling?

Many diseases are related to genetic (inherited) abnormalities. Genes, which are made up of DNA, determine all of our physical characteristics, such as height, eye color, and the shape of our noses. To some extent, genes determine our mental characteristics as well. They can also carry a wide range of inherited diseases, such as sickle cell disease, cystic fibrosis, and many others.

Sometimes a gene causing an abnormal disease is passed on from parent to child. Several members of a family may have the abnormal gene. In other cases, the abnormal gene (mutation) was not passed on from the parents but seems to be an isolated occurrence in just one family member. Other abnormalities that babies are born with result from abnormal development of the baby during pregnancy and are not genetically inherited.

Genetic counseling may be recommended in a number of situations in which genetic diseases are likely to be present. Examples include when the parents are older during pregnancy, when a routine screening test gives abnormal results, when one parent has a genetic disease that may be passed on to a child, or when a child is diagnosed with a genetic disease. Unfortunately, in some conditions, a specific diagnosis cannot be made. In this situation, different possible diagnoses and their effect on the child are discussed with the parents.

A *medical geneticist* is a doctor specializing in genetic diseases. This specialist can help to make or confirm the diagnosis in patients who appear to have a genetic disease. A *genetic counselor* is a professional who can help you to understand the risks and impact of genetic diseases on your family. The information provided by these experts can help you to understand genetic diseases, the risk of passing them on to future children, and your options for medical treatment and family planning.

Who may need genetic counseling?

Several factors increase the risk of genetic disease. Genetic counseling may be recommended in certain situations:

- If your newborn infant has had an abnormal result on routine screening tests. These are blood tests for multiple genetic diseases that are performed in every infant.

- If your child is diagnosed with some type of congenital disease (present since birth) or birth defect.

- If you had a stillborn baby (one who died before birth) with some type of congenital abnormality.

- If the parents are older when the baby is conceived. Risk is increased when the mother is over 35 years old or the father is over 50.

- If the parents are related to each other. This increases the risk that both parents will carry an abnormal gene.

- If you or others in your family have some form of genetic disease that could be passed on to your child.

- If you were exposed during pregnancy to a drug or toxin that might lead to birth defects.

- Certain racial/ethnic backgrounds are associated with an increased risk of genetic diseases. For example, the risk of sickle cell disease is increased in some African-American families.

What is genetic counseling like?

Genetic counseling may be performed by a genetic counselor, who is a health care professional with special training and expertise in genetic and congenital diseases. Other times, counseling is done by a medical geneticist, who is a doctor specializing in genetic diseases.

There are several steps in the genetic counseling process. The genetic counselor will:

- Ask about your family's medical history (pedigree). The questions will probably be very detailed, including health information on relatives, any stillborn children, and the ages and reasons for death of family members.

- Assemble and talk to you about all relevant medical records, for example, your child's records, if he or she has been diagnosed with a genetic disease; or the mother's prenatal, pregnancy, and delivery history.

- Discuss the results of genetic tests. Further tests may be recommended. For example, if you or your child has been diagnosed with a genetic disease; other members of your family may need testing to see if they also have the abnormal gene.

- Give information to help you make decisions regarding the health of affected children and other family members and the risk of passing the disease on to future children. The counselor doesn't tell you what you should do. Instead, his or her job is to give you accurate factual information so you can make an informed decision about what's best for your family.

● The counselor or geneticist can also provide information on available medical resources such as further tests that may be helpful, medical treatment options, or support groups for families with genetic diseases.

What happens after genetic counseling?

Families often have to make difficult decisions after going through genetic counseling:

● Whether to terminate or continue a pregnancy. If pregnancy screening tests lead to the diagnosis of a genetic disease, some couples may consider terminating the pregnancy (having an abortion). This decision may need to be made urgently because abortions generally have to be performed early in the pregnancy. For couples who decide to continue the pregnancy, the information provided by genetic counseling can help prepare for the birth of the baby.

● Family planning issues. For many genetic diseases, the risk of inheritance is fairly predictable. The genetic counselor may be able to provide information on the likelihood that future pregnancies will be affected by a particular genetic disease.

● However, it's important to realize it's not always easy to predict the risk of passing on a genetic disease. Inheritance of genetic diseases can be complex; an exact gene abnormality is known for only about 10% of genetic diseases. The genetic counselor can provide you with the most accurate information available on risks.

● Options for follow-up and support. Finding out that your family has some type of gene abnormality or genetic disease is a stressful event. The genetic counselor can help put you in touch with support groups and other valuable community resources.

When should I call your office?

Call our office if you have any questions or concerns about genetic counseling. We can help to put you in touch with a qualified genetic counselor.

Where can I get more information?

Here are a few good sources of general information about genetic diseases and birth defects. We may be able to recommend other resources, depending on your child's and family's situation.

● March of Dimes Birth Defects Foundation. On the Internet at *www.marchofdimes.com* or call 1-888-MODIMES (663-4637).

● The National Center on Birth Defects and Developmental Disabilities. Information and publications are available on the Internet at *www.cdc.gov/ncbddd*.

Klinefelter's Syndrome

Klinefelter's syndrome is a relatively common genetic disorder, affecting only boys. One of the main abnormalities is lack of normal growth of the testicles during puberty and smaller than average size of the penis. This is related to problems with making the normal amount of sex-related hormones. Your son may also have difficulties with school performance and behavior, including anger problems. Treatment with testosterone (male hormone replacement therapy) can lessen the impact of Klinefelter's syndrome.

What is Klinefelter's syndrome?

Klinefelter's syndrome is a genetic (inherited) disorder affecting approximately 1 in 500 newborn boys. It is caused by inheritance of an extra X chromosome. Boys with Klinefelter's syndrome have abnormal or slow sexual development. As a result, the condition may not be recognized until your son reaches the age of puberty.

The genetic abnormality can also cause problems with intellectual ability, ranging from learning disorders to mild mental retardation. Behavior problems are common as well, including aggressive or antisocial behavior.

Boys with Klinefelter's syndrome need treatments with the male hormone testosterone to develop more normally. Special education and other services can help your child's intellectual and social development.

What kinds of problems occur with Klinefelter's syndrome?

The most typical features of Klinefelter's syndrome are:

- *Abnormal sexual development.*

  - Your son does not progress into puberty at the expected time: the testicles remain small, the penis is smaller than average, and facial hair doesn't grow normally.

  - Breast enlargement (gynecomastia) may occur.

  - Males with Klinefelter's syndrome have problems with fertility (the ability to have children).

- *Intellectual/social issues.*

  - Most boys with Klinefelter's syndrome do not have major reductions in intellectual ability. However, on average, intelligence is lower than in your child's siblings. Some boys with Klinefelter's syndrome have mental retardation, although it is usually mild.

  - Your child may have problems at school, such as poor grades or learning disorders. Speech and language development may be delayed.

  - Your son may have behavior problems. Many boys with Klinefelter's syndrome are shy and immature. They may also have outbursts of angry or antisocial behavior.

  - Boys with Klinefelter's syndrome tend to be tall and thin, with long legs. Some have problems with physical coordination.

- *Health problems.* Boys with Klinefelter's syndrome are at increased risk of certain medical conditions:

  - Scoliosis (abnormal curvature of the spine).

  - Undescended testicles; this occurs when the testicles don't "drop" (descend) from the abdomen into the scrotum before your child is born.

  - Certain cancers, including male breast cancer.

All of these signs vary a lot. The abnormalities are often quite mild. Klinefelter's syndrome often goes unrecognized until puberty, when sexual development doesn't occur normally. Sometimes, the problem isn't diagnosed until adulthood, when men have trouble producing children.

With modern testing techniques, the genetic abnormality causing Klinefelter's syndrome may be recognized during pregnancy.

What causes Klinefelter's syndrome?

Klinefelter's syndrome is caused by a genetic abnormality. Genetically normal boys have one X chromosome and one Y chromosome (XY).

Boys with Klinefelter's syndrome have two X chromosomes plus one Y chromosome (XXY). Some people prefer the term "XXY males" instead of Klinefelter's syndrome for the disorder.

The extra X chromosome can develop in different ways. It is unrelated to anything the parents did wrong or anything the mother did during pregnancy.

What puts your child at risk of Klinefelter's syndrome?

The risk of having a child with Klinefelter's syndrome is slightly increased for older mothers. In addition, if one child has Klinefelter's syndrome, there is a slightly increased risk for future children (1 in 100).

How is Klinefelter's syndrome diagnosed?

- Klinefelter's syndrome may be suspected because of delayed puberty, your child's appearance, and other problems.

- Genetic testing is needed to confirm the gene abnormality causing Klinefelter's syndrome. Although the XXY pattern is most common, other variants can occur. We will likely recommend a visit to a medical geneticist, a doctor specializing in genetic diseases, who can provide more complete information.

How is Klinefelter's syndrome managed?

Several types of treatment are helpful for boys with Klinefelter's syndrome:

- *Testosterone replacement.* Regular treatments with the male hormone testosterone can help to normalize your son's sexual and physical development. A doctor specializing in hormone problems (endocrinologist) can manage this part of your child's treatment.

- *Treatment for enlarged breasts.* Enlarged breasts (gynecomastia) can be a problem in boys with Klinefelter's syndrome. The problem may improve over time, and the endocrinologist can recommend treatment, if needed.

- *Help with school and behavior problems.* Your son may need extra help in school, particularly with speech/language. Special education services are available in every state. You are entitled to expert evaluation of your child. Based on the results, an Individualized Education Program (IEP) can be developed to meet your child's educational needs.

- *Infertility treatment.* For some men with Klinefelter's syndrome, special infertility treatments may make it possible to have children.

When should I call your office?

Learning that your child has a genetic disorder is a difficult situation for any parent. Call our office if you have any questions about this disorder, especially how to access the expert medical care and other services your son needs.

Where can I get more information?

Information on resources and support for families affected by Klinefelter's syndrome/XXY conditions is available from Klinefelter Syndrome & Associates on the Internet at *www.genetic.org/ks*, or call 1-888-XXY-WHAT (1-888-999-9428).

Marfan's Syndrome

> Marfan's syndrome is an inherited disorder resulting from an abnormality of the connective tissue, which helps to hold the various tissues of the body together. In Marfan's syndrome, the connective tissue abnormality leads mainly to problems in the skeleton (bones), heart and blood vessels, and eyes. There is no cure, but regular medical care can reduce the rate of serious complications.

What is Marfan's syndrome?

Marfan's syndrome is a genetic (inherited) condition affecting 1 in 5000 to 1 in 10,000 newborns. Your child is born with this disease, even if it isn't recognized until later. Marfan's syndrome is caused by an abnormal gene affecting the body's connective tissue, which works like glue to help hold various tissues together.

Children with Marfan's syndrome may have abnormalities of the bones and joints, heart and blood vessels, eyes, and skin. The high risk of heart problems is the main concern. Children with Marfan's syndrome don't all have the same problems or disease severity. Your child will receive close medical attention to keep him or her as healthy as possible and to prevent complications.

What kinds of problems occur with Marfan's syndrome?

- The typical person with Marfan's syndrome is tall and thin, with long legs, arms, and fingers. The face may also appear long and thin.

- Heart and blood vessel diseases are the most serious complications of Marfan's syndrome. Because of the connective tissue abnormality, the aorta (the main artery through which blood is pumped out of the heart) may become widened and stretched (dilated). This may lead to weakening and bulging of the aorta ("aneurysm") and tearing of its walls ("dissection"). Leaks and other problems of the heart valves can also develop.

- Abnormalities of the skeleton may include a "caved-in" chest (called pectus deformity), abnormal curve of the spine (called scoliosis), and crowding of the teeth. Your child may have loose joints ("double-jointed") that are easily dislocated.

- Various eye problems may occur, including dislocation of the lens of the eye, nearsightedness (myopia), glaucoma, cataracts, and detached retina.

- Loose skin, sometimes with stretch marks.

- Lung problems: as your child ages, he or she will be at increased risk of a problem called "pneumothorax." In this condition, the lungs leak air, putting pressure on them and causing chest pain and difficulty breathing.

- Your child may not have all of these abnormalities. Even when caused by the same genetic abnormality, the disease is more severe in some patients than in others.

What causes Marfan's syndrome?

- An abnormality of the fibrillin gene. Fibrillin is essential for development of connective tissue and is found in nearly every organ of the body.

- Most often, the abnormal gene is inherited from a parent. If one parent has an abnormal fibrillin gene, each child will have a 50% chance of inheriting Marfan's syndrome. Genetic counseling can help you understand your chances of passing on the disease to future children.

- In 25% of people with Marfan's syndrome, the gene mutation (which means a change in genetic material occurred) that made the abnormal fibrillin gene happened when your child was conceived; neither parent has an abnormal gene. In this situation, other children in your family are not necessarily at increased risk of Marfan's syndrome.

How is Marfan's syndrome diagnosed?

- There is no specific test for Marfan's syndrome. The diagnosis is based on the presence of typical abnormalities, including heart and eye problems, and information on your family's medical history. Genetic testing may be possible.

- Once Marfan's syndrome is diagnosed, tests will be performed to check the various organs and body systems:

  - A test called an echocardiogram ("echo"), which uses sound waves to take pictures of the heart.

  - A slit-lamp examination (a test using a special light to examine the inside of the eye).

  - Other tests may be recommended as well.

How is Marfan's syndrome managed?

Various doctors may be involved in your child's care: for example, a cardiologist (heart specialist), an ophthalmologist (eye doctor), a medical geneticist (specialist in genetic diseases), and an orthopedic surgeon (bone and joint specialist). Our office will help to coordinate your child's care.

Regular, repeated evaluations of all of the organ systems involved are essential to protecting your child's health and to detecting any complications as early as possible:

- *Heart problems.* A key concern is to monitor enlargement of the body's central main artery (the aorta) and the functioning of the heart valves. The cardiologist will determine what tests and possible treatment are needed. Your child may have to follow certain precautions, including:

  - Avoiding overexertion. Gentler forms of exercise, such as bicycling and swimming, are a good choice.

  - Wearing a Medic-Alert bracelet or necklace to alert health care providers that he or she has Marfan's syndrome.

  - If your child has heart valve problems, he or she may need to take antibiotics before dental procedures or surgery. This is done to prevent a serious condition called infective endocarditis (infection of the heart valves and tissues lining the heart).

- *Bone and joint problems.* Scoliosis (abnormal spinal curvature) and other bone and joint problems are possible. The orthopedic surgeon will evaluate and treat these problems.

- *Eye problems.* We will probably recommend visits to an eye doctor (ophthalmologist) for evaluation of possible eye problems. Yearly eye examinations are essential for your child.

- *Pregnancy.* Sexually active women and girls with Marfan's syndrome must be especially careful about birth control. Although it is possible for women with this disease to have successful pregnancies, the risks are a lot higher than for women without it.

Family or individual counseling may help your child and family deal with the stresses of living with Marfan's syndrome.

When should I call your office?

Your child with Marfan's syndrome will be scheduled for regular medical visits, including screening for heart disease and other problems.

Between visits, call our office or go the emergency room if your child develops:

- Signs of problems related to the heart or lungs, such as chest pain or shortness of breath.

- Eye problems—any change in vision.

Where can I get more information about Marfan's syndrome?

The National Marfan Foundation on the Internet at *www. marfan.org*, or call 1-800-8-MARFAN (1-800-862-7326).

Turner's Syndrome

Turner's syndrome is a congenital syndrome caused by a genetic abnormality in girls. Girls with Turner's syndrome are short and do not go through normal sexual changes at puberty. Intelligence is usually normal, but there is an increased risk of certain health problems. Hormone therapy can increase height and promote sexual development. However, most women with Turner's syndrome are unable to have children.

What is Turner's syndrome?

Turner's syndrome is a relatively common genetic (inherited) disorder, affecting about 1 in 2500 girls. Girls with Turner's syndrome have a chromosomal abnormality that interferes with the normal development of the ovaries.

Turner's syndrome results in certain physical abnormalities, most noticeably short height (stature). Other malformations may be present as well, including heart defects. Turner's syndrome may not be recognized until the early teen years, when affected girls don't go through the normal changes of puberty.

Growth hormone therapy may allow your daughter to achieve near-normal height. Treatment with the hormone estrogen can allow development of normal female sex characteristics but cannot restore fertility. Although close medical follow-up is needed to detect health problems, most girls with Turner's syndrome have a normal life span.

What kinds of problems occur with Turner's syndrome?

Physical problems. Girls with Turner's syndrome have certain physical characteristics, some of which may be present at birth:

- Swelling of the hands and feet.
- Loose skin at the base of the neck.
- Low birth weight/small size.
- Later in childhood, other signs may develop:
  - Short stature; this is sometimes the only abnormality until puberty.
  - Webbed neck; it looks wider at the base.
  - Low hairline at the back of the head.
  - Small jaw; prominent ears.
  - Broad chest.
  - Narrow fingernails.

For some girls with Turner's syndrome, the condition goes unrecognized until the early teen years.

- Most girls with Turner's syndrome don't go through the normal sexual changes at puberty (for example, breasts enlarging, menstrual periods starting).
- Females with Turner's syndrome are usually infertile (unable to bear children).
- *Medical problems.* Certain medical problems are possible, either in childhood or later in life:
  - *Heart problems.* Some girls with Turner's syndrome are born with heart defects, especially an abnormality of one of the heart valves (the aortic valve). A defect called aortic coarctation (narrowing of the aorta, the body's main artery) is more serious but less common. Aortic coarctation is more common in girls who have the typical "webbed neck" appearance of Turner's syndrome.
  - *Kidney problems.* Various kidney defects can be present at birth. These may cause problems with kidney function or contribute to problems with high blood pressure (hypertension).
  - *Thyroid problems.* Girls with Turner's syndrome can develop hypothyroidism (not making enough thyroid hormone).
  - *Ear and hearing problems.* Middle ear infections (otitis media) may be a recurrent problem. Risk of hearing loss is higher as your daughter gets older.
- *Developmental difficulties.* Certain types of learning disorders may occur in girls with Turner's syndrome. However, intelligence is usually normal.

What causes Turner's syndrome?

- Normally, girls have two X chromosomes (XX). In most girls with Turner's syndrome, one of those X chromosomes is missing. Less often, just part of the X chromosome is missing. Other girls have some cells in their bodies with two X chromosomes and others with one (mosaicism).
- In most cases, the chromosomal abnormality occurs at the time of conception; it is not passed on from the parents. In this situation, there is not a high increase in the risk of Turner's syndrome in future children.

How is Turner's syndrome diagnosed?

In most cases, the doctor first suspects Turner's syndrome because of abnormalities on physical examination, such as short stature or delayed puberty. A specific genetic test called karyotyping can show the absent or missing X chromosome that causes Turner's syndrome. It may also provide important information for medical treatment and genetic counseling.

How is Turner's syndrome managed?

Medical testing and follow-up

- When Turner's syndrome is diagnosed, your child undergoes tests to detect other possible birth defects and abnormalities. These tests usually include an echocardiogram ("echo"), which uses sound waves to take pictures of the heart, and ultrasound scans to look for possible abnormalities of the kidneys and ovaries.

- We will probably recommend visits to some medical specialists, such as a medical geneticist (specialist in genetic diseases), a cardiologist (heart specialist), and an endocrinologist (specialist in hormone problems).

- Your child will have regular checkups to look for medical problems that can occur with Turner's syndrome, such as hearing problems, high blood pressure, high cholesterol, or scoliosis (abnormal curvature of the spine).

Hormone therapy

- For most girls with Turner's syndrome, treatment with human growth hormone can help them to reach a more normal adult height. For very short girls, growth hormone treatment may start in early childhood.

- Around the time of normal puberty, treatment with the female hormone estrogen may be recommended. This will help to provide a more normal female appearance (such as normal breast development). However, it cannot restore fertility.

- The endocrinologist will discuss issues with you related to when these two types of hormone therapy should be started.

Support

- Support groups and other forms of support can be helpful for girls with Turner's syndrome. Contact the Turner Syndrome Society at 1-800-365-9944, or on the Internet at *www.turner-syndrome-us.org/*.

When should I call your office?

Call our office, or the specialist managing your child's care, if you have any questions about Turner's syndrome or your child's treatment.

Section XIV ▪ Genitalia

SECTION XIV ■ GENERAL

Epididymitis

Epididymitis is an infection or inflammation of the epididymis, a structure that carries sperm from the testicles. Epididymitis can be a sexually transmitted disease, but not always. The main symptoms are pain and swelling of the scrotum (the sac containing the testicles). It is important to get medical help for this condition. Rest and antibiotics are the usual treatments.

What is epididymitis?

Epididymitis is a painful condition caused by inflammation of the epididymis, which carries and stores sperm. It is located in the scrotum next to the testicle. Epididymitis is most common in young men. It may be caused by a sexually transmitted infection, although other sources of infection are possible. Once epididymitis is recognized, it usually improves quickly with antibiotics and other simple treatments.

Epididymitis is uncommon in boys before puberty. In this age group, swelling of the scrotum is more often caused by a condition called testicular torsion. Immediate treatment is needed—this condition can permanently damage the testicles.

Boys with pain in the testicles always need prompt medical attention.

What does it look like?

- Pain and swelling of the scrotum, often involving the testicle.
- Pain develops over a few days and may be severe.
- There may be redness on the skin of the scrotum.
- There may be a painful lump (the epididymis) on the affected testicle.
- Fever may be present.
- Sometimes, pain may occur when your child is urinating or fluid may drain from the penis.
- Can look like *testicular tortion* because of pain and swelling of the testicle.

What causes epididymitis?

- The usual cause is infection with bacteria, spreading either from the penis or the bladder. In sexually active boys and men, the main causes are sexually transmitted diseases (STDs). The most common causes of infection are the bacteria *Chlamydia* or *Neisseria gonorrhoeae*.
- However, epididymitis is not always a sexually transmitted disease. For example, it can occur in boys or men who have had a bladder infection. In boys before puberty, epididymitis may be associated with abnormalities of the reproductive system (testicles) or urinary system (bladder and kidneys).

What are some possible complications of epididymitis?

- With proper treatment, complications are uncommon.
- Without treatment, the infection may spread. This can cause damage to the reproductive organs, possibly including infertility.

What increases the risk of epididymitis?

- When epididymitis is from a sexually transmitted disease, the main risk factors are having a lot of partners and not using a condom every time you have sex.
- Bladder infections and other infections of the reproductive organs may also lead to epididymitis. Other abnormalities or previous surgery of the reproductive or urinary organs also increases the risk.

Can epididymitis be prevented?

- Not having sex is the best way to prevent epididymitis and other STDs. If you are sexually active, limit the number of your sex partners.
- Use a condom every time you have sex.

How is epididymitis diagnosed?

- Your doctor can usually tell whether epididymitis is present based on symptoms and a physical examination.
- If there is any doubt, an ultrasound examination may be performed. This is done to make sure there isn't another cause of pain and swelling, especially testicular torsion.
- Urinalysis and tests for STDs are done.

How is epididymitis treated?

- *Eliminating the infection.*
  - Antibiotics are prescribed. The exact antibiotic depends on the identified or most likely cause of the infection.
  - Make sure to finish the antibiotic prescription, even if symptoms have gotten better. Stopping treatment too early may allow the infection to come back.
  - If the epididymitis is from a STD, sexual partners may need to be tested and treated as well.

- *Treating pain and swelling.*
  - Rest.
  - Support for the scrotum: wear briefs rather than boxer shorts.
  - Take medications for pain, such as acetaminophen or ibuprofen.
  - Pain and swelling usually improve within a few days after the start of treatment. If not, call our office.

When should I call your office?

- Call our office if symptoms of epididymitis (swelling of the scrotum, pain of the testicles) do not improve within a few days, or if they get worse.
- Call our office if symptoms of testicular torsion develop, especially sudden, severe, or increasing pain and tenderness of the scrotum. *This is an emergency!*

Foreskin Problems

Most uncircumcised boys have no problems related to the intact foreskin—the skin covering the tip of the penis. In infants and toddlers, it is normal for the foreskin not to slide back over the end of the penis. In older boys, the foreskin may be too tight to slide back (phimosis), but this is usually not a serious problem. If the tight foreskin is forced over the head of the penis and cannot be pulled back, this may cause a serious condition called paraphimosis.

What kinds of foreskin problems may occur?

Phimosis means tight foreskin. In this condition, the foreskin cannot easily be pulled over the head of the penis. This is normal in toddlers and infants. Usually, the foreskin becomes loose enough to be pulled back as your child gets older. In older boys, phimosis can make it difficult to clean the head of the penis. Occasionally it causes problems with urination.

Balanoposthitis refers to inflammation to the head of the penis and foreskin that results from irritation or infection. Infection can be either bacterial or yeast. Poor hygiene can be part of the problem.

Paraphimosis is a problem in which the foreskin gets pulled over the head of the penis and cannot be pulled back. This can cause problems with blood flow in the head of the penis, and there is a risk of permanent damage.

(!) • *Paraphimosis can be an emergency requiring immediate treatment.*

What do they look like?

• *Phimosis.*

  • "Tight" foreskin that cannot easily be pulled back over the head of the penis.

  • This is normal in infants and young boys. Usually by age 3, the foreskin becomes loose enough to be pulled back easily.

  • Never force the foreskin back over the head of the penis. This actually increases the risk of problems with tight foreskin/phimosis.

  • Phimosis sometimes causes problems during urination. The foreskin may fill up like a balloon before the urine finally comes out. *If this occurs, see your doctor.*

  • In older boys, phimosis may cause pain when the penis is erect.

• *Balanoposthitis.*

• Redness, tenderness, or swelling of the foreskin or head of the penis.

• Pus or other fluid draining from the tip of the penis.

• May be pain with urination.

• *Paraphimosis.*

  • Tight foreskin pulled back over the head of the penis.

  • Head of the penis becomes swollen and very painful.

  • Paraphimosis requires immediate treatment to avoid damage to the head of the penis caused by problems with insufficient blood supply. *Call the doctor immediately.* (!)

What causes foreskin problems?

• Phimosis is usually a normal condition. However, it can occur as a result of infection or injury, including injury from forcing the foreskin back.

• Phimosis usually occurs in boys who are not circumcised. (Circumcision is a minor operation to remove the foreskin, usually performed in infant boys.)

• Infections usually result from poor hygiene. Your doctor can show you (or if he is older, your son) how to clean the uncircumcised penis properly. Push the foreskin back gently until you first feel resistance. Then cleanse the penis with a damp, soft cloth.

• Paraphimosis may occur when the tight foreskin is forced back. This sometimes happens when attempting to clean the head of the penis.

Can foreskin problems be prevented?

• Circumcision, if properly performed, prevents phimosis and other foreskin problems.

• Never force the foreskin back over the head of the penis, especially in infants and young boys.

• Keep the genital area clean.

How are foreskin problems treated?

• *Phimosis:*

  • In infants and boys younger than 3, a tight foreskin is normal. Never force the foreskin over the head of the penis. In most boys, the foreskin will become looser over time.

  • Phimosis generally needs treatment only when it is causing pain or problems with urination.

- Your doctor may recommend using a steroid cream to loosen the foreskin. Apply the cream as prescribed. This gradually loosens the tight foreskin in most boys.

- If necessary, circumcision can be performed.

- *Balanoposthitis:*

  - Antibiotics may be needed if infection is present. The antibiotic used depends on the cause of the infection.

  - Your doctor may recommend antibiotic pills or cream. Steroid cream or ointment may also be used for the inflammation.

  - Circumcision is sometimes recommended if the problem occurs repeatedly.

- *Paraphimosis:*

  - *Paraphimosis can be a medical emergency.* Immediate treatment is needed to prevent permanent damage to the penis.

- In the emergency room, the doctor will take steps to put the foreskin back in its proper position. This is successful most of the time. If not, surgery may be needed.

- Swelling and tenderness of the penis may take a few days to clear up.

- The doctor will provide you, or your son, with instructions for keeping the penis clean.

- Your doctor may recommend a visit to a specialist (surgeon or urologist) for further evaluation. Circumcision may be recommended to prevent future problems with paraphimosis.

When should I call your office?

Call our office whenever symptoms related to the foreskin develop, especially pain, tenderness, or swelling of the foreskin or head of the penis.

Hydrocele

Hydrocele is a relatively common condition in newborn boys. The scrotum (sac containing the testicles) becomes enlarged because of excessive fluid. Most of the time, hydrocele is a minor problem that clears up on its own. In more severe cases, or if your son has an inguinal hernia, a minor operation may be needed.

What is hydrocele?

Hydrocele is a collection of fluid in the scrotum. It is present in 1% to 2% of newborn boys. It occurs because of an abnormal opening between the scrotum and the abdomen. Most of the time, the opening closes by the time your baby is born, but occasionally it does not. This is called "noncommunicating" hydrocele; it generally clears up on its own by age 12 months.

If the opening is still present after 1 year ("communicating" hydrocele), the problem is less likely to clear up on its own. Some boys with communicating hydrocele also have a problem called an inguinal hernia, in which part of the intestine slips from the abdomen into the scrotum.

Minor surgery may be needed for hydroceles that are large or do not clear up on their own. Surgery is also needed if an inguinal hernia is present.

What does it look like?

- Swelling of the scrotum.
- Swelling may appear on one or both sides. It is usually painless.
- If the opening that caused hydrocele is still present, the swelling may seem small in the morning but get larger during the day.
- A bulge or lump may appear elsewhere in the groin area. This may be a sign of inguinal hernia.
- Hydroceles are usually relatively small and painless. *If the swelling becomes large or painful, get medical help as soon as possible.*
- Rarely, older boys may develop hydrocele as a complication of another problem of the reproductive organs, such as:
- Testicular torsion (twisting of the spermatic cord leading to the testicles).
- Epididymitis (inflammation or infection of the epididymis, which carries and stores sperm).

What are some possible complications of hydrocele?

- An inguinal hernia may be present in boys with hydrocele that does not get better or changes in size.
- Otherwise, hydroceles rarely cause complications unless they grow very large.

What puts your child at risk of a hydrocele?

There are no known risk factors, and there is no known way to prevent hydrocele.

How is hydrocele treated?

- Most boys with hydrocele don't need treatment. The hydrocele gradually goes away on its own, usually by age 1. The doctor will monitor your child's hydrocele at regular medical visits.
- The doctor will examine your child to make sure that that hydrocele is the cause of the swelling and to check for an inguinal hernia.
- *Surgery* is recommended in certain situations:
  - If an inguinal hernia is present.
  - If the hydrocele is very large. This is because large hydroceles are unlikely to clear up on their own, and they make it difficult to be sure that an inguinal hernia isn't present.
  - If the hydrocele is still present by ages 12 to 18 months.
  - During the operation, the surgeon will also repair an inguinal hernia if it is present.
- Hydrocele repair is a fast and safe operation with a low complication rate. Most children can go home from the hospital the same day as the procedure.
  - Children usually recover very quickly after hydrocele surgery. While your child is recovering, give pain medication and follow other instructions provided by the surgeon.

When should I call your office?

Call our office if:

- Your child still has hydrocele at age 12 months.
- The size of the hydrocele changes from day to day. (An inguinal hernia may be present.)

- Your child develops swelling or tenderness in the groin area.

- After hydrocele surgery, call the surgeon's office (or our office) if your child develops:

- Significant pain or swelling in the groin area.

- Vomiting.

- Fluid draining from the surgical wound.

Hypospadias

Hypospadias is a minor birth defect of the penis in boys. The urethra (the opening that lets urine pass out of the body) is located somewhere other than the tip of the penis. The most common location is on the underside of the penis, at some distance from the tip. Usually, hypospadias can be repaired by a fairly simple operation.

What is hypospadias?

Hypospadias is a congenital abnormality (present since birth) that occurs in about 1 in 250 newborn boys. The opening of the urethra is located away from the tip of the penis (called the *glans penis*), its normal location.

Hypospadias is usually mild and can be repaired by a fairly simple operation. If the opening is not far from the tip of the penis, surgery may not be needed. Surgery may be delayed until your child is 6 to 12 months old. After healing, there are usually no further problems related to hypospadias.

What does it look like?

- The opening of the urethra is found on the underside of the penis rather than at the tip. Hypospadias located near the scrotum (the sac containing the testicles) is less common and more severe.

- The abnormality is usually discovered during the physical examination after birth, or when it is noticed that urine doesn't flow from the tip of the penis.

- The penis may have an obvious curve (called *chordee*), and an abnormality of the foreskin may be present.

- Most boys with hypospadias have no other birth defects. However, some have other malformations, such as undescended testicle or inguinal hernia, which also require treatment. Additional malformations are more likely when hypospadias is located near the scrotum.

What causes hypospadias?

The cause of hypospadias is unknown.

What are some possible complications of hypospadias?

- Without surgery to correct hypospadias, it may lead to problems with urination or fertility.

- Surgery has a high success rate in correcting hypospadias. There is a low risk of complications after surgery.

What puts your child at risk of hypospadias?

If someone else in your family has had hypospadias, your child may be at higher risk. Otherwise, there are no known risk factors.

Can hypospadias be prevented?

There is no known way to prevent hypospadias. Surgery to repair the abnormality will avoid complications later in life.

How is hypospadias treated?

- After initial evaluation, your doctor will recommend a visit to an expert in treating hypospadias, usually a pediatric urologist (a specialist in urinary-tract diseases).

- Usually, no x-rays or other special tests are needed. If your child's hypospadias is found near the scrotum, tests for other abnormalities may be recommended.

- *Surgery* is the usual treatment for hypospadias.

- The surgeon may recommend waiting to perform the surgery until your son is 6 to 12 months old. This helps further reduce the small risks of anesthesia. Your child will receive anesthesia during the operation and medication to reduce pain afterward.

- If your child has hypospadias, circumcision (minor surgery to remove the foreskin of the penis) should be delayed, as the foreskin is often used in repairing the hypospadias.

- If hypospadias is located near the tip of the penis, the operation is simple. Success rates are high, and complications are few.

- If hypospadias is very mild—that is, if the opening is very near the tip of the penis—it may be possible to avoid surgery. The pediatric urologist can explain the advantages and disadvantages of performing or avoiding surgery in this situation.

- For more severe hypospadias, that is—if the opening is located near the scrotum—surgery is more complicated. Success rates are still high, but complications are somewhat more common.

- Any related abnormalities, such as abnormal curvature of the penis or an inguinal hernia, will probably be corrected during the same operation.

- Your child should heal quickly after surgery. Most boys have no further problems related to hypospadias.

When should I call your office?

- Call your surgeon's office or our office if there are any signs of healing problems, infection (redness, tenderness, fever), or abnormal urination after surgery for hypospadias.

Testicular Torsion

Testicular torsion is the most serious cause of pain of the scrotum (the sac containing the testicles) in boys. This causes interruption of the blood supply, which can rapidly lead to permanent damage to the testicle. Immediate surgery is required. Boys who are having pain in the testicles always need prompt medical attention.

What is testicular torsion?

Testicular torsion occurs when the spermatic cord leading to the testicles becomes twisted. It causes sudden pain and swelling of the scrotum. Loss of blood supply to the affected testicle can rapidly cause damage.

Boys with pain and swelling of the scrotum need immediate medical attention. If your child has testicular torsion, he will probably need emergency surgery. In severe cases, surgery should be performed within 4 to 6 hours to prevent permanent damage to the testicle. In less severe cases, the testicle can still be saved if surgery is performed within a day or two.

What does it look like?

- Sudden pain and swelling of the scrotum. Pain may be severe. The scrotum may appear red and very tender.

- Vomiting, sweating, and other symptoms related to severe pain.

- Your son may have recently (but not necessarily) had an injury to the scrotum.

- Testicular torsion most commonly occurs during the teenage years. It can also be present at birth in newborn boys. In newborns, the scrotum appears enlarged and bruised on one side, usually not red and tender.

What causes testicular torsion?

- In some boys, the testicles are not well attached in the scrotum, allowing them to move around more than they should. This can result in twisting (torsion) of the spermatic cord.

- Torsion sometimes occurs after an injury or exercise. However, at other times there is no noticeable injury or other responsible event.

What are some possible complications of testicular torsion?

- Damage to the testicle can occur within hours. Emergency surgery can reduce this risk if it is performed within 6 hours or so.

- The testicle's ability to produce sperm may be impaired. This does not necessarily mean your son will be infertile (unable to have children). Fertility may still be normal as long as the other testicle is unharmed.

- In severe cases, the testicle may die. If this occurs, surgery may be needed to remove it.

What puts your child at risk of testicular torsion?

- Torsion is most common in boys ages 12 and older. It rarely occurs in boys under 10.

- There are no known risk factors. However, if torsion occurs in one testicle, there is a risk that it may occur in the other testicle. When your son has surgery for testicular torsion, the surgeon will place a few stitches in the second testicle to prevent it from becoming rotated.

Can testicular torsion be prevented?

There is no known prevention. Immediate surgery is usually needed to prevent permanent damage to the testicle.

How is testicular torsion diagnosed?

- Your son will be examined to see if testicular torsion is the cause of his pain and swelling. There are some other conditions that can cause similar symptoms, such as epididymitis (inflammation or infection of the epididymis, which carries and stores sperm) or inguinal hernia (part of the intestine slipping through an opening between the abdomen and groin).

- The doctor may recommend tests, such as ultrasound, to confirm the diagnosis before surgery.

- Another, less serious condition, called *torsion of the appendix testis,* can cause similar symptoms. This occurs when a small bit of tissue attached to the testicle (the "appendix testis") becomes twisted.

  - Torsion of the appendix testis also causes pain and swelling of the scrotum. The pain usually develops gradually, not suddenly.

  - It is more common in younger boys (ages 2 to 11).

  - Torsion of the appendix testis does not usually require surgery. However, it can be difficult to distinguish between torsion of the appendix testis and testicular torsion. If there is any doubt about the diagnosis, the doctor may recommend surgery.

How is testicular torsion treated?

Before surgery.

- If the pain has been present for only a few hours, the doctor may attempt to untwist the testicle by hand. If this maneuver is successful, it can provide rapid pain relief. However, your son may still need further evaluation and possible surgery.

Emergency surgery.

- For many boys with testicular torsion, emergency surgery is needed. Your son will be asleep (under general anesthesia) for the surgery.

- The surgeon will untwist the spermatic cord, returning blood flow to the testicle. He or she will then place a few stitches to make sure the testicle doesn't become rotated again. This part of the operation is called *orchiopexy*. The same will be done to the opposite testicle.

- During the operation, the surgeon will look for any signs of permanent damage to the testicle. If torsion is severe and/or has been present for a long time, the testicle may have been badly damaged or may even have died. If so, it will need to be removed. As long as the other testicle is undamaged, your son may still be fertile (able to have a child).

In newborns.

- Some boys are born with testicular torsion. This is usually obvious at birth.

- In most babies born with this condition, the torsion occurred weeks earlier. By the time the baby is born, the testicle is permanently damaged.

- Especially for the first month, your son will be at high risk for torsion of the other testicle. Your doctor will arrange a visit to a specialist (pediatric urologist) for evaluation. This expert can recommend the most appropriate treatment for your son's condition.

When should I call your office?

Boys with severe pain in the testicles always need prompt medical attention.

- After surgery for testicular torsion, call the surgeon (or our office) if the following occur:
  - Continued pain and swelling.
  - Redness or fluid oozing from the surgical wound.

Undescended Testicles

Undescended testicles are a common problem in newborn boys. In this condition, one or both testicles did not drop down (descend) from the abdomen into the scrotum before your child was born. In most babies, the testicles normally descend by 3 months of age. If this does not happen by 6 months, an operation may be needed to bring them down.

What are undescended testicles?

During development of boy babies, the testicles normally drop from the abdomen into the scrotum (the sac containing the testicles) during the last few weeks of pregnancy. Sometimes, this doesn't happen before the baby is born. Usually just one testicle doesn't drop, but sometimes both are affected. Undescended testicle(s) is sometimes called *cryptorchidism.*

In most babies, the testicle eventually descends, usually during the first 3 months of life. If this doesn't happen by age 6 months, it is unlikely to happen on its own. A simple operation can be done to bring the testicle down. As an adult, your son will be at increased risk of cancers of the originally undescended testicle

What does it look like?

- The testicle cannot be seen or felt in the scrotum.

- Usually just one testicle is undescended. In about 10% of babies with this problem, both testicles are undescended.

- Sometimes the testicle can be felt in another location, such as the groin.

- At other times the testicle cannot be felt at all. In about half of these boys, the testicle is absent—it either didn't develop normally or it was injured some time during the pregnancy.

- In some boys, a testicle may be located in the scrotum. This is called "retractile testicles" and is sometimes confused with undescended testicles. Usually, retractile testicles require no treatment. However, medical follow-up is needed because the testicles may rise again and remain "undescended."

- Less often, testicles are found in the scrotum at birth but later move back up out of the scrotum. This is called "acquired" undescended testicles. It is most common between ages 4 and 10. If the testicles do not come back down, treatment is required.

What causes undescended testicles?

- The cause of undescended testicles is unknown.

- If neither of the testicles can be felt, tests will be done to make certain of the sex of your newborn.

What are some possible complications of undescended testicles?

- *Infertility.* With proper treatment, most boys with undescended testicles remain fertile (able to have children). The risk of infertility is higher for boys with two undescended testicles.

- *Testicular cancer.* As a teenager and young adult, your son will be at increased risk of cancer of the testicles. This risk is highest from ages 15 to 40.

  - Cancer risk remains higher even if your son has surgery to bring the testicle down.

  - As an adult, your son should receive regular checkups and perform self-examination to detect testicular cancers as early as possible.

  - Boys with rectractile testicles are not at increased risk of infertility or testicular cancer.

What puts your child at risk of undescended testicles?

- Over 4% of boys have undescended testicles at birth.

- For premature babies, the risk increases to 30%.

Can undescended testicles be prevented?

- There is no known way to prevent undescended testicles.

- If testicles remain undescended after the first few months of life, surgery may help to prevent infertility later in life.

How are undescended testicles treated?

- If your child is born with undescended testicles, he will receive regular examinations to check their position. In most cases, the testicles drop to their normal position in the scrotum by the age of 3 months.

- If your son has retractile testicles, he probably will not need any treatment. However, follow-up examinations are necessary to make sure the testicles stay down.

- If your son's testicles have not dropped on their own by the time he is 6 months old, they probably never will. We will probably recommend a visit to a urologist or other specialist for evaluation and treatment.

- As time goes on, the undescended testicles are gradually damaged. This occurs because the testicles become too warm when they remain inside the body. They need the relatively cooler location of the scrotum to develop normally.

- *Surgery for undescended testicles.*

  - Surgery for undescended testicles is a relatively minor procedure called *orchiopexy*. Most likely, your son won't even have to stay in the hospital overnight. The operation is highly successful in bringing the undescended testicles down to their normal position in the scrotum and keeping them there.

  - In some boys with undescended testicles, the position of the testicles cannot be felt. In about half of these boys, the testicle is found inside the abdomen. If the testicle is otherwise normal, it can still be brought down to the scrotum and develop normally there.

  - In other boys whose testicles cannot be felt before surgery, the testicles may turn out to be missing or shrunken. This is sometimes called "vanishing" testicle.

- Vanishing testicle probably occurs because the testicle was injured during pregnancy. In this case, the testicle has been severely and permanently damaged, and only a remnant is left.

  - If the testicle has been damaged badly, the surgeon will probably remove it. Your son may still be fertile as long as the other testicle has not been harmed.

- *After surgery.*

  - Your son should recover quickly and completely after the orchiopexy procedure.

  - If surgery for undescended testicle is required, your son will be at increased risk of testicular cancer. He will need regular medical examinations beginning in the teenage years. He should also learn to perform regular testicular self-examination to detect any cancers as early as possible.

When should I call your office?

Call our office if:

- Your son is born with undescended testicles. The doctor will monitor this condition at each regular checkup. Call our office if you have any questions or concerns.

- The testicles have not dropped to their normal position by age 6 months. We will probably recommend a visit to a urologist or other specialist for further evaluation and treatment.

Varicocele

Varicocele is a dilated (enlarged) group of veins in the scrotum (the sac containing the testicles) in teenage boys and young men. Varicoceles are usually painless, although your child may feel a lump around one testicle—usually the left one. Varicoceles can lead to reduced fertility. Surgery may help to prevent this complication.

What is a varicocele?

A varicocele is an abnormality of the blood vessels in the scrotum, usually developing in teenage boys and young men. Varicoceles are a common cause of reduced fertility (the ability to have children) in men. They do not lead to any other health problems.

Varicoceles are usually painless. Your son may feel a lump near one of his testicles. Over time, the testicle with a varicocele may start to shrink. By the time this happens, the testicle's ability to produce sperm may be affected. Surgery to remove the varicocele may help to prevent problems with fertility.

What does it look like?

- Varicocele is usually painless but can cause a dull ache in the affected testicle.

- Your child (or the doctor) may feel a lump or mass around the testicle. The lump is sometimes described as feeling like a "bag of worms." It may be felt only when your child is standing, and it may go away or feel smaller when he lies down.

- Varicoceles nearly always occur on the left testicle. Sometimes both sides have varicoceles.

- The testicle on the side with the varicocele may be smaller than the other testicle.

- Varicoceles most commonly develop in the middle teen to young adult years. They rarely develop before puberty.

What causes a varicocele?

Varicoceles develop when a valve in one of the veins connected to the testicles does not work properly. Too much blood builds up, causing the veins to widen (dilate). Over time, this damages the affected testicle. The testicle may shrink, and its ability to make sperm may be reduced.

What are some possible complications of varicocele?

Reduced fertility is the main complication. About 15% of men with varicoceles will have trouble fathering a child.

What puts your child at risk of varicocele?

About 15% of men have a varicocele. There are no specific risk factors.

Can varicocele be prevented?

- There is no known way to predict varicoceles from developing.

- Surgery to remove the varicocele may prevent later fertility problems.

How is varicocele treated?

- We may recommend a visit to a urologist, a specialist in treating diseases of the reproductive organs.

- If varicocele is present only on the right testicle or if it develops before age 10, further evaluation is needed to search for the cause. There could be a mass somewhere in the abdomen causing the varicocele.

- Surgery may be recommended to remove the varicocele in certain situations:

  - If varicocele is present on both sides of the scrotum, near both testicles.

  - If the testicle on the side with the varicocele is smaller than the other testicle.

  - If pain is present.

  - If the varicocele is very large.

  - The operation to correct varicocele (called varicocelectomy) is very simple. A small incision is made and the abnormal blood vessel is blocked off. Usually, there is no need for your child to stay overnight in the hospital.

  - Anesthesia will prevent your son from feeling any pain during the procedure. Afterward, ice packs and medications can be used to reduce pain and swelling.

  - Your child should recover quickly after the operation. There is a small risk of complications; the urologist can advise you of these risks.

  - Surgery to correct varicocele can still be successful later in life if your son has fertility problems. However, performing surgery at a younger age reduces the chance of ever developing such problems.

When should I call your office?

Call our office if:

- Your son develops pain or swelling of the scrotum or testicles. Although varicocele is usually painless, pain can occur. There are other possible causes of pain in this area, some of which are serious.

- Boys with pain in the testicles always need prompt medical attention.

Section XV ▪ The Heart

Arrhythmias and Palpitations

Arrhythmias are abnormal heart rates or rhythms. The heart rate may be too fast, too slow, or irregular. Arrhythmias requiring treatment are not common in children. When present, they can usually be treated with medications. Palpitations simply mean that a person feels or is aware of the heartbeat. Although palpitations are occasionally a symptom of arrhythmias, most of the time they are harmless.

What are arrhythmias?

Arrhythmias are abnormal heart rates or rhythms. The heart rhythm is the pattern of the heart rate—usually a consistent, regularly timed beat. When the rhythm is variable—not in a regular pattern—an arrhythmia may be present. *Tachycardia* means fast heartbeat, while *bradycardia* means slow heartbeat.

Medically important arrhythmias are relatively common in adults but uncommon in children. Some arrhythmias are normal and of no concern. For example, "sinus arrhythmia" is normal in children. This arrhythmia consists of normal changes in heart rate that occur with each breath. Athletes may have "sinus bradycardia," which means that their heart rate is slow because of their good physical condition. Occasional extra beats are also usually harmless but may occur in certain diseases. Arrhythmias are important to diagnose because the abnormal heart rate or rhythm may affect how well the heart is able to pump blood and oxygen to the brain and other organs.

Palpitations refer to the person's awareness of their heartbeat. Although they can be a symptom of an abnormal arrhythmia, most palpitations are not a sign of disease. They may be caused by exercise, stress, certain drugs (like caffeine or cold medications), anxiety, or many other causes. A doctor needs to determine whether palpitations are a medical problem.

What do they look like?

Palpitations. Your child is aware of his or her heartbeat, whether it is slow, fast, or irregular. Sometimes it seems like the heart skips a beat, or a few beats occur quickly together. Beats may be "pounding" or "fluttering." These descriptions may help the doctor to determine whether palpitations are a medical problem.

Arrhythmias. Some possible symptoms include:

- Light headeness or tiredness may occur.
- Palpitations.
- Fainting can occur. Get medical attention.
- Chest pain can occur but is uncommon.

- Occasionally, heart failure may be present. Symptoms include difficulty breathing and swelling of the feet and other areas.

What causes arrhythmias?

A number of causes are possible:

- For some arrhythmias, the cause is unknown.
- Some are caused by drugs, such as caffeine, cold medicines, or asthma medications. Arrhythmias may also be caused by drugs of abuse, like cocaine.
- Some arrhythmias are related to heart problems. They may occur after surgery for congenital heart defects, infection or inflammation of the heart (such as myocarditis or rheumatic fever), or abnormal electrical pathways in the heart.
- Some result from medical conditions that don't affect the heart directly but cause a fast heart rate (for example, anemia or hyperthyroidism).

Other causes are possible.

What puts your child at risk of arrhythmias?

- Various congenital heart defects or heart surgery.
- Rare genetic conditions such as long QT syndrome.
- Certain drugs and medications.

How are arrhythmias diagnosed?

Some arrhythmias are detected when the doctor hears an abnormal heart rate or rhythm through the stethoscope (an instrument used to amplify the heart sounds). Others will require further testing and evaluation.

We may recommend a visit to a doctor specializing in treatment of heart diseases (a cardiologist). The cardiologist may perform additional tests, including:

- An electrocardiogram (ECG) to measure the electrical activity during your child's heartbeat. This provides a lot of information about your child's heart rate, including whether it is irregular, too fast, or too slow, and other information about how the heart is working.
- In some situations, the doctor may recommend 24-hour (ambulatory) ECG monitoring. This provides a full day's worth of information about your child's heart rate and rhythm. The cardiologist may also recommend a stress ECG, which monitors heart activity during exercise.
- An echocardiogram ("echo") uses sound waves to take pictures or your child's heart while it is beating. This is especially important for determining whether your child was born with any congenital heart defects.

For some patients, the cardiologist may perform special electrical conduction studies. These are done to map abnormal electrical pathways that may be causing an arrhythmia.

How are arrhythmias treated?

Most palpitations don't indicate a medical problem, but they do need to be checked by a doctor. The doctor will evaluate your child to look for any other signs of heart disease or other conditions that can cause palpitations. If none are found, then occasional episodes of palpitations are nothing to worry about. Simply knowing this may help to reduce anxiety for both the child and parents. In some situations, evaluation and treatment for anxiety may be helpful.

Most arrhythmias are not medically significant. The doctor will determine whether there is any heart-related or other medical cause that can be treated. If no specific heart-related problem is found, different treatments may be required, depending on the type of arrhythmia. This will be determined by the cardiologist.

Treatment depends on your child's diagnosis and the specific abnormality causing the arrhythmia but may include:

- *Medications.* Most arrhythmias can be controlled using medications. Different types of arrhythmias may require different medications.

- *Ablation.* After thorough testing to identify the source of abnormal electrical signals, the cardiologist can do a procedure to destroy (ablate) that small area of heart tissue. This procedure is done through a catheter placed through the blood vessels into your child's heart. It may be needed if medications aren't enough to control your child's arrhythmia or if the problem is severe or possibly life-threatening.

- *Pacemaker.* In more severe arrhythmias, a pacemaker may be placed. This is an electronic device that helps control your child's heartbeat. Pacemakers are only used when there is a risk of potentially serious or fatal episodes of arrhythmias, such as ventricular fibrillation.

  - Another option may be an implantable cardioverter/defibrillator. This is a device that detects arrhythmias, especially ventricular fibrillation, a life-threatening arrythmia. The device delivers an electrical shock to return the heartbeat to normal.

- In emergency situations, a treatment called *electrical cardioversion* may be needed. In this procedure, an electrical charge is delivered to the body. The "shock" ends the abnormal heartbeat, returning the rhythm to normal.

Obviously, these more serious arrhythmias require expert medical care and follow-up. Some of these conditions require lifelong medical care. With modern medical treatment, including use of a pacemaker if necessary, most arrhythmias in children can be successfully managed.

When should I call your office?

During your child's treatment for arrhythmias, call your cardiologist (or our office if necessary) if medications or other treatments don't seem to be effective in controlling episodes of abnormal heartbeat.

During episodes of arrhythmia, the following symptoms may signal an emergency! Get medical help immediately (call 911 or go to the emergency room):

- Fainting/unconsciousness.

- Chest pain.

- Rapid or difficult breathing.

Heart Murmurs (Innocent Murmurs)

Heart murmurs are an extra sound the heart makes when pumping blood. By far, most heart murmurs are innocent, meaning there is no heart disease present. However, some heart murmurs are pathological, meaning they are a sign of disease. If the doctor has any reason to suspect a pathological heart murmur, further testing will be done.

What are heart murmurs?

A heart murmur does not necessarily mean that your child has heart disease! It's the medical term for a type of extra sound made by the heart.

The heart has four chambers through which blood flows. The chambers are connected by valves. Heart sounds are caused by opening and closing of the valves and movement of blood through the heart chambers. Heart murmurs are the sound of blood flowing through the chambers or out from the heart. Most murmurs sound like a hum or like water rushing through a hose.

Heart murmurs are commonly found in children during regular checkups, most often between the ages of 3 and 7. By far, most heart murmurs are "innocent"—not a sign of heart disease. Temporary conditions affecting your child's heartbeat may increase the likelihood of an innocent murmur, for example, if your child is sick (such as with a fever) or anxious.

Other heart murmurs, known as "pathological" murmurs, are an important sign of heart disease. If the doctor has any reason to suspect a pathological heart murmur, your child will be sent for further tests.

How are heart murmurs diagnosed?

- In many cases, the doctor can be pretty sure a heart murmur is innocent just by listening to it with a stethoscope (an instrument that amplifies the heart sounds). If the doctor diagnoses an innocent heart murmur, no testing is needed, and there is no increased risk of future heart problems.

- If there is any reason for concern, the doctor may arrange for further tests, such as an electrocardiogram (ECG), which measures the electrical activity during your child's heartbeat; an echocardiogram ("echo"), which uses sound waves to take pictures of your child's heart while it is beating; or chest x-rays. We may also recommend a visit to a heart specialist (a *cardiologist*).

- We are more likely to recommend further evaluation in infants, or if your child has any other symptoms of heart disease, for example, slow growth or blue color of the skin (cyanosis).

How are innocent heart murmurs managed?

- If your child has an innocent heart murmur, he or she needs no treatment! Innocent murmur means there's nothing wrong with the heart and no increased risk of future heart disease.

- There is no need to limit your child's activity because of an innocent heart murmur. He or she can run, play, go to gym class or camp, and do any other type of normal childhood activity.

- The heart murmur may or may not go away as your child grows. (It doesn't really matter, because it's a harmless condition.) The murmur may become more noticeable in some situations, such as when your child has a fever.

Remember to tell other doctors and health care providers about your child's heart murmur. This will help to avoid unnecessary concern and testing.

When should I call your office?

Call our office if you have any additional questions or concerns about your child's heart murmur. Remember, an innocent murmur indicates no heart disease!

High Blood Pressure (Hypertension)

There are many possible causes of high blood pressure in children. In young children, high blood pressure is most often caused by other diseases, particularly kidney disease. In adolescents, high blood pressure often occurs without other diseases; this is called essential hypertension. It may be related to other factors such as obesity and family history and occurs most often in obese teens. Treatment to reduce high blood pressure is needed to prevent long-term damage to organs such as the heart, brain, and kidneys.

What is high blood pressure?

Hypertension is the medical term for high blood pressure. You probably know that high blood pressure is a common problem in adults, but it can also occur in children and teens. Hypertension is *not* diagnosed from a single blood pressure measurement (unless it is very high or if other symptoms are present) but after a number of measurements over time.

In younger children, high blood pressure is usually "secondary" or caused by other diseases. The most common causes are diseases of the kidneys and/or blood vessels. Treating the underlying cause usually corrects the high blood pressure.

In adolescents, like adults, high blood pressure can occur on its own. This is called "essential" or "primary" hypertension, and it is most common in obese teens. Treatment is needed. For many teens, high blood pressure can be reduced through diet and exercise.

What does it look like?

High blood pressure usually causes no symptoms. Most of the time, it is detected on routine medical checkups.

- *Essential hypertension* (no underlying disease) is rare in preteen children. Most teens with high blood pressure are overweight or obese, but not all. Many teens with essential hypertension have parents with high blood pressure too.

- *Secondary hypertension* (increased blood pressure caused by other diseases) also usually causes no symptoms. Although symptoms may be present, they are generally caused by whatever disease is causing your child's hypertension.

Although uncommon, symptoms such as headache, fainting, or seizures may occur if blood pressure is very high.

- Get medical help if your child has any of these symptoms.

What causes high blood pressure?

- *Essential hypertension.* In teens as in adults, the cause of high blood pressure is usually unknown. The most important cause is genetics—high blood pressure tends to run in families. Other factors, such as weight, diet, and stress, also play a role.

- *Secondary hypertension.* Many causes are possible, including:

  - Kidney disease. This is the most common cause of high blood pressure in children. Specific causes include problems with repeated infection (pyelonephritis) or inflammation caused by an immune system reaction (glomerulonephritis).

  - Drugs and medications. Many substances can cause high blood pressure, including medications, drugs of abuse (especially cocaine), and oral contraceptives (birth control pills).

  - Endocrine diseases, such as hyperthyroidism.

What are some possible complications of high blood pressure?

- High blood pressure is a major contributor to heart disease, stroke, and kidney failure. These complications occur because high blood pressure gradually causes damage to the heart, brain, and kidneys.

- When hypertension develops in the teen years, there is a high risk it will continue into adulthood. Prevention and treatment of high blood pressure in teens and young adults is a key goal of efforts to prevent heart disease and stroke.

What puts your child at risk of high blood pressure?

For *essential hypertension* in teens, the main risk factors are:

- Genetics. If one or both parents have high blood pressure, the child may be at higher risk. Children of parents with hypertension have increased blood pressure and heart rate. This is especially true of African-American children.

- Obesity. Like adults, teens who are overweight or obese are most likely to develop high blood pressure.

For *secondary hypertension,* risk factors depend on the specific disease causing high blood pressure.

Can high blood pressure be prevented?

The most important steps in reducing the risks of high blood pressure in teens (and adults) are:

- Not smoking. If you are already a smoker, our office can give you advice on how to quit.

- Keeping weight under control by exercising regularly and eating a sensible diet.

How is high blood pressure diagnosed and treated?

Most of the time, repeated measurements of blood pressure are needed to diagnose hypertension. Some people get nervous at the doctor's office, causing blood pressure to increase. This is sometimes called "white coat hypertension." In this case, blood pressure may be measured at home by the parents to get an idea of the true blood pressure. For some patients, especially teens with borderline hypertension, we may recommend 24-hour (ambulatory) blood pressure monitoring. This provides a full day's worth of information about your child's blood pressure.

If your child is diagnosed with hypertension, the doctor will perform an examination and tests to determine the cause and appropriate treatment. This may include tests for kidney disease or other conditions that can cause high blood pressure, especially in children under 10.

If your child has even mild hypertension, the doctor will likely recommend treatment in order to lower the blood pressure to normal.

- *Nondrug Treatment.* For many teens with hypertension, exercise, weight loss, and cutting back on salt in the diet are enough to reduce high blood pressure. It's also important to avoid smoking and alcohol use. We may recommend avoiding medications that could contribute to high blood pressure, such as cold medicines or birth control pills. If these measures do not reduce your child's blood pressure, the doctor will likely recommend medications.

- *Drug Treatment.* There are many types of blood pressure–lowering medications. Your doctor will recommend the best kind for your child's type of blood pressure. Options include diuretics ("water pills," which work by increasing the amount of urine made by the kidneys) or certain types of medications that affect the cardiovascular system, such as beta-blockers, ACE inhibitors, or calcium channel blockers. This part of your child's care may be directed by a kidney specialist (nephrologist) or another specialist.

- Your child will need regular follow-up visits to be sure treatment is effective. Sometimes a few medications have to be tried to get the blood pressure to go down.

- Side effects can occur. These will be checked as part of medical follow-up. Be sure to tell your doctor if you think your child may be having medication side effects.

- It is important that your child follow his or her prescribed treatment. This may be difficult for teens (and adults) with high blood pressure; they usually feel fine and don't want to take medications. You and your child must understand that uncontrolled high blood pressure greatly increases the risk of heart disease, stroke, and other serious diseases later in life.

When should I call your office?

Call our office if your child has:

- Any symptoms that may be related to high blood pressure, like severe or frequent headaches, fainting, or seizures.

- Possible side effects of blood pressure–lowering drugs.

Kawasaki Disease

Kawasaki disease is a condition involving inflammation of the blood vessels in young children. Children with this disease develop a high fever lasting five or more days, rash, red eyes and lips, and other symptoms. The main danger is a risk of damage to the blood vessels in the heart. Treatment is needed to reduce the chances of this complication. With treatment, most children with Kawasaki disease recover completely.

What is Kawasaki disease?

Kawasaki disease is a potentially serious disease involving inflammation of the blood vessels (vasculitis) in children, mainly under age 5. The cause is unknown. Children with Kawasaki disease can become very ill for a week or two, then take a long time to recover if untreated.

Although most children recover completely, there is a risk of damage to the coronary arteries supplying blood to the heart. This complication occurs in about 20% of children with Kawasaki disease if not treated. With appropriate treatment, the risk drops to 5%. The longer the initial fever lasts, the higher the risk.

Children with Kawasaki disease need timely treatment and close follow-up during the recovery period. If there are no complications, your child should recover completely over a period of several weeks.

What does it look like?

The first symptom of Kawasaki disease is fever:

- Fever may be very high—up to 104°F (40°C).
- Fever comes and goes.
- It usually lasts 1 to 2 weeks, if untreated.
- It does not improve with antibiotics.

Other typical symptoms are:

- Red eyes.
- Red, dry, cracked lips; red, swollen mouth and throat, including "strawberry tongue."
- Redness and swelling of the palms and soles, followed by peeling of the skin on the fingers and toes.
- Various skin rashes.
- Swelling of the lymph nodes in the neck, usually on one side.
- During the illness, children are usually very fussy. Other, less common symptoms include:

- Joint swelling.
- Vomiting.
- Inflammation of the urethra (opening where urine comes out).
- Swollen gallbladder.

The early, acute phase of Kawasaki disease lasts 1 to 2 weeks. Illness becomes less severe for about a month afterward. The risk of coronary artery disease is highest during this period. Your child then slowly gets better over another month or two. All symptoms are much shortened by appropriate treatment.

Heart involvement is the most serious problem. Various parts of the heart may be affected. However, permanent damage can result from inflammation of the coronary arteries, which supply blood to the heart muscle.

What causes Kawasaki disease?

The exact cause is unknown.

What are some possible complications of Kawasaki disease?

Heart problems are the main complication of Kawasaki disease. Most of the symptoms result from inflammation of the blood vessels.

- *Myocarditis or pericarditis.* Inflammation of the heart muscle or heart lining. Early in the illness, these complications may cause fast heartbeat or reduced heart function.

- *Coronary artery aneurysms.* Inflammation of the vessels that supply blood to the heart muscle can lead to "weak spots" in the vessel walls, causing them to balloon out or dilate. These weak spots, called aneurysms, can develop a blood clot (thrombosis). The clot can prevent enough blood from getting to the heart muscle, causing problems such as myocardial infarction (MI, or "heart attack").

- *Without treatment,* about one fifth of children with Kawasaki disease develop aneurysms. The risk is highest in the second or third week of illness.

- *With treatment,* the risk of coronary artery damage is reduced to less than 5%.

As long as heart and blood vessel damage does not occur, most children with Kawasaki disease recover completely. Even without treatment, about 50% of aneurysms go away. There may still be some mild abnormalities, such as narrowing of the blood vessels.

What puts your child at risk of Kawasaki disease?

- Kawasaki disease almost always occurs in infants and children under age 5.
- The risk is highest in Asian children, but any racial/ethnic group can be affected.

Can Kawasaki disease be prevented?

There is no known way to prevent Kawasaki disease.

How is Kawasaki disease diagnosed?

There is no specific test for Kawasaki disease. The diagnosis is based on symptoms, with the help of some blood tests, especially tests for inflammation such as the erythrocyte sedimentation rate (ESR). Increased platelet counts (blood particles that help stop bleeding) may be present.

Because of the risk of heart and blood vessel complications, it's important to diagnose Kawasaki disease promptly. Unfortunately, Kawasaki disease can be difficult to recognize; at first, it may be confused with viral infections, strep infections, or others. Diagnosis is especially difficult if your child doesn't have the typical symptoms.

Once the disease is recognized, a test called echocardiography ("echo") may be done to check for damage to the heart and blood vessels. This painless test uses sound waves to take pictures of your child's heart. It may be repeated a few times to look for aneurysms and other abnormalities. A specialist in children's heart diseases (a pediatric cardiologist) will supervise this part of your child's care.

How is Kawasaki disease treated?

Once Kawasaki disease is recognized, your child will be admitted to the hospital for treatment.

- Treatment consists of giving *immune globulin*, which is the part of our blood that contains our antibodies. When given intravenously it is called IVIG. Antibodies are made by our immune system to fight infection. *Aspirin* is also given, at first for inflammation and then to prevent any clots from forming on aneurythms that might be present.

  - For most children, this treatment quickly reduces fever and other symptoms.

  - Treatment greatly reduces the risk of heart and blood vessel complications.

  - Treatment is most effective if started within 10 days after the start of your child's illness. Treatment is usually still given if Kawasaki disease is recognized later on, but it is not known how effective it is.

  - Your child's doctors will closely monitor his or her condition during treatment. If the response is not as good as expected, treatment may be repeated or other drugs (such as steroids tried).

- If your child's tests find no heart or blood vessel abnormalities, aspirin treatment should continue at a lower dose for 6 to 8 weeks from the start of illness. It may take several more weeks before your child recovers completely.

- If heart or blood vessel abnormalities are present, your child will need further treatment. Echocardiograms will be done to check on your child's condition.

  - Medications such as aspirin and warfarin (coumadin) are used to prevent clotting. Blood clots can be removed if necessary.

  - Small aneurysms usually clear up in a year or two, but some abnormalities may remain. If your child has a small aneurysm, he or she may have to continue taking aspirin for a long time.

  - If your child has a large aneurysm or more than one aneurysm, other treatments may be needed.

  - With close medical follow-up, the risk of death from complications of Kawasaki disease is low.

When should I call your office?

Call the pediatric cardiologist, or our office, if your have questions regarding Kawasaki disease and your child's treatment and recovery.

Rheumatic Fever and Rheumatic Heart Disease

> Rheumatic fever results from infection with bacteria called group A streptococci, usually "strep throat." Illness begins 2 to 3 weeks after strep throat and can involve the heart (carditis), joints (arthritis), skin, and brain (uncontrolled movements called chorea). If carditis is present, it can cause later damage to the heart valves; this is called rheumatic heart disease. Your child may need antibiotics to keep rheumatic fever from coming back.
>
> This is a potentially serious condition requiring close medical follow-up.

What are rheumatic fever and rheumatic heart disease?

Rheumatic fever is much less frequent in the United States than it once was, although outbreaks can still occur. It remains a common problem in poor countries.

Rheumatic fever is not an infection but the body's response to the group A streptococci bacteria that cause strep throat. By the time rheumatic fever develops, the infection is usually no longer present. However, antibodies to the bacteria can still be found in your child's blood. It's not clear exactly how the reaction to strep bacteria causes problems with the heart, joints, and other organs. It may result from some toxic effect of the bacteria, or from the way your child's immune system reacts to the bacteria.

Rheumatic fever can cause inflammation of the heart (carditis), inflammation of the joints (arthritis), small lumps under the skin (subcutaneous nodules), a skin rash (erythema marginatum), and uncontrolled body movements, especially of the arms (chorea). Inflammation of the heart can cause permanent damage to the heart valves, called *rheumatic heart disease*. This damage shows up fairly long after the initial attack of rheumatic fever. Not everyone who gets rheumatic fever has heart involvement or rheumatic heart disease.

Antibiotic treatment for strep throat greatly reduces the risk of rheumatic fever. With close medical follow-up, most children recover completely. Your child may need to continue taking antibiotics indefinitely to prevent future attacks of rheumatic fever.

What does rheumatic fever look like?

The symptoms of rheumatic fever vary a lot. Rheumatic fever *always* occurs a few weeks after an episode of strep infection, usually strep throat. However, the infection may have been a mild one.

A few weeks after the infection, symptoms of acute rheumatic fever develop. Symptoms usually include fever—102°F (39°C) or higher—along with one or more of the following:

- *Carditis.* Occurs in at least half of patients. Inflammation of the heart valves (valvulitis) or the inside lining of the heart (endocarditis) is usually present. Inflammation can cause damage to the heart valves, which shows up years later. This later damage to the heart valves is rheumatic heart disease. Symptoms of carditis include:

  - Chest pain; difficulty with activity.

  - Heart rate may seem fast. The doctor will listen for abnormal heart sounds and murmurs (extra sounds the heart makes; sometimes normal, sometimes not), which may reflect heart involvement.

  - Heart involvement ranges from a mild, temporary problem to severe heart failure.

- *Arthritis.* Occurs in most children with rheumatic fever. Not just joint pain, but painful, swollen joints. Pain is worse with movement.

  - Usually affects large joints, such as knees, ankles, wrists, and elbows.

  - Joints are hot, red, swollen, and very tender.

  - Pain and swelling tend to move from one joint to another. This is called *migratory polyarthritis,* and it is a major symptom of rheumatic fever.

- *Chorea* (pronounced "korea"). Nervous system involvement causing uncontrolled movements of the arms and other parts of the body. Behavior changes may be present as well.

- *Rash.* Children with rheumatic fever have a typical red, "squiggly" skin rash, called *erythema marginatum.*

- *Bumps under the skin,* called subcutaneous nodules.

What are some possible complications of rheumatic fever?

- *Rheumatic heart disease* is the main complication of rheumatic fever. Damage to the heart valves typically shows up years after the attack of rheumatic fever and can be a lifelong problem. Antibiotics and other treatment reduce this risk.

- Other symptoms, like arthritis and chorea, generally get better and cause no further problems.

- After recovery, there is a risk that rheumatic fever will occur again. Your child will receive antibiotics to prevent repeated strep infection that could lead to recurrences of rheumatic fever.

What puts your child at risk of rheumatic fever?

- Rheumatic fever, and therefore rheumatic heart disease, is uncommon in the United States. The main risk factor is getting strep throat. The group A strep bacteria are usually passed from person to person. The risk of rheumatic fever is very low if strep infection is treated with appropriate antibiotics. Even without treatment, most cases of strep throat don't lead to rheumatic fever.

- Rheumatic fever occurs most commonly between early school age and the teen years. Although strep infections may occur at any time of year, they are most common in winter and spring.

Can rheumatic fever be prevented?

Most of the time, there is no practical way to prevent strep infection. If your child has strep throat, antibiotic treatment is essential to reduce the risk of rheumatic fever. Be sure to continue taking antibiotics for the total time prescribed—usually 10 days. Amoxicillin and penicillin are the most commonly used antibiotics.

After an episode of rheumatic fever, your child will need to take antibiotics to prevent strep infections from occurring again. The length of treatment depends on whether the heart was involved, among other factors. Preventive antibiotic treatment will continue for at least 5 years, probably into adulthood, and possibly for the rest of your child's life.

How is rheumatic fever treated?

Once rheumatic fever is recognized, treatment starts immediately. Depending on your child's situation, we may recommend visits to a heart specialist (a cardiologist) or a specialist in rheumatic diseases (a rheumatologist).

Immediate treatment.

- *Antibiotics* against strep infection are given even if the bacteria are no longer present. Antibiotics may be given as a shot or orally for 10 days. Your child needs to continue taking antibiotics for a prolonged period of time to prevent future episodes of rheumatic fever (see under "Can rheumatic fever be prevented?").

- *Anti-inflammatory drugs:*
  - If your child has mild carditis or arthritis, he or she will likely be started on aspirin. Treatment will continue for 1 month.
  - If your child has more severe carditis, he or she will be started on steroid drugs, such as prednisone. Treatment usually continues for several weeks, with the dose gradually being reduced.
  - After your child finishes anti-inflammatory treatment, the symptoms may return. This reaction is usually mild and temporary.
  - *Call your doctor's office if symptoms are severe.*

- If chorea is present, your child may be treated with sedatives or other drugs, if necessary.

Follow-up treatment.

- Arthritis, chorea, skin rash, and bumps under the skin usually clear up completely, with no complications.
- Even when carditis is present, most children recover completely.
- Rheumatic heart disease can be a chronic problem. The more severe your child's initial heart involvement, the higher the risk of permanent damage.
- As mentioned previously, your child will need long-term antibiotic treatment to prevent future strep infections. If rheumatic heart disease was present, antibiotics may also be needed before surgery or certain dental procedures.
- If your child has permanent damage to the heart valves, he or she will need close follow-up care by a heart specialist (cardiologist). Valve damage can get worse over time and may eventually require valve replacement surgery.

When should I call your office?

Rheumatic fever is a serious medical condition, requiring treatment to prevent complications. Your child should receive close medical follow-up until he or she has recovered completely. After recovery, the doctor will discuss the need for long-term preventive antibiotics.

Section XVI ▪ Infections

Acute Diarrhea (Gastroenteritis)

Diarrhea is a common problem in children, and one of the most frequent reasons for visits to the doctor's office. Infections with viruses or bacteria are the main causes of acute diarrhea, but other causes are possible. Regardless of the reason for the diarrhea, your child must be watched carefully to avoid dehydration, especially in infants.

What is acute diarrhea?

Diarrhea means loose bowel movements, usually causing to move his or her bowels frequently. Vomiting may be present as well.

Acute diarrhea means the diarrhea lasts for only a limited time; this is also called *gastroenteritis*. There are many possible causes of gastroenteritis, including infections with bacteria, viruses, or parasites. Diarrhea may also be a symptom of other diseases, but this is less common.

Gastroenteritis is a leading cause of illness in children worldwide, especially in places where children are living in unsanitary conditions. Acute diarrhea usually clears up within a few days to a week.

Your child may need antibiotics or other treatments if the cause is infection with a bacteria or parasite. If the cause is a virus (commonly called "stomach flu"), antibiotics are not effective. You'll need to watch your child closely to make sure the diarrhea isn't causing him or her to become dehydrated and to give fluids to replace what is being lost.

What does it look like?

- Acute diarrhea may start suddenly. Your child begins having frequent bowel movements; it may seem like he or she simply can't stop going to the bathroom.

  - Bowel movements are loose and watery.

  - Blood may be present in the bowel movements. This may be more common if bacteria are the cause of acute diarrhea. *Call your doctor's office if your child has bloody stools.*

- Vomiting may be an early symptom but usually doesn't continue for more than a few days.

- Other symptoms may include abdominal cramps and fever.

What causes acute diarrhea?

There are many possible causes of gastroenteritis. Some of the most common are:

- *Viruses.* Infections caused by viruses are the most common cause of acute diarrhea. These infections are sometimes called stomach flu, although they are not caused by the influenza virus. Diarrhea caused by viruses usually clears up within a few days, with no need for antibiotics.

- *Bacteria.* Diarrhea can be caused by infections with bacteria, such as *Salmonella, Shigella,* or certain types of *Escherichia coli.* These germs may be spread by means of contaminated foods or water or by your child's getting germs from an infected person into his or her mouth. Some of these infections are treated with antibiotics, but others are not.

- *Parasites.* Diarrhea may be caused by certain parasites; the most common is *Giardia lamblia.* These infections are more likely if your child has recently traveled or come from an area where these parasites are common. However, outbreaks can occur in other areas as well. Specific drugs are given to kill the parasite.

- *Many other causes are possible,* including allergies, food poisoning, and gastrointestinal or other diseases. If your child's diarrhea doesn't clear up as expected, your doctor may recommend tests to help pinpoint the cause.

What are some possible complications of acute diarrhea?

Dehydration is the main complication of diarrhea in children. It occurs when your child doesn't drink enough liquids to replace the fluids his or her body is losing because of diarrhea. Your child may become dehydrated even if he or she doesn't feel thirsty. Dehydration can develop quickly, especially in infants.

Signs of *early dehydration* are:

- Urinating less often, in smaller amounts.

- Dryness or stickiness inside the mouth.

- Decreased appearance of tears when crying.

Signs of *more severe dehydration* are:

- No tears.

- Dry or sunken eyes.

- In babies, sunken "soft spot" on top of the head (fontanelle).

- Doughy-looking skin.

- Extreme sleepiness.

To avoid dehydration, give fluids, including special preparations such as Pedialyte.

Call our office if your child develops symptoms of dehydration.

What puts your child at risk of acute diarrhea?

- Diarrhea is a very common symptom. Nearly all children develop at least mild diarrhea at one time or another.

- Certain factors increase your child's risk of acute diarrhea, including going to day-care facilities, living in unsanitary conditions, and travelling to areas where parasites are common.

- Children who have diseases that impair the ability of the immune system to fight off germs are at higher risk of getting infections that lead to acute diarrhea, including some viruses and parasites that would not cause diarrhea in healthier children.

Can acute diarrhea be prevented?

Have your child wash his or her hands frequently and take other steps to avoid spreading the infection causing your child's diarrhea.

How is acute diarrhea treated?

Determining the cause. The doctor will examine your child and ask questions to help determine what is causing his or her diarrhea. Your child's other symptoms, in addition to information on what he or she has eaten, can provide important clues. Your doctor may also have an idea of what diarrhea-causing germs are "circulating" in your community. A sample of your child's bowel movement may be examined or tested for clues to the possible cause.

Treatment. If infection with a certain type of bacteria is the cause, your child may receive antibiotic treatment. Antibiotics are given to help your child recover more quickly, reduce the chances of spreading the infection, and prevent complications. Make sure your child finishes his or her prescribed antibiotic; don't stop giving the medication because he or she seems better.

- If infection with a parasite is suspected, your child will undergo further tests. Special medications may be needed to kill the parasite.

- If infection with a virus is the cause, antibiotics will not be helpful—these medications kill only bacteria, not viruses. Most viral causes of diarrhea clear up within a few days.

Preventing dehydration. Regardless of what is causing your child's diarrhea, the most important treatment is fluids to replace what is being lost to prevent dehydration. This is especially true in infants, who can lose body fluids very rapidly.

- Special solutions, such as Pedialyte, are available to replace lost body fluids. These products provide not only water but also sugars and electrolytes (salts) that your child's body needs. These preparations help your child's body to absorb as much water as possible.

- For older children who won't drink Pedialyte, Gatorade and Crystal Light are good liquids to give. Don't give fruit juices because they can make diarrhea worse. Milk is allowed. Most children with mild diarrhea who can drink milk don't need special fluid solutions.

Treating dehydration. If your child is dehydrated, he or she may need large amounts of fluids. The fluids may be given in small amounts over short periods of time. If necessary, give as little as a teaspoon every minute or two. After a while, you can gradually give larger amounts of fluid replacement over longer intervals. Your child can eat other foods too, if he or she can tolerate them.

- Fluids to replace what has been lost is important even if your child is vomiting. Give as much fluid as possible, even if it's just a teaspoon or two, at frequent intervals. Vomiting usually decreases with time.

If vomiting is continued or severe, and your child is not "holding down" any fluids, he or she may need to go to the hospital. There intravenous (IV) fluids will be given, along with other needed treatments.

- After your child is rehydrated (no longer dehydrated), resume feeding as soon as possible, including breast-feeding for infants. For older children, start with foods such as rice or bread, lean meats, yogurt, or vegetables.

- Usually, children shouldn't use over-the-counter antidiarrheal medicines, such as Imodium or Kaopectate. These products may decrease the number of bowel movements but not reduce the amount of diarrhea.

- The duration and severity of your child's diarrhea will depend mainly on the cause. Most cases of diarrhea should start to get better in a few days.

When should I call your office?

Call our office if:

- Your child's diarrhea doesn't start getting better within 3 to 5 days.

- Your child has severe or continued vomiting that makes it impossible to replace missing fluids.

- You are having trouble advancing your child's diet, especially if he or she can't eat for more than 1 day.

Call our office immediately if:

- Your child has symptoms of dehydration.

- He or she has little or no urination; in babies, no wet diaper for 6 to 8 hours.

- Dryness inside the mouth.

- Unusual sleepiness.

- Sunken eyes or soft spot (fontanelle).

- Diarrhea with visible blood.

Bacterial Vaginosis

Several types of vaginal infections can occur in sexually active women and girls. The most common is bacterial vaginosis, which causes an abnormal odor and fluid or discharge coming from the vagina. Other causes of vaginal infection are possible as well. Testing by your doctor can identify the cause of the infection and the most effective treatment.

What is bacterial vaginosis?

Bacterial vaginosis is the most common vaginal infection in teenage girls and women. These infections occur more often in sexually active women and girls, although they can occur in sexually inactive females. The main symptom is an abnormal discharge from the vagina.

Bacterial vaginosis clears up rapidly with treatment. However, there are numerous causes of vaginal infection, including infections with yeast (*Candida*) and sexually transmitted diseases. The doctor can make the diagnosis by looking at a sample of the vaginal discharge under the microscope. Since other infections may be present (for example, gonorrhea or infection with the bacteria *Chlamydia*), your doctor may recommend additional tests.

What does it look like?

The main symptoms of bacterial vaginosis are:

- Whitish-gray fluid coming from the vagina.
- Abnormal odor from the vagina, sometimes described as a "fishy" smell. The odor may be more noticeable after sexual activity.

Other types of infections may cause different symptoms. For example:

- Infection with the parasite *Trichomonas* may cause a larger amount of yellowish discharge.
- Yeast (*Candida*) infections may cause pain or itching with a white, creamy discharge.

What causes bacterial vaginosis?

Bacterial vaginosis is caused by abnormal growth of certain bacteria. Several types of bacteria are normally present in the vagina. Bacterial vaginosis occurs when the normal balance among these bacteria is disrupted. Although bacterial vaginosis isn't always spread or contracted by sex, it usually occurs in sexually active women.

- Other vaginal infections may be caused by bacteria (such as *Chlamydia*) or by the parasite *Trichomonas*. These infections are transmitted only by having sexual relations. Yeast infections can also occur.

What are some possible complications of bacterial vaginosis?

- Bacterial vaginosis has been linked to a more serious infection deeper inside the reproductive system, including the uterus (womb), ovaries, and ovarian tubes. This is called pelvic inflammatory disease (PID), and it may lead to an increased risk of infertility. Teenage girls are at highest risk of PID.
- Irregular menstrual periods.
- In pregnant women, an increased risk of premature labor or ruptured membranes.

What increases your risk of bacterial vaginosis?

- Having a new sexual partner, or having more than one sexual partner.
- Douching.

Can bacterial vaginosis be prevented?

- If you are sexually active, limit the number of sexual partners.
- Use a condom every time you have sex.

How is bacterial vaginosis treated?

Any time you have symptoms of bacterial vaginosis or any type of vaginal infection (abnormal fluid or odor coming from the vagina, itching), seek medical care. To ensure proper treatment, it's important for the doctor to identify the cause of the infection.

- *Antibiotics* are needed to kill the germs that are causing the infection. Flagyl (generic name: metronidazole) is the most commonly used drug. It can be used as a cream placed in the vagina or as a pill. A single oral dose can be used but is less effective than a 7-day course of pills.
  - Make sure to finish your antibiotic prescription, even if your symptoms have gotten better. Stopping treatment too early may allow the infection to come back.

When should I call your office?

Call our office if your symptoms (vaginal fluid or odor, itching, or pain) do not get better with treatment or if they return after treatment.

Bronchiolitis

Bronchiolitis is caused by infection and inflammation of the small airways in the lungs. It is very common in infants and toddlers and occurs most often in winter. Bronchiolitis can be a frightening illness and sometimes can become severe enough to require hospitalization of your child. Most children with bronchiolitis recover completely.

What is bronchiolitis?

Bronchiolitis is infection and inflammation (swelling and blocking) of the very smallest breathing tubes in your child's lungs, called the bronchioles. It is caused by infection with a virus, most often the very common respiratory syncytial virus (RSV). As the small airways become narrowed or blocked, you may hear wheezing (high-pitched sounds coming from the lungs) as your child breathes.

If bronchiolitis becomes severe, your child may have difficulty getting enough air. If this happens, he or she may need to be admitted to the hospital for oxygen and other treatments.

What does it look like?

Bronchiolitis starts off with the symptoms of a typical cold, with sneezing and a runny nose. Your child may recently have been exposed to an older child with a cold. He or she may also have a fever.

After a few days, your child may develop more severe breathing-related problems, such as:

- *Coughing or wheezing* (high-pitched sounds coming from the chest, especially when your child is breathing out).

- *Shortness of breath* (as if your infant is having trouble getting enough air).

- *Fast breathing*, which may make it difficult for your infant to nurse or feed.

- *Dehydration* (not drinking enough fluid), which may result from feeding difficulties. Symptoms of dehydration include:
  - Decreased urination.
  - *Dryness* inside the mouth.

- *Agitation or irritability* may be a sign that your child is not getting enough oxygen. Get medical help as soon as possible.

- *More severe signs* of difficulty breathing (respiratory distress). Take your child to the emergency room immediately if any of the following symptoms occur:

- Chest caves in, ribs stick out, belly goes up and down, and nostrils flare (called retractions).

- Skin turns blue (called cyanosis). This is an emergency—call 911.

What causes bronchiolitis?

- Bronchiolitis in infants is caused by viruses, most commonly RSV. Nearly all infants have been exposed to RSV by age 2. In older children and adults, RSV usually causes a cold. Only in infants and toddlers does the infection get into the small breathing tubes, causing bronchiolitis.

- Bronchiolitis is not caused by infection with bacteria, so antibiotic treatment probably won't be prescribed. Antibiotics may be recommended if your doctor suspects that a bacterial infection is present in addition to bronchiolitis.

What puts your child at risk of bronchiolitis?

- Bronchiolitis usually occurs in infants under 2 years of age. Severe bronchiolitis requiring hospitalization is more likely in infants under 6 months old.

- It often occurs after exposure of your infant to older children with colds.

- It mainly occurs during "cold season," that is, late fall and winter.

- Premature infants and those with other lung diseases are more likely to develop severe bronchiolitis.

Can bronchiolitis be prevented?

- The best prevention for bronchiolitis is taking whatever steps you can to avoid spreading colds. Avoid exposing your infant to older children with colds if possible. Wash your hands frequently, especially during cold season.

- Premature infants and those with certain lung diseases may be treated with infection-fighting bodies called immunoglobulins to prevent RSV disease.

What are some possible complications of bronchiolitis?

- Even when bronchiolitis is severe enough to require hospitalization, most children recover completely. However, it may take a couple of weeks before all of your child's symptoms clear up.

- Rarely, severe bronchiolitis can lead to respiratory failure (severe difficulty in breathing). Proper medical care can reduce this risk.

- Children who have had bronchiolitis seem more likely to develop asthma later in childhood.

How is bronchiolitis treated?

Like colds caused by RSV and other viruses, bronchiolitis goes away on its own with time. Your child's symptoms may seem to get worse for a few days but should start to get better after a week or so.

Treatment for bronchiolitis generally aims to help get your child over the worst of his or her symptoms. If your child develops symptoms of respiratory distress, such as wheezing, difficulty breathing, or dehydration, he or she may have to be treated in the hospital.

In the hospital, your child's treatment may include:

- *Oxygen.* If your child's blood oxygen levels are low, he or she will receive additional oxygen. Oxygen is usually given through a mask placed over the child's nose and mouth or through tubes going into the nostrils. Your child will be monitored carefully to make sure that he or she is getting enough oxygen in the blood.

- Although it is very uncommon, your child may need *mechanical ventilation* if breathing problems become severe. A tube is placed in your child's airway and connected to a machine called a ventilator. The ventilator helps to make sure your child receives enough oxygen until he or she is well enough to breathe on his or her own without difficulty.

- *Fluids.* If your infant has become dehydrated or unable to drink enough liquids, he or she may need additional fluids. Fluids may be given through a tube placed in a vein (intravenously or IV).

- *Monitoring.* Your infant may be placed on special equipment to monitor his or her breathing, oxygen level, and heart rate.

- *Medications.* Your infant may receive various medications, including bronchodilators (such as albuterol), to help open the breathing tubes; steroids, to help reduce inflammation; or antiviral drugs (such as ribavarin). However, these medications have not been found to be very helpful in most patients.

When should I call your office?

Call our office if any of the following occurs:

- Your child has signs of difficulty breathing, rapid breathing, or increased wheezing.

- Your child seems irritable or anxious.

- Your child has signs of dehydration (decreased urination, dryness inside the mouth).

If your child has more severe signs of respiratory distress, especially cyanosis (blue skin color), call 911 or another emergency number. *This is an emergency!*

Cat-Scratch Disease

Cat-scratch disease is a common infection in children causing swollen lymph nodes, especially in the underarm and neck areas. It is caused by infection with bacteria called *Bartonella*, most often spread by a bite or scratch from a cat. Most children recover completely, even without treatment. Some complications are possible.

What is cat-scratch disease?

Cat-scratch disease is an infection of the lymph glands caused by the bacteria *Bartonella henselae*. It usually occurs after a bite or scratch by a cat, particularly a kitten. Infected cats spread the disease to humans.

Cat-scratch disease causes swollen glands and other relatively minor symptoms. However, the symptoms may take weeks or even months to clear up completely. Cat-scratch disease occurs in thousands of people each year. Because children love to play with cats, they are often affected.

What does it look like?

The main symptom of cat-scratch disease is swollen lymph glands:

- Swollen glands may be found in the underarm area, in the head and neck, or in the groin area. Sometimes more than one area is affected.

- The glands are tender and slightly red. The area of swelling is usually no bigger than a few inches but can become larger.

- Glands usually remain swollen for 1 to 2 months.

Other symptoms of cat-scratch disease include:

- One or more small red bumps (papules) appearing at the place where the cat bite or scratch occurred. Because these papules are small, they are easily overlooked. They may go unnoticed until the doctor suspects cat-scratch disease and starts to look for them.

- Fever sometimes occurs, along with other symptoms such as loss of appetite, tiredness, headache, and "feeling sick."

Less commonly, cat-scratch disease may affect the eyes. Your child may have inflammation (redness and swelling) of one eye, along with swollen lymph glands. This form of cat-scratch disease probably results from rubbing the eyes after contact with an infected cat.

Rarely, cat-scratch disease causes more severe illness, including high fever, abdominal pain, and weight loss.

What causes cat-scratch disease?

Cat-scratch disease is caused by infection with *Bartonella henselae* bacteria. The bacteria usually spread to humans who are bitten or scratched by an infected cat.

Kittens may be more likely to spread the infection than older cats. The infected cat may not appear sick.

Papules usually develop at the site of the bite or scratch after about 1 or 2 weeks. Swelling of the glands located near the scratch develops 1 to 4 weeks later.

What puts your child at risk of cat-scratch disease?

Playing with cats, especially kittens. Although the infection is often spread by strays, it can also come from pet cats.

Can cat-scratch disease be prevented?

- Except for avoiding contact with cats, there is no way to prevent cat-scratch disease. Even a healthy-looking cat can be infected with the *Bartonella* bacteria.

- Cat-scratch disease does not spread from person to person.

What are some complications of cat-scratch disease?

Although they are uncommon, some complications of cat-scratch disease can occur. Most are not serious, although recovery may take some time.

- Up to 5% of patients may develop neurologic symptoms (encephalopathy), such as seizures, behavior changes, or confusion. Recovery may take several months to occur.

- Other complications are possible but rare, including:

  - Other nerve-related complications, such as temporary paralysis of facial muscles.

  - Eye complications, sometimes including temporary loss of vision.

  - Anemia and other blood abnormalities.

How is cat-scratch disease diagnosed and treated?

There are many possible causes of swollen lymph glands. Usually a simple blood test that checks for a specific antibody can determine whether your child is infected with *Bartonella* bacteria.

Cat-scratch disease generally clears up on its own, with or without treatment. It may take several weeks before your child's symptoms go away completely.

- Your child may receive antibiotics, such as azithromycin. However, medical studies have not proven that antibiotics will help your child recover any more quickly. In fact, cat-scratch disease is sometimes diagnosed only after antibiotics have failed to cure other suspected causes of swollen lymph glands.

- Rest and simple treatments will help to make your child more comfortable.

- If lymph glands become very swollen and painful a simple surgical procedure to drain away some of the pus inside the gland may be recommended.

- Your doctor will probably recommend follow-up visits to monitor your child's recovery from cat-scratch disease.

When should I call your office?

Call our office if:

- Your child's symptoms don't get better over time. However, be aware that it may take a few months for symptoms to clear up completely.

- Your child's lymph glands become very swollen and painful.

- Your child develops any changes in vision, behavior, or feeling (for example, tingling or numbness) or has difficulty moving the muscles of the face.

Chickenpox (Varicella)

Chickenpox is a common childhood disease caused by the varicella zoster virus and producing a rash and other symptoms. Although there is a risk of serious complications, these rarely occur. Vaccination against chickenpox is now recommended for most children. Infection with the varicella virus can cause severe disease in newborns and young infants.

What is chickenpox?

Until recently, chickenpox was one of the most common infectious diseases of childhood. It is caused by a widespread and highly contagious virus called the varicella zoster virus. Once your child has had chickenpox, he or she usually won't be infected again. The virus can be "reactivated" later in life, causing a disease called herpes zoster, but this is less common in children than adults.

The virus spreads by means of respiratory secretions (such as coughing or sneezing), or by contact with fluids from the rash. In the past, nearly all children in a family caught chickenpox in childhood. An effective varicella vaccine is now available and is recommended for most children. Although vaccinated children occasionally get chickenpox, the disease is usually very mild.

Chickenpox is generally mild in children, but there is a risk of serious complications. Chickenpox in pregnant women or in newborns may result in serious illness.

What does it look like?

Symptoms of chickenpox develop about 2 weeks after your child is exposed to someone with the varicella zoster virus. Initial symptoms, more common in older children, include:

- Fever, usually about 100°F to 102°F (38°C to 39°C), but sometimes higher.
- Loss of appetite, sometimes with abdominal pain.
- Headache and "feeling sick."

A few days later, your child starts to develop the typical chickenpox rash:

- The rash starts as small red spots, which can be extremely itchy.
- The spots develop into small raised blisters, which eventually break open and turn crusty.
- Meanwhile, new "crops" of rash continually develop, so that all stages are present at once.
- The rash usually occurs on the face and trunk at first, then spreads to the arms and legs.

- Some children develop ulcers or blisters in other areas, such as the mouth and throat, vagina, or the eyes and surrounding area.

If your child has received varicella vaccine:

- The chances of catching chickenpox are greatly reduced.
- If he or she does catch chickenpox, the symptoms will likely be mild. However, vaccinated children with chickenpox can still spread the disease to others.

What causes chickenpox?

- Chickenpox is caused by a virus called varicella zoster virus. Before the varicella vaccine was available, nearly everyone was infected with this virus sometime during childhood.
- The virus spreads very easily by direct contact with someone who is infected. If your child has chickenpox, any other children or adults who have not had the disease or vaccination will probably be infected as well. Chickenpox may also spread through contact with other children at school. It takes 10 to 21 days after exposure for the skin rash to begin.
- Chickenpox is contagious starting a day or two before the skin rash appears. It continues to be contagious until 5 days after the rash began, or as long as there are still blisters.

What are some possible complications of chickenpox?

Serious complications of chickenpox are uncommon but can occur.

- *Pneumonia* is rare but can occur. Symptoms include coughing and difficulty breathing.
- *Infections involving the brain* are also rare. Your child may have unsteady walking, severe headaches, or a stiff neck and may not be acting normally.
- *Bacterial infection of the skin* may cause the skin rash to become more red or tender. You may see pus coming from the sores.
- *Scarring of the skin* may occur if your child scratches too much.
- Severe abdominal pain and bleeding from skin blisters are important warning signs of severe infection. *If either of these symptoms occurs, call our office immediately!*
- Varicella during pregnancy can cause severe problems. The fetus or infant may develop severe disease before or shortly after birth. If you are pregnant, have never had chickenpox, and believe you may have been exposed

to someone infected with varicella, inform your doctor immediately!

- *Herpes zoster.* Sometime after your child recovers from chickenpox, he or she has a small risk of developing *herpes zoster.* The main symptom is a group of blistres in just one area of the body. It is usually not very serious.

What puts your child at risk of chickenpox?

- If your child has not been vaccinated, he or she will be at increased risk for chickenpox. Chickenpox can occasionally occur in a vaccinated child but is likely to be mild.

- Children with diseases that interfere with normal immune function (for example, human immunodeficiency virus [HIV] or cancer) are more likely to become infected with varicella and to develop severe chickenpox.

Can chickenpox be prevented?

- Varicella vaccination is recommended for nearly all children. A first dose of vaccine is given after age 1 and a second dose at 4 to 6 years of age. (If your child has definitely had chickenpox, he or she doesn't need this vaccine.) Two more doses are needed after age 13.

- Avoid contact with other children who have chickenpox. This may be difficult, however, as the virus can spread before the skin rash appears. Have your child wash his or her hands frequently.

- If your child has been exposed to chickenpox before getting the varicella vaccination, the vaccine may still be effective in preventing the disease.

- A special preparation of antibodies taken from blood (called VZIG) may help to prevent disease in certain high-risk patients who are exposed to varicella, including children with reduced immune function, pregnant women, and newborns of mothers with chickenpox.

How is chickenpox treated?

- If your child has the typical rash and other symptoms of chickenpox, it will probably be obvious to your doctor.

- Acyclovir, an antiviral drug, may be used in certain situations. However, for most otherwise healthy children with

chickenpox, this drug doesn't make that much difference. Your doctor may not recommend it.

- Acyclovir may be recommended for other family members, such as:

  - Children with skin or lung diseases.

  - Children using oral or inhaled steroid medications.

  - Children taking aspirin regularly.

- Otherwise, give home treatments to keep your child comfortable:

  - Use a washcloth soaked in cool water to reduce itching, which can become quite severe. Keep your child's nails short to avoid damage to the skin from scratching. Antihistamines may be prescribed to control itching.

  - *Do not* give aspirin to children with chickenpox, because it may lead to a serious complication called Reye's syndrome. If needed, other pain relievers (such as acetaminophen or ibuprofen) may be used.

- Once the rash has crusted over, chickenpox is no longer contagious. Your child can return to school or day care 5 days after the rash began, as long as there are no more blisters.

- Your child should get better, with complete clearing of the skin rash, within 7 to 10 days. If not, or if other symptoms develop, call your doctor's office.

When should I call your office?

Call our office if:

- Your child's skin rash and other symptoms of chickenpox haven't cleared up within 7 to 10 days or if new symptoms develop.

- Chickenpox sores show signs of infection: soreness, redness, warmth, or pus.

- Your child has a severe cough or difficulty breathing.

- Your child shows unsteady walking, severe headaches, or a stiff neck or is not acting normally.

- *If your child has severe abdominal pain or bleeding from the blisters, call our office.*

- *If you are pregnant, never had chickenpox, and believe you may have been exposed to someone infected with varicella, inform your doctor immediately.*

Chronic Diarrhea

Diarrhea lasting longer than 2 weeks is considered chronic diarrhea. Your child should have an examination and possibly tests to find out why he or she is having continued problems with diarrhea. Many causes of chronic diarrhea are possible but most are not serious.

What is chronic diarrhea?

Diarrhea simply means loose bowel movements, usually frequent. Most of the time, the problem resolves on its own. Chronic diarrhea means diarrhea lasting for at least 2 weeks. (Acute diarrhea means the diarrhea lasts for only a limited time and is most often caused by an infection.) Over time, continued diarrhea can lead to problems with nutrition.

There are many possible causes of chronic diarrhea. Often, however, no specific cause can be found. Careful evaluation will help to determine what is causing your child's chronic diarrhea and to identify the best form of treatment.

What does it look like?

- Weight loss or other symptoms may be present, or diarrhea may be your child's only symptom.
- Chronic diarrhea can occur in children at any age, from infancy through the teenage years.

What causes chronic diarrhea?

There is a long list of possible causes:

- *Infection.* It may result from an infection that has never cleared up or has caused damage to the intestines.
- *Foods/dietary causes.* It may be caused by something in your child's diet, for example, food allergy or lactose intolerance. Toddlers sometimes get diarrhea from drinking too much fruit juice. It may also result from medications, for example, as a side effect of antibiotics or from overuse of laxatives.
- *Other diseases.* Diarrhea may be caused by certain diseases, including inflammatory bowel disease (ulcerative colitis or Crohn's disease), celiac disease, or malformations of the intestines.
- Even less commonly, diarrhea may be a symptom of more serious diseases (such as cystic fibrosis or immune disorders such as HIV infection).
- Finally, in many children with chronic diarrhea, no specific cause can be found. This is called *idiopathic* diarrhea, which simply means that the cause is unknown. Treatment, including nutritional support, may help to maintain your child's nutrition while giving the diarrhea time to resolve.

What are some possible complications of chronic diarrhea?

Adequate nourishment is the main challenge in children with chronic diarrhea. Regardless of the cause of your child's diarrhea, he or she may need nutritional support.

Can chronic diarrhea be prevented?

There is no practical way to prevent all possible causes of chronic diarrhea. Getting prompt evaluation and treatment may prevent diarrhea from becoming a persistent problem.

How is the cause of chronic diarrhea diagnosed?

- Your child will undergo evaluation and possible testing in an attempt to find out what is causing the diarrhea. Your child may be referred to a *gastroenterologist*, an expert in diseases of the intestines. Your doctor will ask you to provide information on what your child eats and drinks. You may be asked to make a detailed record of everything your child eats over a 3-day period. Samples of your child's bowel movements may be tested for infection and other possible abnormalities. Some routine blood tests may be performed.
- If the cause is still unknown after examination and initial tests, further tests may be carried out. The goal of these tests is to make sure your child doesn't have some of the more serious, less common diseases that can cause chronic diarrhea. Your doctor is more likely to recommend these tests if your child has been losing weight or not gaining enough weight.
- X-rays and other tests may be done. These may include endoscopy, in which an instrument like a small telescope is used to examine your child's gastrointestinal tract. This is done by a gastroenterologist.

How is chronic diarrhea treated?

Treatment for chronic diarrhea depends on the results of examination and testing:

- If a specific cause is identified, treating the problem will eliminate the diarrhea. In many cases, the cause of diarrhea is relatively simple:
  - *Infections with bacteria or parasites.* May be treated with antibiotics.
  - *Food/dietary factors.* Your child may be allergic to or unable to tolerate something in his or her diet (for example, lactose intolerance). In that case, the diarrhea should improve once that food is removed from your child's diet.

- *Fruit juice.* Drinking too much fruit juice is a common cause of chronic diarrhea in toddlers. Cutting back on the amount of fruit juice your child drinks may improve the problem with diarrhea.

- *Malabsorption.* Another possible cause is a malabsorption syndrome. This means that your child's intestines are not working properly to absorb the nutrients from foods. The doctor will try to treat the cause of malabsorption.

- *Medications.* If a medication is causing the diarrhea, then the medication will be stopped if possible. Chronic diarrhea in teenagers is sometimes caused by overuse of laxatives, which may be a sign of an eating disorder.

- Chronic diarrhea can be the first symptom of a more serious underlying disease, such as pancreatitis, cystic fibrosis, or HIV disease.

- Even if no cause for your child's diarrhea can be identified, your doctor can still offer some helpful treatments. A special diet may be easier for your child to digest, while providing a chance for the intestines to heal. Less frequently, some type of artificial (parenteral) nutrition may be needed to provide temporary nutritional support. This type of nutritional support will be used for as short a time as possible.

When should I call your office?

During evaluation and treatment for chronic diarrhea, your child will be seen regularly to keep track of his or her weight and growth. Call our office if:

- Your child has continued diarrhea despite treatment.

- Your child is losing weight or not gaining enough weight.

Cold Sores (Herpes Simplex)

Cold sores are a common and painful problem for children just as for adults. They are caused by a virus called herpes simplex virus type 1 (HSV-1). Although this virus can cause the sexually transmitted disease genital herpes, the two diseases are not the same.

What are cold sores?

Cold sores are common and painful sores occurring in or around your child's mouth. The virus that causes them, herpes simplex virus type 1 (HSV-1), is very common and spreads very easily. Although the virus is commonly spread by kissing, it may also spread by more casual contact.

Cold sores usually go away on their own within a week or so, but they may come back repeatedly. Treatment with a drug called acyclovir may offer some help for more severe cases.

What do they look like?

Two kinds of herpes simplex outbreaks may occur: primary and recurrent.

- *Primary.* When your child is first infected with HSV-1, it causes a more severe outbreak. In addition to cold sores, there may be other symptoms such as fever, swollen gums, enlarged lymph nodes, and sore throat.

- *Recurrent.* Cold sores may come back once in a while. Recurrent outbreaks are much less severe than the primary outbreak. Your child will probably have no fever or other symptoms. However, HSV-1 can cause sores elsewhere on the body.

Cold sore symptoms.

- Your child may notice tingling, mild pain, or itching in or around the mouth for a few days before a cold sore appears.

- The sore initially looks like a small blister, which eventually crusts over and breaks open. The blister may be quite painful and may make it difficult to eat. The sores can also be embarrassing for your child as they are unsightly looking.

- More than one blister may occur at a time. The corners of the mouth are the most common location, but sores may also occur on the lips or inside the mouth.

- Cold sores usually go away in a week or so. They may come back frequently, only once in a while, or never.

What causes cold sores?

Cold sores are caused by infection with a very common virus called herpes simplex virus type 1 (HSV-1).

- HSV-1 is *not* the same as the HSV-2 virus that usually causes the sexually transmitted disease genital herpes, although HSV-1 can also cause genital herpes. Having cold sores does *not* mean your child has caught the virus by having sex or being sexually abused.

- Although many people have HSV-1, it does not always cause symptoms.

- Once your child is infected with HSV-1, he or she will probably carry the virus for life. The virus may become "reactivated" from time to time, causing repeated cold sores. Although HSV-1 can cause more serious disease, this is relatively uncommon.

What are some complications of cold sores?

- The herpes simplex viruses are widespread viruses that can cause a number of diseases. Many of us are infected with HSV-1. Fortunately, however, unless we have some type of disease that interferes with our immune system's ability to fight off germs, the HSV-1 causes only minor problems, such as cold sores. Rarely it may cause infection of the brain (encephalitis meningitis).

- *Bacterial infections.* Cold sores may become infected with bacteria or may lead to ulcers that take a long time to heal. Sores may become more crusted (yellow or oozing pus).

- The rate of recurrent cold sores is highly individual. As your child gets older, recurrences are likely to be less frequent.

What puts your child at risk of cold sores?

- If your child has had cold sores previously, damage to the lips from sunburn or dryness can increase the risk of a new outbreak.

- Cold sores and other diseases caused by HSV-1 may be more frequent or severe if your child has any condition that interferes with normal immune function.

Can cold sores be prevented?

- Many people have the HSV-1 virus. Having your child avoid contact with people who have cold sores may be helpful but is not always very practical.

- When your child is in contact with people who have cold sores, encourage him or her to wash hands frequently and avoid sharing things like glasses or towels. The virus can still be passed on for a while after cold sores have disappeared.

How are cold sores treated?

Most of the time, the doctor will recognize cold sores caused by HSV-1 without the need for any special tests. In some situations, your doctor may recommend testing for HSV-1.

For primary herpes simplex outbreaks, the doctor will probably recommend an antiviral medication. These medications are helpful only if the infection is caught early.

For recurrent outbreaks of cold sores:

- Remind your child not to pick at the sores. Keep the area clean and dry. Your doctor may recommend an antiseptic mouthwash.

- Topical antiviral creams may help cold sores clear up more quickly. Your doctor may recommend oral medications if more severe or extensive HSV-1 is present. However, these medications are usually not used for simple cold sores.

- Cold sores usually clear up on their own within 7 to 10 days, with or without treatment.

- If sores are very painful, pain relievers such as acetaminophen or ibuprofen may help.

- Ice-cold drinks or popsicles may make the mouth feel better, especially if the sores make it very painful for your child to eat or drink. Make sure infants, in particular, are getting enough fluids to avoid dehydration.

- Anesthetic sprays or lozenges may help to reduce pain temporarily.

When should I call your office?

Call our office if:

- Your child has a cold sore accompanied by a high fever or other symptoms that might mean primary herpes simplex infection.

- Your child's cold sores haven't cleared up within 7 to 10 days.

- Your child has any signs of an infected cold sore (redness, pus).

- Your child has signs of possible dehydration (not drinking enough fluids: decreased urine, decreased tears, dryness inside the mouth).

Colds

Nearly all children get colds once in a while, especially during winter. Particularly for young children in day care, it's normal to "catch a cold" about every other month. There is no cure for the common cold. Hand washing is the best way to prevent colds. If your child's cold doesn't get better in a week or so, call our office.

What are colds?

Colds are a very common illness caused by infection with a virus. Symptoms may include a sore, scratchy throat; a stuffy, runny nose; and sometimes a cough. Young children get a lot of colds, sometimes every month or two. As your child gets older, he or she gets colds less often.

Colds are almost always harmless and go away within a week or so. If your child seems to have more than the usual cold symptoms, if the cold gets worse after 5 to 7 days, or if it doesn't start to get better within 10 days, call our office. Your child may actually have some other kind of illness.

What do they look like?

- Colds usually start with a sore or scratchy throat, runny or stuffy nose, or sneezing. This begins 1 to 3 days after your child is exposed to the virus causing the cold.

- After 2 or 3 days, the sore throat gets better. The nasal drainage may change color or become thickened during the cold.

- Your child may have coughing and fever. He or she may "feel bad" but not seem terribly ill. If other symptoms are present, or if your child looks or feels very sick, the problem may be something other than a cold.

- Your child's cold should start to get better by 5 to 7 days.

What causes colds?

- Colds are caused by viruses. We will probably not treat your child's cold with antibiotics because these medications only kill bacteria, not viruses.

- The most common viruses causing colds are called rhinoviruses (which simply means "nose viruses").

- Other types of viruses, including influenza ("flu") virus, can also cause colds. Some of these other viruses may cause more severe cold symptoms.

What increases your child's risk for colds?

- Children have a lot of colds, especially when they are young. Young children average six to seven colds per year; some have more.

- Colds are less frequent in older children; adults average only two or three colds per year.

- Colds can occur any time but are most common during early fall through late spring.

- Children in day care catch more colds than children cared for at home full-time because of exposure to other sick children. This risk decreases somewhat after age 3.

Can colds be prevented?

- Many colds, particularly those caused by rhinoviruses, are spread by direct contact with mucous membranes and secretions. Colds are also spread by droplets in the air, caused by coughing or sneezing.

- Teaching your child to wash his or her hands frequently and to cover his or her mouth when coughing or sneezing is probably the best way to help prevent colds.

- Dietary supplements such as zinc, vitamin C, and echinacea don't appear to have much effect on treatment and prevention of colds. However, the research is unclear.

What are some possible complications of colds?

- *Sinusitis* (infection of the sinuses located behind the nose). Symptoms include runny nose and cough that are not improving after 10 days or symptoms that get worse. Other symptoms may include fever and facial pain (usually in older children).

- *Asthma attacks.* If your child has asthma, colds may be an important trigger for asthma attacks. A cough that doesn't get better may be caused by asthma, not the cold.

- *Other diseases* can look like colds at first. These include allergic rhinitis (hay fever) or even a foreign body that has gotten stuck in your child's nose.

How are colds treated?

Currently, there is no treatment that can cure colds. Some treatments may make your child feel better by reducing the symptoms. If your child is feeling particularly bad, he or she may have to rest more and drink extra liquids.

- *Fever.* Fevers that accompany colds usually don't require any treatment. However, if fever seems to be making your child uncomfortable, give him or her acetaminophen.

- *Stuffy nose.* Saline (saltwater) nose drops placed down each nostril will improve stuffy nose for a short time. This treatment is safe and can be repeated as often as needed. You can buy saline drops or make them at home by stirring one-half teaspoon of salt into 16 ounces of water.

- *Decongestants* such as Sudafed (generic name: pseudo-ephedrine) have not been found to be helpful. Nasal sprays can help to reduce stuffy nose but should not be used in children under 2. Don't use nasal sprays for more than 2 or 3 days because they can actually make a stuffy nose worse.

- *Runny nose.* Antihistamines such as Benadryl (generic name: diphenhydramine) may help to reduce a runny nose. These medications may cause drowsiness. Avoid using antihistamines in young children.

- *Sore throat.* Pain relievers (such as acetaminophen or ibuprofen) may help to reduce sore throat, headache, or muscle aches.

- *Cough.* Antihistamines may help to reduce cough early in your child's cold. "Cough syrups" are usually not that helpful. Drinking extra liquids makes it easier to cough up secretions.

- *Other treatments* have been suggested for treatment of colds, such as vitamin C, zinc lozenges, and echinacea. Thus far, medical studies have not found these treatments to be consistently effective.

- *In general, most medicines for colds are not very effective and may have side effects.* (The exception is saline nose drops, which reduce stuffy nose with no side effects.) If your child is comfortable, it may be just as well not to give him or her any medications at all.

When should I call your office?

Call our office if any of the following occurs:

- Your child's cold seems to be getting worse, not better, after 5 to 7 days.

- Your child's cold isn't getting better after 10 days.

- Your child develops a fever late in the illness, or the fever comes back after going away for a few days.

Call our office if your child develops any other symptoms, such as:

- Abnormal smelling or bloody fluid or pus coming from the nose.

- Swelling or pain of the face, or severe headache.

- Persistent or severe cough.

- Persistent runny nose, especially in infants.

Croup

Croup is a respiratory infection with symptoms of a "barking" cough, hoarseness, and, at times, some difficulty breathing. The child usually improves after a few days of home treatment, but may need to see a doctor if the symptoms are severe enough.

What is croup?

Croup is a respiratory infection involving the voice area (larynx) and windpipe (trachea). It is usually caused by a virus, including some of the same viruses that cause a cold. Croup usually occurs in younger children—about age 4 or less. It can be scary because of the sound of the "barking" cough, one of the main symptoms. Although most children recover in a few days, often there is some difficulty breathing. The medical term for croup is *laryngotracheitis*.

What does croup look like?

- Your child may have symptoms of a cold (runny nose, sore throat, or cough) for a few days before the typical symptoms begin.
  - A "barking" cough is the most common symptom.
  - It usually involves hoarseness.
  - A harsh sound when breathing in is common. This is called *stridor*. This stridor can be mild or severe and cause difficulty breathing.
  - If there is a lot of difficulty breathing, the ribs may stick out and the chest may get sucked in with each breath. This type of breathing is called *retraction*. Retractions can also occur where the neck meets the collar bones.
  - Fever may be present.
- Symptoms, especially stridor, are worse when the child is upset or crying.
- Symptoms are usually worse at night and last a few days, but should be gone within a week.

What puts your child at risk of croup?

- Croup most often occurs in younger children, under age 3 to 4. When croup occurs in older children, it is usually less severe.
- Croup is most common in the winter months but can occur year round.

- Children who have had croup before are more likely to have additional attacks.
- Infants or older children with narrowing of their airways (voice box) resulting from other conditions, such as being on a respirator with a breathing tube in place as a premature baby.

Can croup be prevented?

There is nothing specific you can do to prevent your child from developing croup.

How is croup diagnosed?

- Diagnosis is usually made from symptoms and physical examination.
- Occasionally an x-ray of the neck is needed to be sure the illness is croup.

How is croup treated?

Home treatment. If symptoms are mild, treatment can be done at home without seeing a doctor. The child must *not* have stridor (harsh sound when breathing in), retractions, or difficulty breathing. They also must not appear to be acting very sick and must be taking enough liquids.

- For some children, cool mist with a vaporizer or moist air with a humidifier may help.
- If a vaporizer or humdifier is not available, turning on a hot shower and sitting in the bathroom with your child may help.
- Lots of liquids.
- Acetameophen (Tylenol) or ibuprofin (Advil) may be needed for fussiness or fever.

Other treatments at the doctor's office, hospital, or emergency room:

- Steroids have been shown to be helpful and are often given except for very mild cases. Usually just one dose is needed, either orally or as a shot.
- If your child is having a lot of problems breathing, a drug called *epinephrine* may be given as a mist to breathe through a mask.
- Antibiotics are not given unless the doctor think a bacterial infection is now a problem.
- If your child is not taking enough liquids or is dehydrated, fluids may have to be given intravenously (IV).
- Oxygen may be needed if found to be low.

- Your child may have to stay in the hospital if there is still a lot of trouble breathing after the first treatments or if the problem returns.

What are some possible complications of croup?

- Most children recover from croup without problems.

- Although uncommon, breathing problems may become severe enough that a tube will be placed down your child's airway (windpipe) so he or she can breathe more freely. This is called *intubation*.

- Infection can spread to the smaller breathing tubes (bronchioles) or lungs and cause wheezing or pneumonia.

When should I call your office?

You should call our office or seek medical attention if:

- You are concerned that your child is having difficulty breathing.

- Stridor (harsh sounds when breathing in) occurs when your child is resting or calm.

- Your child shows evidence of stridor (chest caving in and ribs sticking out when breathing).

- Your child drools excessively.

- Your child turns blue (cyanosis) at any time. *This is an emergency—call 911.*

- Symptoms do not improve after a few days.

Fifth Disease

Fifth disease is a common childhood disease, caused by infection with parvovirus B19. The main symptom is a rash, sometimes accompanied by other symptoms such as fever. Fifth disease is usually mild and clears up without treatment. In healthy children, complications of parvovirus B19 infection are rare.

What is fifth disease?

Fifth disease (sometimes called *erythema infectiosum*) has long been known as a common childhood infection. (It got its unusual name because it was listed fifth in an old classification of childhood rashes.) However, it's only in the past two decades that the true cause of fifth disease has been recognized: infection with a virus called parvovirus B19.

Fifth disease is usually a mild illness that clears up in a week or so. By the time your child develops the typical rash of fifth disease, he or she probably isn't contagious anymore. Once your child has been infected with parvovirus B19, he or she will be immune for life. Fifth disease can be more dangerous in children who have other diseases, such as sickle cell anemia or human immunodeficiency (HIV) disease. Parvovirus B19 infection can also be more serious in pregnant women.

What does it look like?

The main symptom of fifth disease is a typical rash. The rash may not look exactly the same in every child, however.

- Usually the disease starts with a bright red rash on the face, sometimes described as a "slapped-cheek" rash.

- The rash may rapidly spread to your child's body, arms, and legs.

- As the rash begins to clear up, it may have a fine, "lacy" appearance—it looks like "squiggly" lines on your child's skin.

- The rash may get worse if your child is exposed to sunlight or heat or from excessive exercise or stress.

- The rash usually clears up within 7 to 10 days but sometimes takes up to 3 weeks to go away completely. It may clear up and reappear.

Besides rash, other symptoms of fifth disease may include:

- A mild illness, like a cold, with a low-grade fever and headache. This often happens right before the rash appears.

- The rash may itch a little, especially in older children.

- Sometimes, pain and swelling may develop in the joints, such as the hands, wrists, and knees. This is more common in older teens and adults than in younger children with fifth disease. Females are more likely than males to have joint pain.

What causes fifth disease?

- Fifth disease is caused by infection with parvovirus B19, a common virus that spreads easily from one person to another. If one person in your home is infected, the chances of spreading the infection to others are about 50–50. However, not all people who are infected with parvovirus B19 develop fifth disease.

- Fifth disease develops 1 to 4 weeks after the virus is spread. Once your child has been infected with parvovirus B19, he or she will likely be protected against future infection with this virus.

What are some possible complications of fifth disease?

- Complications of fifth disease are rare in healthy children, especially younger children. Some people develop other unusual rashes.

- Older children and adults with fifth disease are more likely to develop joint pain and swelling. The joint pain usually clears up in a few weeks. Some patients develop more lasting arthritis.

- Parvovirus B19 interferes with the production and survival of red blood cells. In patients with certain types of anemia (such as sickle cell anemia), this can lead to a complication called aplastic crisis, in which the body is not making enough new red blood cells.

- Parvovirus B19 disease is also more serious in children with conditions that interfere with the immune system, such as HIV disease or cancer chemotherapy.

- In pregnant women, parvovirus B19 may pose a risk to the developing fetus. If you are pregnant and your child has fifth disease, mention this situation to your obstetrician.

What puts your child at risk of fifth disease?

- Parvovirus B19 is very common. About one half of people are infected during childhood or adolescence.

- Besides exposure to an infected person, there are no specific risk factors for parvovirus B19.

- Parvovirus B19 is mainly contagious before the rash occurs. By the time your child develops the typical rash of fifth disease, he or she can probably no longer spread the virus.

Can fifth disease be prevented?

There is no specific way to prevent the spread of parvovirus B19.

How is fifth disease treated?

- No specific treatment is needed for fifth disease.
- Fifth disease is contagious only before the rash develops. Keeping your child home from school or day care does not prevent the spread of parvovirus B19.
- Pain relievers (such as acetaminophen or ibuprofen) may be helpful, especially if your child has joint pain.

When should I call your office?

Call our office if:

- Your child's rash and other symptoms of fifth disease don't improve within 7 to 10 days.
- Your child develops joint swelling.
- Your child's symptoms get worse instead of better or if new symptoms develop.

Food Poisoning

Food poisoning is most often caused by bacteria growing in food that has not been prepared or stored properly. Vomiting, diarrhea, and other symptoms may occur within hours after your child eats the contaminated food. The problem usually clears up within a day or two. In some types of food poisoning, symptoms take longer to develop.

What is food poisoning?

Food poisoning is a general term that describes an illness that comes from eating food that contains toxins—usually made by bacteria—or germs that cause infection. Most often, the symptoms occur soon after eating food contaminated with bacteria, such as the common "staph" (*Staphyococcus*) bacteria. Nausea, vomiting, and other symptoms occur because of toxins produced by the bacteria. Once the toxins leave the body, your child should feel better.

In other types of food poisoning, symptoms develop more slowly. These include contamination of food with *Salmonella or Shigella* bacteria, or with certain viruses. It is sometimes difficult to tell if food is what made your child sick. Symptoms develop at different times, depending on what bacteria are the cause. If symptoms don't clear up in a day or two, or if certain symptoms such as bloody diarrhea occur, call our office.

What does it look like?

Common symptoms of food poisoning include:

- Nausea and vomiting.
- Abdominal pain and cramps.
- Diarrhea.
- Symptoms may develop within a few hours after eating contaminated food or may take a day or two to develop.
- Rarely, more serious symptoms may develop, such as bloody diarrhea or muscle weakness. *Seek medical care immediately if these conditions occur.*

What causes food poisoning?

There are many different types/causes of food poisoning:

- For food poisoning developing within 4 to 12 hours, the usual cause is bacteria such as *staph* bacteria or *Bacillus cereus*. The symptoms aren't caused by the bacteria themselves but rather by toxins produced by the bacteria.
- Symptoms developing after a day or two may be related to different types of bacteria, such as *Salmonella*. Sometimes the cause may be a virus. For these slower developing

types of food poisoning, you may not even realize the infection came from food. Instead, it may be called *gastroenteritis* or "stomach flu."

Some more serious food-related infections are possible, but less common. *These are more serious conditions requiring immediate medical care.*

- Bloody diarrhea may be caused by a bacteria called *Escherichia (E.) coli* 0157:H7. This infection can sometimes cause a disease called *hemolytic-uremic syndrome*, which can lead to anemia and kidney damage.
- Muscle weakness and other neurologic symptoms may be caused by bacteria called *Clostridium botulinum* (botulism) or by toxins found in certain foods, especially in shellfish and mushrooms/toadstools. Botulism in infants usually causes constipation; in adults, it can cause either constipation or diarrhea.
- Food allergies may be mistaken for food poisoning. The most serious types of allergic reactions include sudden itching, hives, difficulty breathing, and low blood pressure. This is called *anaphylaxis* or allergic shock.

What are some possible complications of food poisoning?

- Food poisoning usually clears up within a few days. The main problem to watch out for in your child is dehydration (not enough liquids). This may occur if your child is having a lot of vomiting or diarrhea.
- Certain types of food poisoning are less common but more serious, requiring medical care (for example, botulism, *E. coli* 0157:H7).

What puts your child at risk of food poisoning?

Eating foods that have been improperly prepared or stored. See preventive measures below.

Can food poisoning be prevented?

- Wash your hands before cooking or preparing food.
- Keep kitchen surfaces and utensils clean.
- Make sure meats are fully cooked. Don't let raw meat come into contact with other foods.
- Keep foods refrigerated. Outbreaks of food poisoning most often occur when food is left out for a long time, such as at picnics.
- Don't use any foods that are outdated (expired) or smell "off." Don't use food from bulging cans.

How is food poisoning treated?

- For the most common types of food poisoning, no treatment is needed. Vomiting, diarrhea, and other symptoms get better in a few days.

- Antibiotic treatment may or may not be needed, even if the cause is bacteria. Symptoms are usually caused by toxins produced by the bacteria. Once the toxins are gone, your child should feel better.

- If the doctor does recommend antibiotics, make sure your child finishes his or her prescription; don't stop giving the medication because he or she seems better.

- The doctor may recommend tests to determine what is causing your child's vomiting, diarrhea, or other symptoms. On the other hand, if your child has typical symptoms that are clearly related to eating contaminated food, no testing may be needed.

- Regardless of the cause of nausea and vomiting, the most important treatment is fluid replacement to prevent dehydration. This is especially true in infants, who can lose body fluids very rapidly.

- Special solutions, such as Pedialyte, are available to replace lost body fluids. These products provide not only water but also necessary sugars and electrolytes (salts).

- If your child becomes dehydrated, he or she may need larger amounts of these fluids. The fluids can be given in small amounts frequently: as little as a teaspoon every minute or two. Over time, you can gradually give larger amounts of fluid replacement less often. Your child can eat other foods too, if tolerated.

- Giving fluids is important, even if your child is vomiting. Vomiting usually decreases with time.

If vomiting continues or is severe, and your child is not "holding down" any fluids, he or she may need to go to the hospital. There he or she can receive intravenous (IV) fluid replacement, along with other needed treatment.

- Usually, children shouldn't use over-the-counter antidiarrheal medicines, such as Imodium or Kaopectate. These products don't help much and may cause side effects.

- If your child has any of the more serious food-related infections, other treatments will be recommended. If your child hasn't recovered in the expected time or if new symptoms develop, call our office.

When should I call your office?

Call our office if:

- Your child's vomiting, diarrhea, and other symptoms don't clear up within 2 or 3 days.

- Your child has severe or continued vomiting that makes it difficult to give enough fluids.

If any of the following appear, *call our office immediately*:

- Diarrhea with visible blood.
- Muscle weakness or other neurologic symptoms.
- Symptoms of dehydration:
  - Dry mouth.
  - Decreased tears.
  - Weight loss.
  - Little or no urine produced.
  - Fast heartbeat.
  - Irritability or extreme tiredness.
  - In infants, going 6 to 8 hours without wetting a diaper; sunken eyes or soft spot at the top of the head (fontanelle)

German Measles (Rubella)

> German measles used to be one of the most common childhood diseases. It is now very uncommon because of effective vaccination programs. Today, German measles in children is rarely a serious problem. It can be serious if it occurs in pregnant women who have not been vaccinated.

What is German measles?

German measles, or rubella—sometimes called "three-day measles"—is an easily spread illness that is relatively mild, causing a rash and swollen lymph glands. In the past, it was a widespread childhood disease, with outbreaks affecting millions of children. Today, nearly all infants are vaccinated, and German measles has become rare.

However, outbreaks still occur, especially in children from other countries or in groups of people who have not been vaccinated.

In pregnant women who have not been vaccinated, German measles can cause serious problems to the developing fetus.

German measles is different from another childhood infection called simply measles, or rubeola.

What does it look like?

- German measles begins with a few days of a mild illness, similar to that of a cold.

- The child then develops swollen, tender lymph glands, mainly in the head and neck.

- A day or so later, small red spots appear, often with a bump in the center. This rash occurs first on the face and then spreads over the entire body. Your child may have mild itching.

- The rash develops, spreads, and fades very rapidly. By the third day, it is usually gone completely.

- Joint pain and swelling may occur, especially in girls.

What causes German measles?

- German measles is caused by the rubella virus. This virus is very common around the world and is highly contagious; it may be spread even if the infected person does not appear sick. With the development of effective vaccines against rubella, German measles has nearly been eliminated in the United States.

- Once your child has had or been vaccinated against German measles, he or she will likely be protected against this disease in the future.

What are some possible complications of German measles?

- *Congenital rubella syndrome* is the most serious complication of German measles. It occurs when a pregnant women is infected with the rubella virus early in pregnancy and passes it on to her developing baby. The disease can be severe, causing serious illness, brain damage, and death. Fortunately, because of the widespread use of rubella vaccination, congenital rubella is now rare in the United States.

- In children with rubella, complications are rare. There is a small chance of rubella infection involving the brain (encephalitis).

Can German measles be prevented?

Yes. Rubella vaccination greatly reduces your child's chances of getting the disease. Measles, mumps, rubella (MMR) vaccination is recommended for nearly all children: one dose at age 12 to 15 months; a second dose at age 4 to 6 years. There is a low risk of some mild symptoms occurring after MMR vaccination, such as fever and a rash.

How is German measles treated?

- Usually, no specific treatment is needed for rubella. The rash develops and clears up quickly, most often within a few days.

- If your child is uncomfortable or has a very high fever, give him or her acetaminophen or ibuprofen.

- As much as possible, have your child's avoid contact with other people until he or she is well. Rubella can spread quickly among people who have not been vaccinated.

When should I call your office?

Call our office if:

- Your child has not received all recommended vaccinations.

- You are pregnant and have been in contact with someone who has rubella.

Hand-Foot-and-Mouth Disease and Related Infections

Hand-foot-and-mouth disease is a distinctive rash caused by a family of viruses called enteroviruses, which spread easily. The viruses can cause a blistering rash in the throat, hands, and feet. Your child's rash may not appear in all of these areas. The infection is rarely serious and usually clears up without treatment.

What is hand-foot-and-mouth disease?

Hand-foot-and-mouth disease is a common childhood infection causing a distinctive rash and other symptoms. It is unrelated to "foot-and-mouth disease" in farm animals.

The illness is usually mild, although the rash forming in the throat, hands, feet, and other areas may look alarming. Your child should recover in a week or so. Serious complications are rare.

What does it look like?

- Illness may begin with fever, loss of appetite, and sore throat. Younger children are more likely to have a high fever.

- A rash develops in and around the mouth. The rash starts out as small red spots, which may turn into blisters (vesicles) or shallow ulcers.

- A rash also develops on the skin, especially the hands, fingers, and feet and sometimes also on the buttocks and groin. This rash may appear as blisters or reddish or pink bumps or spots.

- Your child's rash may appear in all or only some of these areas and is usually not very itchy.

- Rash and other symptoms usually clear up in a week or so, with no further problems.

What causes hand-foot-and-mouth disease?

- Your child's rash and other symptoms are caused by a family of viruses called enteroviruses. Common subgroups include the coxsackieviruses and echoviruses. Some enteroviruses cause more severe disease than others.

- Enteroviruses can cause other types of disease, including a condition called herpangina that also causes ulcers in the mouth. Sores are more likely to appear at the back of the mouth.

- Enterovirus infection may also involve the lungs, eyes, heart, and nervous system, but these conditions are less common.

- Enteroviruses can spread easily to people your child comes into contact with at home or school. The infection is most contagious during the early stages.

What are some possible complications of hand-foot-and-mouth disease?

- Serious complications are uncommon. The infection usually clears up in a week or so, without further problems.

- Some enteroviruses cause more severe infection than others.

- On occasion, enterovirus infection can spread to the nervous system. These conditions, such as meningitis or encephalitis, are more serious and require medical evaluation, but children usually recover without problems.

  - Call our office if your child develops any nervous system symptoms, such as headache, stiff neck, or back pain.

What increases your child's risk of hand-foot-and-mouth disease?

- Hand-foot-and-mouth disease is most common in infants and children under 10 years old but can occur at any age.

- Enteroviruses are most likely to spread in the summer and fall.

Can hand-foot-and-mouth disease be prevented?

- Enteroviruses are very common and spread easily through oral secretions and cough. Wash your hands frequently to reduce the risk of spreading the disease to others. Be especially careful to clean up after changing your baby's diapers.

How is hand-foot-and-mouth disease treated?

Usually, no specific treatment is needed for hand-foot-and-mouth disease. The infection clears up on its own, with or without treatment.

- Antibiotics are not needed. These medications kill only bacteria, not viruses.

- Give your child pain relievers (acetaminophen or ibuprofen) for high fever or painful mouth sores, if needed. Placing an anesthetic gel (such as Anbesol) on the sores can temporarily reduce pain.

- Encourage your child to drink lots of liquids. Avoid orange juice or other acidic drinks, as these can irritate the throat.

When should I call your office?

Call our office if:

- Your child's skin rash and other symptoms of hand-foot-and-mouth disease do not begin to clear up after 3 or 4 days.

- Your child develops any nervous system symptoms, such as headache, stiff neck, or back pain.

Hepatitis (Hepatitis A, B, or C Virus)

> Viral hepatitis is a major health problem worldwide. There are several different hepatitis viruses, which cause different diseases. The most common type of hepatitis in children is caused by hepatitis A virus. This virus usually causes a mild illness that goes away in a few weeks. Other viruses, especially hepatitis B or C virus, can be lifelong infections that cause permanent liver damage.

What is hepatitis?

Hepatitis is an infection or inflammation of the liver. Various causes are possible, but infection with hepatitis viruses is the most common cause. The main difference between the various hepatitis viruses is the type of disease they result in:

- *Hepatitis A virus.* Disease is usually not severe, and the infection goes away completely within several weeks.

- *Hepatitis B and C viruses.* Can cause permanent, lifelong infection, with potentially serious complications.

All of the hepatitis viruses cause similar symptoms, including jaundice (yellow color of the skin). Or, they may cause no symptoms at all. Hepatitis B or C virus may lead to chronic infection with liver disease and other complications.

What does it look like?

Hepatitis A virus:

- Your child may develop a sudden illness, including fever, nausea and vomiting, loss of appetite, and abdominal pain. In infants and preschoolers, you may not even notice these symptoms.

- Later, your child's skin may begin to turn yellow or orange (jaundice). This happens because the infection makes it difficult for the liver to get rid of a normally produced substance called bilirubin. Jaundice is sometimes called "hyperbilirubinemia."

- Your child's urine may be dark-colored.

- Symptoms go away gradually over several weeks. Most children recover completely within 1 month. Rarely, the symptoms return.

Hepatitis B and C viruses:

- Your child may develop symptoms similar to those of hepatitis A virus infection.

- With hepatitis B virus, the initial illness may be more severe, including symptoms such as joint pain and a rash. Hepatitis C virus usually causes less severe symptoms at the outset.

- Often, the initial symptoms are mild, or there are no symptoms at all. Your child may have hepatitis B or C virus for years before the infection is discovered.

- Both hepatitis B and C viruses may lead to chronic hepatitis (continuing infection). Although it may not happen until adulthood, chronic hepatitis can eventually lead to serious complications. Your child may be infected with these viruses for life.

- Pregnant women may pass hepatitis B and C viruses on to their newborns.

How is viral hepatitis spread?

Although many different viruses may infect the liver, hepatitis A virus is the most common in children, followed by hepatitis B and hepatitis C viruses. Other hepatitis viruses exist but are less common.

Hepatitis viruses spread in different ways:

- *Hepatitis A virus* is found in the stool (bowel movements) of infected people. The virus spreads by means of hand-to-mouth contact or through contaminated food or water.

- *Hepatitis B and C viruses* are spread through direct contact with blood or body fluids from an infected person. There are relatively few ways that this can happen:

  - Having sex with an infected person.

  - Being exposed to blood from an infected person, for example, being stuck with an infected needle or other sharp object.

- If a pregnant woman is infected, she can spread hepatitis B or C virus to her baby.

What are some possible complications of viral hepatitis?

- *Hepatitis A virus.* Serious complications are rare. In some people, hepatitis symptoms go away, then come back again.

- *Hepatitis B or C virus.* Infection with hepatitis B or C virus may remain present for life.

  - Hepatitis C virus is the most common cause of *chronic hepatitis* (long-term). Both hepatitis B and C may lead to permanent liver damage, including *cirrhosis* (scarring of the liver) and other complications.

- These complications may take many years to develop. Treatment can help to keep your child as healthy as possible but cannot cure the infection.

What puts your child at risk of viral hepatitis?

- *Hepatitis A virus.* If someone in your family is infected with hepatitis A virus, there is a high risk that the virus will be passed on to others. Hepatitis A virus is more common in certain regions of the United States and in poor countries.

- *Hepatitis B and C viruses.* Hepatitis B and C viruses are transmitted by contact with blood and other body fluids and by sexual activity. Your teenager will be at high risk if he or she engages in activities such as having multiple sex partners or injecting drugs. If you are infected with hepatitis B or C virus and are pregnant, there is a risk that you will pass the infection on to your baby.

Can viral hepatitis be prevented?

Vaccines. Effective vaccines can protect against infection with hepatitis A or B virus. There is no vaccine for hepatitis C virus.

- Hepatitis A vaccine is recommended for all children ages 1 to 18 and some high-risk groups, such as people living in or traveling to areas where hepatitis A is common. People with hepatitis B or C infection should be vaccinated against hepatitis A virus.

- Hepatitis B vaccine is recommended for all infants. The first dose is given soon after birth. Two more doses are given between 1 and 18 months. Vaccination is also recommended for certain high-risk groups: if you or your child is infected, all other family members should be vaccinated.

Preventing the spread of hepatitis A. If your child has hepatitis A, the disease will be contagious for 2 weeks before and about 1 week after symptoms develop.

- *Wash your hands frequently to reduce the risk of spreading infection.* Be especially careful to clean up after changing diapers and before preparing meals.

- We will probably recommend injections of immunoglobulin (antibodies) for you and other members of your family to reduce your risk of catching the virus. After being infected with hepatitis A virus, your child will be immune to future infection.

Preventing the spread of hepatitis B and C viruses. Hepatitis B and C viruses cannot be spread by casual contact.

Teenagers should learn safe sex and other practices to reduce the risk of spreading the virus to others. Pregnant women should be tested for the virus.

How is viral hepatitis diagnosed and treated?

- If we suspect that your child has hepatitis, we may recommend blood tests for hepatitis A, B, or C virus. Treatment will depend on which of these viruses, if any, your child is infected with.

- *If your child has hepatitis A,* the disease will clear up gradually over several weeks. There are no specific treatments that will help your child get better faster. Make sure your child drinks plenty of fluids.

  - Symptoms get better then come back in about 15% of patients with hepatitis A. If this happens, it may take several months before your child's hepatitis finally clears up permanently.

  - Very rarely, more serious complications resulting in severe liver damage may develop.

- *If your child has chronic hepatitis B or C,* he or she will need thorough medical evaluation and follow-up. The goal is to determine the best treatment and reduce the long-term risk of complications. We may recommend a visit to a specialist in treating liver diseases.

  - Your child is likely to need lifelong medical follow-up as well as health education to learn to live with chronic hepatitis B or C. He or she should avoid high-risk behaviors, especially drug use, and learn to practice safe sex, especially using condoms. People with hepatitis should avoid alcohol, as it can make their liver disease worse.

  - Although chronic hepatitis B and C are not curable, they are treatable. Doctors, nurses, and other health care professionals can help your family to live with these diseases.

When should I call your office?

Call our office if you have any questions about your child's hepatitis, its treatment, or how to prevent the spread of hepatitis viruses.

As your child is recovering from an episode of viral hepatitis, call our office if your child has any of the following symptoms:

- Bleeding.

- Continued vomiting or abdominal pain.

- Swelling of the hands, feet, or elsewhere in the body.

- Behavior changes.

- Decreased responsiveness, grogginess.

HIV/AIDS

HIV stands for "human immunodeficiency virus." This is the virus that causes AIDS, or "acquired immunodeficiency syndrome." In AIDS, the immune system doesn't work normally to fight off disease-causing germs. With current treatments, people with HIV infection can lead relatively normal lives. Practicing safe sex reduces the chances of catching HIV. Pregnant women with HIV need treatment to keep from spreading the virus to their baby.

What are HIV and AIDS?

HIV is the virus that causes AIDS. HIV slowly destroys the body's immune system. Not all patients with HIV infection have AIDS. AIDS occurs when the HIV infection has become severe. AIDS is a serious disease that reduces the body's ability to fight off infections. Germs that cause mild or no illness in people with normal immune systems can be dangerous in people with AIDS, who are highly susceptible to them.

The global epidemic of HIV/AIDS is a major health problem. Millions of people around the world are infected with this currently incurable disease. For infants, the main risk is that HIV will be passed on from an infected mother, although effective treatments can reduce this risk. Teenagers may get HIV infection through unsafe sex or from being exposed to blood from an infected person.

In the United States and other developed countries, effective medications are available to control HIV and reduce the chances of AIDS. These treatments cannot eliminate HIV, but they can help infected people lead nearly normal lives. All patients with HIV infection need lifelong medical follow-up.

What are the facts on HIV/AIDS?

- It's estimated that about 1 million people in the United States were living with HIV infection by the end of 2003, according to the Centers for Disease Control (CDC). About one fourth of these may not even know they have HIV.

- A person with HIV infection can look perfectly healthy. The virus may be present for 5 to 6 years before any symptoms develop.

- Infants and young children can catch HIV from an infected mother during pregnancy, birth, or breast feeding. Almost all children with HIV/AIDS are infected in this way. Fortunately, simple treatments can greatly reduce the risk of passing HIV on from mother to child. If you are pregnant, it's a good idea to be tested to make sure you don't have HIV.

- In the past, children and adults sometimes were infected with HIV through blood transfusions. However, with current testing procedures, this is now rare.

- Older children and teenagers may be infected with HIV by having sex with an infected person. Having several sexual partners and not using condoms when having sex are the main risk factors.

- Being exposed to blood from an infected person can also spread HIV. This most often occurs when drug users share needles used to inject drugs.

- HIV is *not* passed by more casual contact, such as sharing eating utensils or toilet seats.

- *Symptoms may not develop for months or even years after HIV infection is transmitted.* However, the virus is still present, and the infected person can still pass it on to others.

What are some possible complications of HIV/AIDS?

- The main complication of HIV infection is AIDS. In AIDS, the body's immune system has been damaged and can't work effectively to fight off germs. This leads to dangerous infections and other health problems. For people with HIV infection, effective treatment can reduce the chances of developing AIDS.

- When children have HIV, the mother and others in the family may be infected too. This can make it difficult to provide a stable environment for the family. If needed, community resources may be able to help the family deal with the difficult challenges of living with HIV.

What increases the risk of HIV/AIDS?

- Unsafe behaviors, especially having unprotected sex with many partners and using injectable drugs and sharing needles.

- Living in an area with a high rate of HIV/AIDS, including developing countries and certain U.S. cities.

Can HIV/AIDS be prevented?

If you are infected with HIV and are pregnant, it is very important that you get treatment to reduce the chances of passing the virus to your baby. Treatments such as azathioprine (AZT) can greatly reduce your baby's chances of becoming infected with HIV.

- Practice safe behaviors that reduce your chances of becoming infected with HIV or, if you are infected, of passing the virus to others:

- Do not use injectable drugs or share needles.
- Limit the number of sexual partners.
- If having sex, always use a condom (protected sex).

How is HIV/AIDS treated?

- The treatment of HIV/AIDS can be very complicated and require the use of various kinds of medications. Usually an expert in HIV infections—typically a specialist in infectious diseases—will be involved in the care of your child. Treatment can't completely cure HIV infection, but it can help to keep the infection under control. Many people whose HIV infection is not severe can live nearly normal lives with proper treatment.

- HIV/AIDS has a major impact on the lives of many families. Fortunately, with good medical care and community support, these families can lead healthy, active, and productive lives.

When should I call your office?

Call our office or an HIV specialist if you have any questions about HIV/AIDS, including prevention, testing, and treatment.

Impetigo

> Impetigo is a very common skin infection in children. Caused by bacteria, the infection usually causes a crusty rash. Less commonly, it causes a blistering rash. Both types of impetigo are usually not serious and clear up within a week or two.

What is impetigo?

Impetigo is a common skin rash in children. It is usually caused by infection of the very top layer of the skin with *Staphylococcus* or less often with *Streptococcus* bacteria. The rash rarely causes serious problems and usually clears up with or without antibiotic treatment. However, the infection is contagious and may spread to other people your child comes into contact with.

What does it look like?

The most common type is *nonbullous* (nonblistering) impetigo:

- Your child develops a rash, usually beginning on the face or limbs. The rash often starts in areas where a minor injury has occurred, such as a scrape, burn, or insect bite.

- Small pimples form, soon changing into a crusty, orange-yellow rash. The rash spreads easily to other areas of the skin.

- The rash is usually not painful but is sometimes itchy.

Bullous (blistering) impetigo usually occurs in infants and young children:

- Small blisters develop on your child's body, most commonly on the face, buttocks, and trunk. In babies, the blisters may first appear in the diaper area.

- The blisters pop easily.

- The blisters may or may not be itchy.

Your child may have a mix of the two types of impetigo. Both types usually clear up in a week or two.

- Antibiotic treatment may help your child's impetigo heal faster. Unless there are complications, healing usually occurs without scarring.

What are some possible complications of impetigo?

- If impetigo is caused by *Streptococcus* bacteria, there is a small risk of a kidney problem called glomerulonephritis, which causes blood in the urine.

- Very rarely, the infection can spread to the deeper skin layers (cellulitis).

What puts your child at risk of impetigo?

- The bacteria that cause impetigo spread on close contact with another person. If your child has impetigo, there is a chance the infection will spread to others in your family.

- Impetigo can follow minor scrapes.

Can impetigo be prevented?

- Washing your hands frequently is probably the best way to prevent the infection.

- Do not share towels or similar items.

How is impetigo treated?

- Your child may receive antibiotics to fight the infection causing impetigo, which may help it to clear up more quickly. A common medication is an antibiotic ointment called Bactroban (generic name: mupirocin). Apply the ointment frequently as instructed by your doctor, usually three times daily for 7 to 10 days.

- Oral antibiotics may be prescribed if your child has widespread impetigo or in other situations.

- Keep the area of the rash clean.

When should I call your office?

Call our office if:

- Your child's impetigo doesn't start to get better within 3 days after treatment.

- Your child develops new impetigo lesions, or the rash seems to be spreading.

- The skin surrounding the rash is becoming red, swollen, or painful.

- Your child's urine becomes red colored.

Influenza

Influenza is an infection mainly affecting the respiratory tract, including the throat and airways. It is caused by a family of related viruses and can become quite severe. Most children with influenza recover completely. However, full recovery may take several weeks, and complications may occur. Getting a yearly "flu shot" helps prevent influenza.

What is influenza?

Influenza is an infectious illness caused by a certain family of viruses. Worldwide outbreaks of influenza occur each year, with young children being at high risk of infection. Influenza is highly contagious and can spread rapidly through communities, especially in places like schools or hospitals.

Influenza can develop suddenly, become quite severe. Although most children with influenza recover completely, there is a risk of further infection such as ear infections and pneumonia.

What does it look like?

The symptoms and severity of influenza depend on several factors, including the characteristics of the influenza virus that is being spread in your community. Illness may develop quite suddenly: within 2 or 3 days after your child is exposed to the influenza virus.

Some common symptoms of influenza are:

- Fever and chills, usually lasting 2 to 4 days.
- Dry cough, which may continue for a long time.
- Sore throat.
- Headache and muscle aches.
- Runny nose and eyes.
- Malaise; "feeling sick."
- Diarrhea.

Other members of your family may be sick at the same time. Infants and young children may develop more severe symptoms, including high fevers.

What causes influenza?

Influenza is caused by a family of related viruses, with slightly different viruses "going around" each year.

Once your child has been exposed to a specific influenza virus, he or she will usually become immune to it. Because babies and young children have not been exposed to as many influenza viruses, they may be more likely to catch influenza.

What are some possible complications of influenza?

- Ear infections (otitis media) occur in up to one fourth of children with influenza.
- Pneumonia (infection of the lungs).
- Other complications such as myositis (inflammation of the muscles) or myocarditis (inflammation of the heart muscle) are possible but uncommon.

What puts your child at risk of influenza?

- Infants and young children are more likely to be infected with influenza virus and may have more severe symptoms.
- Influenza is most common during the winter months.
- Influenza is more likely to cause more problems in children with pre-existing health problems (such as heart disease, asthma, or cystic fibrosis).

Can influenza be prevented?

- Getting a yearly influenza vaccination ("flu shot") can help prevent influenza. Currently, influenza vaccination is recommended for all children between 6 months and 5 years old. It is also recommended for children with certain high-risk diseases, such as diseases of the heart or lungs (including asthma), cancer, or HIV or other conditions causing reduced immune function.
- Influenza vaccination is also recommended for adults who are in close contact with "high-risk" children, and for women who will be in the second or third trimester of pregnancy during "flu season." Ask your doctor whether your child, you, or other family members should get vaccinated.
- Certain antiviral drugs may be used to treat or prevent influenza in children and adults who have been exposed to influenza outbreaks at home, school, or work.

How is influenza diagnosed and treated?

- Diagnosis is based on symptoms and whether a lot of cases are occurring in the community at the time. If necessary, tests on mucous from the nose and throat can be done.
- Make sure your child gets plenty of rest and drinks extra liquids.

- Pain relievers (such as acetaminophen or ibuprofen) may help to lower fever and reduce pain from sore throat, headache, or muscle aches. *Do not* give aspirin to children with influenza, because it may lead to a serious complication called Reye's syndrome.

- We will probably not treat your child's influenza with antibiotics, because these medications only kill bacteria, not viruses. However, if your child develops another infection, such as an ear infection or pneumonia, antibiotics may be recommended.

- Certain antiviral medications such as Tamiflu (generic name: oseltamivir) may be used. These drugs may help your child to feel better and get better faster. However, they are only effective if treatment begins within 2 days after the first symptoms of influenza.

- Most children with influenza recover completely. However, it may take up to several weeks until your child's cough disappears completely and he or she is completely back to normal.

When should I call your office?

Your child's symptoms of influenza should start to get better within 4 or 5 days. If not, or if symptoms get worse, call our office.

Call our office if your child has fever lasting longer than 3 or 4 days, or if the fever gets better and then returns.

Call our office if your child develops other symptoms, including:

- Earache.

- Severe headache.

- Any difficulty breathing, or fast breathing.

- Bloody sputum.

- Muscle weakness or pain developing a week or more after the initial illness.

- Any signs of dehydration (dryness inside the mouth, decreased urination).

Laryngitis

Laryngitis is a viral infection of the larynx, or voice box. Older children with laryngitis may become hoarse or lose their voices completely. However, the illness is rarely severe and usually gets better within a few days. In younger children, infections of the larynx and trachea ("windpipe") may cause a barking cough, called croup.

What is laryngitis?

Laryngitis is infection of the vocal cords and surrounding area, usually caused by a virus. It is a very common, usually mild infection, especially in older children. Your child may be unable to speak above a whisper, or to speak at all. Laryngitis is generally mild and starts to clear up within 4 to 7 days.

What does it look like?

- Your child's voice becomes hoarse or disappears completely.

- Sore throat and cough may also be present, but hoarseness is the main symptom. Your child may "sound sicker" than he or she feels.

- Other symptoms, such as noisy or difficult breathing, are uncommon.

- In younger children, especially under age 3, an infection of the larynx and trachea is called *croup* and may cause a distinctive, "barking" cough.

What are some possible complications of laryngitis?

- Laryngitis in older children has few complications. Your child should start to feel better in 4 to 7 days.

- Sometimes, laryngitis is a symptom of a more severe infection. If your child has other symptoms, such as a high fever or difficulty breathing, call our office.

Can laryngitis be prevented?

Have your child wash his or her hands frequently and try to avoid contact with people who have coughs or colds.

How is laryngitis treated?

- Just as for colds, there is no specific treatment for laryngitis. Antibiotics are usually unnecessary.

- Your child should rest his or her voice as much as possible for a few days.

- If your child is feeling particularly ill, he or she may have to rest more and drink extra liquids.

- Pain relievers (such as acetaminophen or ibuprofen) may help to reduce sore throat. Drinking plenty of liquids may also help your child's throat feel better. Have your child avoid exposure to anything that may irritate the throat, especially cigarette smoke.

When should I call your office?

Laryngitis should start to improve within a few days. If your child's hoarseness or sore throat doesn't get better within 1 week, or if symptoms get worse, call our office.

Call our office if your child develops any of the following symptoms:

- High fever.

- Difficulty breathing or wheezing (high-pitched sounds coming from the lungs).

Lyme Disease

> Lyme disease is a bacterial infection spread by ticks. It is especially common in the northeastern United States but can occur in other areas as well. Lyme disease can cause lasting symptoms, especially if it is not recognized and treated promptly. With appropriate and timely treatment, nearly all patients with Lyme disease recover completely.

What is Lyme disease?

Lyme disease is an infectious disease caused by bacteria carried by deer ticks. People can only get Lyme disease when they are bitten by an infected tick. The disease begins with a circular, red rash that continues to expand over days. Some patients have more general symptoms.

Without treatment, arthritis and other symptoms can eventually develop. Once Lyme disease is diagnosed and treated, the infection generally clears up with no further harmful effects.

Lyme disease causes a lot of concern in areas where it is common, especially in New England and the Middle Atlantic states. (The disease is named after Lyme, Connecticut, where it was first discovered.) However, the risk of catching the infection is relatively low, even in those areas and even after tick bites. Wearing protective clothing while in wooded areas is a simple way to prevent tick bites and Lyme disease.

What does it look like?

Symptoms of Lyme disease vary but are usually divided into early and late phases.

Early phase:

- The usual first symptom of Lyme disease is a red rash (typically called *erythema chronicum migrans*). The rash usually appears at the area of the tick bite a week or two following the bite. The typical rash is a red ring around a white central area that sometimes looks like a target.

- The rash may be itchy and painful and may occur anywhere on the body. Without treatment, the area of the rash may become quite large.

- While the rash is spreading, your child may have other symptoms, such as fever, sore muscles, headache, and just "feeling sick."

- After a few days or weeks, the rash may spread to other parts of the body. Fever and aches may occur, and your child may have red, irritated eyes and swollen lymph glands. Involvement of the heart (carditis) is rare but may occur.

- Nervous system abnormalities may occur, such as:

  - Meningitis, causing symptoms like headache and stiff neck.

  - Bell's palsy, causing temporary difficulty moving some of the facial muscles.

Late phase:

- Later on, Lyme disease may cause other symptoms, especially when no treatment has been given.

- Arthritis is the most common late symptom. Swelling and soreness of the knees is most common, although any joint may be affected. Joint swelling may go away after a week or two. Then it may return, sometimes in a different joint. Without treatment, arthritis attacks may last for a longer time.

- Later, neurologic symptoms can occur. This is rare in children.

What causes Lyme disease?

Lyme disease is caused by bacteria called *Borrelia burgdorferi*. The bacteria is spread to your child when bitten by a tick infected with the bacteria.

What are some possible complications of Lyme disease?

Serious complications of Lyme disease are uncommon, especially with treatment. There is a small chance of infection involving the heart or of more serious infections involving the nervous system.

What puts your child at risk of Lyme disease?

- Living in areas where ticks infected with the bacteria are common.

- Going into woody or grassy areas, where those ticks may be present, without wearing protective clothing.

Can Lyme disease be prevented?

The most important step in preventing Lyme disease is to make sure your child's skin is covered when walking or playing in areas where ticks might be present:

- Have your child wear long pants and long-sleeved shirts. Tuck the bottom of your child's pant leg into his or her socks or boots.

- Apply insect repellant containing "DEET" to your child's clothes.

- Examine your child's body for ticks after spending time outdoors ("tick checks").

- If you see a tick, remove it using tweezers. Be careful not to leave the head. Removing ticks within 48 hours will prevent the child from catching the disease.

- Most tick bites do not cause Lyme disease.

How is Lyme disease diagnosed and treated?

- The first step in effective treatment is recognizing that Lyme disease is present. Many possible conditions can look similar to Lyme disease, and tests to detect antibodies to *Borrelia* bacteria have important limitations.

- Because testing is not that accurate, it should be used only when Lyme disease is possible, based on your child's symptoms and whether the disease is present in your area. Even if your child tests positive for *Borrelia* antibodies, this doesn't conclusively prove that Lyme disease is the cause of his or her symptoms.

- Early recognition allows prompt treatment of Lyme disease. This may shorten the duration of symptoms. However, no studies have specifically looked at Lyme disease treatment in children.

- The usual treatment for Lyme disease in children over 8 is an antibiotic called doxycycline. Younger children may be given a different antibiotic.

- The antibiotic is usually given three times daily for 2 to 3 weeks. Make sure your child finishes the entire prescription, even if he or she is feeling better.

- Doxycycline can make the skin very sensitive to sunlight. Keep your child's skin covered when he or she is outdoors during treatment.

- While your child is recovering, use medications such as acetaminophen or ibuprofen to reduce headaches and muscle aches.

When should I call your office?

Call our office if your child develops any of the following symptoms:

- Stiff neck; severe headache.

- Other signs of nervous system abnormality, such as muscle weakness, numbness, difficulty moving the facial muscles, confusion.

- Joint pain and swelling (arthritis).

Measles (Rubeola)

Measles was once a common and potentially dangerous childhood disease, and it remains so in many parts of the world. In the United States and other developed countries, the risk has been greatly reduced by the use of effective vaccines. Measles is very contagious and can cause outbreaks, especially among groups who have not been vaccinated.

What is measles?

Measles is a disease caused by infection with the rubeola virus, producing a high fever and a red rash all over the body. Measles was once widespread, with occasional outbreaks affecting thousands of children. Although vaccines have made measles uncommon in developed countries, it can still occur and can be serious.

Most cases of measles in the United States occur in people who have come from countries where measles is still a major problem. Although most children with measles recover completely, there is a small risk of serious complications. Measles (rubeola) is different from another childhood infection called German measles, or rubella.

What does it look like?

- Measles starts with a few days of fever and other symptoms, such as cough, runny nose, and red, irritated eyes (conjunctivitis). The fever can sometimes become very high—up to 104°F (40°C)—usually when the rash appears. Your child may look very ill.

- After 2 or 3 days, the typical rash of measles begins, appearing as red spots often with a "bump" in them. There can be so many spots that an entire area will look red. Your doctor may look for typical grayish-white dots inside the mouth, called "Koplik spots."

- The rash usually begins on the face and neck, then spreads downward over the body, covering the arms and legs. By the time the rash reaches the feet, it begins to clear up on the face. The rash usually starts to fade after 2 or 3 days and lasts a total of 5 or 6 days.

- Other symptoms are possible, such as abdominal pain, vomiting, and diarrhea.

How is measles spread?

Measles spreads very easily by means of coughing, sneezing, or contact with mucous or saliva.

If your child has not been vaccinated and is exposed to the rubeola virus, the chances that he or she will get measles are very high.

After your child is exposed to measles, there is about a 2-week incubation period before symptoms begin.

What are some possible complications of measles?

- There are several possible complications, some of them serious:
  - Ear infections (otitis media).
  - Pneumonia (bacterial infection of the lungs).
  - Nervous system complications, including encephalitis (inflammation of the brain) or seizures (involuntary movements).

- With good medical care, few children die of measles in the United States.

- The risk of complications is highest for children under 5 years old.

What puts your child at risk of measles?

- *Not receiving the recommended vaccinations increases your child's chances of getting measles!* If your child is vaccinated, he or she will be almost completely protected against this disease.

- Children who have immigrated from or traveled to countries where measles is common may be at higher risk.

Can measles be prevented?

- *Yes.* Measles vaccination greatly reduces your child's chances of getting the disease. Measles, mumps, rubella (MMR) vaccination is recommended for nearly all children: one dose at age 1; a second dose at ages 4 to 6 years. There is a low risk of some mild reactions after MMR vaccination, such as fever and a rash.

- If you or others in your family have not been vaccinated and are exposed to someone with measles, vaccination may still help to prevent the disease. This is especially important for pregnant women and infants under 1 year old.

- Immune globulin (a blood product that contains antibodies to measles) is used to prevent infection after exposure in certain cases.

How is measles treated?

- No specific treatment can cure measles or kill the rubeola virus. The disease has to run its course. Your child's fever should go down by the time the rash reaches his or her feet. The rash usually clears up completely after 5 or 6 days.

- Your child will probably not receive antibiotics, because they are not effective against rubeola or other viruses. If your doctor suspects secondary infection with bacteria (such as an ear infection or pneumonia), antibiotics will be prescribed.

- Your doctor may order tests to confirm that your child has measles.

- If your child is uncomfortable or has a very high fever, give him or her acetaminophen or ibuprofen.

- Make sure your child gets plenty of fluids.

- The rubeola virus spreads very easily: avoid contact with others who may not have been vaccinated against measles.

When should I call your office?

Call our office if your child's rash doesn't start to get better within 2 or 3 days or if your child develops any of the following symptoms:

- Difficulty breathing along with cough.

- Worsening cough.

- Diarrhea.

- Earache.

- Seizures (involuntary movements).

- Extreme sleepiness or behavior changes.

- Fast or difficult breathing.

Meningitis—Viral and Bacterial

Meningitis is an infection of the membranes lining the brain and spinal cord. When the infection is caused by bacteria (bacterial meningitis), it is a dangerous medical problem requiring immediate treatment. Infection caused by a virus (viral meningitis) is more common but usually less severe. Symptoms of meningitis (fever, stiff neck, irritability, abnormal sleepiness) should always be checked by a doctor and given medical attention!

What is meningitis?

Meningitis is an inflammation of the membranes lining the brain or spinal cord. Although other causes are possible, meningitis is usually produced by bacteria or viruses.

- Meningitis caused by bacteria is a dangerous infection with a high risk of complications, even death. Because *bacterial meningitis* is so dangerous, your doctor may recommend a test (lumbar puncture or "spinal tap") if there is even a small chance that your child has it. The earlier bacterial meningitis is recognized and the earlier treatment begins, the better the chances of your child's recovery.

- Meningitis caused by a virus can spread in outbreaks. *Viral meningitis* is usually less dangerous than bacterial meningitis; serious complications are uncommon.

- With either type of meningitis, your child will need close medical follow-up until the problem has resolved completely.

What does it look like?

Symptoms of meningitis vary, but the most common are:

- Fever.
- Headache.
- Behavior changes; your child may be irritable, lethargic (abnormal sleepiness), confused, or even unconscious.
- Eyes can become very sensitive to light (photophobia); this can occur in other conditions as well.
- Stiff neck.
- Vomiting.
- Babies with meningitis may be irritable and have vomiting, and you may feel bulging of the "soft spot" (fontanelle) at the top of the head. Babies younger than 18 to 24 months old often don't get a stiff neck.

Other symptoms may occur, including skin rash, muscle aches, back pain, or seizures.

What are some possible complications of meningitis?

- *Bacterial meningitis* can result in a number of serious complications, including hearing loss, seizures, damage to the brain or nervous system, and occasionally death. Even after your child recovers, he or she may have neurologic problems, including poor school performance.

- *Viral meningitis* is less likely to cause serious complications or death.

What puts your child at risk of meningitis?

Bacterial meningitis. The main risk factors for bacterial meningitis are:

- In some cases, such as with the bacteria *Haemophilus influenzae* type B (Hib) or *Neisseria meningitidis,* being exposed to someone who has bacterial meningitis increases the risk of catching the disease. (Because an effective vaccine is available, Hib meningitis is now very uncommon.)

- Some medical conditions, such as lack of a spleen, can increase the risk of bacterial meningitis.

Viral meningitis. Viral meningitis usually occurs in outbreaks. It may be caused by "summer viruses," such as coxsackievirus or echovirus. Other viruses causing meningitis may be spread by ticks or mosquitoes, for example, West Nile virus.

Can meningitis be prevented?

Vaccinations are available and recommended for the most common causes of bacterial meningitis, including:

- *Haemophilus influenzae* type B (Hib) vaccine.
- Pneumococcal vaccine.
- Meningococcal vaccine.
- If your child is exposed to someone with bacterial meningitis, getting vaccinated or taking antibiotics may lower the risk of developing meningitis, depending on which bacteria is the cause.
- There is no vaccination for the "summer viruses" that cause most cases of viral meningitis.

How is meningitis diagnosed?

If your doctor suspects meningitis, he or she may perform a test called a lumbar puncture or "spinal tap." This is done by placing a needle between the bones of your child's spine and removing a small amount of fluid (called cerebrospinal fluid). Your child will receive an anesthetic so that he or she does not feel the needle.

Tests are performed on the fluid sample to help find out whether your child has meningitis and what type it is. If bacteria are discovered, the test results will help determine what kind of antibiotic treatment your child needs. If no bacteria are found, then the meningitis probably results from infection with a virus.

How is meningitis treated?

If your child has bacterial meningitis, he or she will need hospital treatment. Some cases of viral meningitis can be handled at home.

Bacterial meningitis requires hospitalization and treatment with of antibiotics to kill the bacteria causing the infection.

- It is important to treat bacterial meningitis as soon as possible. Your child's treatment may start even before the results of the spinal tap are available. Depending on the results of the test, your child's antibiotic may be changed to kill the specific bacteria found in the spinal tap.

- To be as effective as possible, your child will receive the antibiotics through a vein (intravenous, or IV). Treatment time varies, depending on which bacteria are the cause, but lasts at least a week.

- As your child is recovering, he or she may need to have a repeated spinal tap test to make sure the treatment is working.

- Your child may receive other medications (such as steroids) to fight the inflammation caused by meningitis.

- In the hospital, your child will be watched closely to make sure he or she is getting better and to prevent or detect any complications.

Viral meningitis does not require antibiotics. Antiviral drugs are generally not used. However, the doctor may start antibiotics until he or she is sure of the cause.

- Your child will probably be hospitalized if the doctor is not sure a virus is the cause or if symptoms are severe.

- For most types of viral meningitis, there is no medication that can destroy the virus. The viral infection should start to clear up within a few days.

- Common medications for pain and fever may be used.

- Your child will be monitored closely to prevent or detect any complications.

When should I call your office?

Because meningitis is a potentially serious problem, it is important to make sure your child gets close medical follow-up attention until the meningitis clears up completely.

If your child is recovering from meningitis at home, call our office if his or her condition gets worse. For example:

- He or she develops fever.

- He or she stops drinking fluids and starts vomiting.

- He or she seems confused or very sleepy and difficult to arouse.

- He or she just seems "sicker."

- For babies with meningitis, call your doctor if your child seems more irritable.

Mononucleosis (Infectious Mononucleosis)

Infectious mononucleosis—sometimes known as "mono"—is caused by infection with a virus called Epstein-Barr virus (EBV). Symptoms vary but may include swollen lymph glands, sore throat, and tiredness. There are usually no complications, although it may take several weeks for mononucleosis to clear up completely.

What is mononucleosis?

Infectious mononucleosis is a common, usually mild illness. It is most often caused by infection with the Epstein-Barr virus (EBV). Since EBV is spread by saliva, close contact, such as kissing or young children playing together, spreads the disease. Other viruses can cause similar illnesses. It may take a while before your child recovers fully.

What does it look like?

Symptoms of infectious mononucleosis vary, but the most common are:

- Tiredness and fatigue.
- Sore throat.
- Swollen lymph glands, especially in the neck.
- Fever, headache, stomachache, nausea, rashes, and muscle aches.
- Symptoms often come on gradually.
- Pain in the left upper part of the abdomen that may be caused by enlargement of the spleen.
- Younger children have mild symptoms or none at all.

What causes mononucleosis?

Mononucleosis is usually caused by EBV. The virus spreads by close contact with saliva, such as kissing or sharing food. It may spread in day-care centers or schools.

- Nearly everyone is infected by EBV some time before adulthood. However, not everyone who catches EBV will get mononucleosis. The chances of getting sick seem highest in teens and young adults.
- Once your child is infected with EBV, the virus may be present for life. However, it usually does not cause any further illness.

What are some possible complications of mononucleosis?

Complications of mononucleosis are uncommon.

- There is a small risk that the swollen spleen will rupture or bleed. Your child should avoid contact sports such as football until the doctor gives permission, usually after a few weeks.
- Your child's throat may become very swollen, causing difficulty breathing.
- Other complications, such as involvement of the nervous system, are rare.

What puts your child at risk of mononucleosis?

- Infectious mononucleosis occurs mainly in adolescents and young adults. Although children under 4 years old may catch EBV, they often or mild symptoms or none at all.
- Your child can catch EBV only through close contact with saliva from an infected person. Casual contact does not pass the infection.

How is mononucleosis diagnosed and treated?

Your doctor may recommend blood tests to be sure of the diagnosis. Since "mono" can look a lot like a "strep" throat, often a swab from your child's throat will be tested for the streptococcus bacteria.

- For most cases there is no specific treatment that can help your child's mononucleosis clear up any faster. Antibiotics are not used because they are not effective against viruses like EBV.
- If your child's tonsils become so swollen that they interfere with breathing, he or she may receive steroid treatment.
- Medications such as acetaminophen or ibuprofen may help reduce fever and sore throat.
- Make sure that your child drinks enough liquids to prevent dehydration.
- Your child can be as active as his or her energy level permits.
- Your child can return to school when he or she is feeling better. It may still be possible to spread the virus, so have him or her avoid close contact (for example, kissing, sharing cups or food) with other children.

- He or she should avoid contact sports, or other activities that could result in injury to the abdomen, until the doctor gives permission.

- Your child's symptoms should get better within 2 to 4 weeks. However, it may take several weeks longer until your child's energy level returns to normal.

When should I call your office?

The doctor may want to check your child again in 2 to 3 weeks. Call our office if your child's major symptoms haven't cleared up within 2 to 4 weeks or if your child develops any of the following:

- Increased tiredness and weakness.

- Severe sore throat or difficulty breathing or swallowing.

- Not drinking enough liquids to prevent dehydration.

- Sudden or severe abdominal pain, especially after an injury.

- Jaundice (yellow color of the skin).

- Neurologic symptoms (such as stiff neck, difficulty moving the muscles of the face, reduced strength or feeling).

- New skin rash.

Mumps ■

> Mumps is a disease that causes painful swelling of the salivary glands, along with other symptoms. It was once a common childhood disease. Now most children are vaccinated against mumps, but it can still occur. Although complications are possible, most children with mumps recover completely.

What is mumps?

Mumps was once one of the most common childhood diseases. It is caused by infection of the parotid glands (which are salivary glands) with the mumps virus. Its main symptom is swelling of the parotid glands on one or both sides of the face, near the lower jaw and cheek, and can be very painful. It spreads easily by contact with saliva from an infected person to people who have not been vaccinated or have not had the disease. Infection can spread to the testicles in older boys and men. Other complications are possible as well.

Today, nearly all children are vaccinated against mumps, and the disease is rare.

What does it look like?

The main symptom of mumps is swelling of the parotid glands:

- Swelling can occur on one or both sides of the face. Swelling usually develops first on one side and then the other.

- Swelling starts near the earlobe and spreads downward and forward along the jaw. The earlobe may be pushed upward. The area of swelling can become very large.

- Swelling develops rapidly, sometimes within a few hours, although usually over a period of 1 to 3 days. Then it resolves gradually, usually within a week or so.

- The neck and jaw area are very tender and painful. The pain may be at its worst when your child drinks acidic liquids, such as orange juice.

- Your child may have a low fever.

What are some possible complications of mumps?

- The most common complication in children is infection spreading to the brain or spinal cord (meningitis/encephalitis), causing severe headache and other symptoms. However, the illness is usually mild.

- In older boys and young men, mumps may spread to the testicles, causing painful swelling (orchitis). Although orchitis sometimes causes infertility, this occurs rarely.

- Several other complications are possible but also rare, including hearing loss and arthritis.

What puts your child at risk of mumps?

Not being vaccinated is the main risk factor for mumps. Children adopted from other countries who have not received the vaccine may be at risk.

Can mumps be prevented?

Yes. Mumps vaccine has reduced the rate of mumps among children by more than 99%. Measles, mumps, rubella (MMR) vaccine is recommended for nearly all children: one dose is given at 12 to 15 months; a second dose at 4 to 6 years. If your child has missed the second dose of mumps vaccine, it should be given before 11 to 12 years of age.

How is mumps treated?

- There is no specific treatment for mumps. The disease usually goes away on its own in a week or so.

- Medications (such as acetaminophen or ibuprofen) can help to reduce fever and pain.

- Facial pain and swelling make it difficult for your child to chew and swallow. Give soft foods or liquids until the swelling begins to go down.

- To avoid spreading the virus, have your child avoid contact with others for 9 days after the swelling has started.

When should I call your office?

Call our office if your child's swelling doesn't start to get better within a few days or if your child develops any new symptoms, such as:

- Severe headache, confusion or behavior changes, stiff neck.

- Pain and swelling of the testicles or groin.

- Abdominal pain and tenderness.

- Vomiting.

- Chest pain.

- Joint pain.

- Reduced hearing or vision.

Pertussis (Whooping Cough)

Pertussis has the potential to be a serious respiratory infection, especially in young infants. It is caused by a family of bacteria called *Bordetella pertussis*. Pertussis frequently causes intense coughing attacks. It is sometimes called whooping cough because children may "whoop" as they gasp for breath after a coughing attack. Infants with pertussis may need hospital treatment.

What is pertussis?

Pertussis can be a serious childhood disease. Each year, it affects millions of children around the world and causes thousands of deaths. Fortunately, because of the availability of effective vaccines, pertussis is now relatively rare in the United States and other developed countries.

However, pertussis may still occur, even in vaccinated children. The main symptom is attacks of relentless coughing, usually preceded by a runny, stuffy nose. Antibiotics may improve your child's condition and will prevent spreading the disease to others. Family members and others in close contact with a child with pertussis should receive antibiotics as well.

What does it look like?

Pertussis usually starts out with symptoms of a cold. Your child may have a stuffy or runny nose, sometimes with fever, sneezing, and watery eyes. The cold symptoms seem to get better after a few days.

Following these symptoms, your child begins coughing. A dry, hacking cough turns into attacks of coughing. After a coughing spell, your child may "whoop" as he or she gasps for air. The coughing fits may be followed by vomiting. After the coughing spell passes, your child will feel exhausted.

Coughing attacks become worse and more frequent, sometimes occurring as often as once an hour. Gradually, the attacks become less frequent, shorter, and less severe as your child starts to recover, but the cough may last several weeks.

The symptoms may be different in:

- *Children who have been vaccinated against pertussis.* Symptoms are usually milder.

- *Infants with pertussis.* In babies younger than 3 months old, "whooping" is less common. The infant may experience choking or gasping. Symptoms may last a month or longer.

- *Older children and teens.* Pertussis may look like a regular cold, but often the cough last longer—usually two weeks or more.

What causes pertussis?

Pertussis is caused by specific bacteria called *Bordetella percussis*. Other bacteria and viruses may cause similar attacks of coughing and other symptoms.

What are some possible complications of pertussis?

- Especially in infants who are less than 3 or 4 months old, pertussis can be a serious disease. Apnea (periods without breathing) may occur. Pertussis is especially dangerous in premature infants.

- Many babies with pertussis need hospital treatment, occasionally including the use of mechanical ventilation to help them breathe. Although death is rare with proper medical care, it can occur.

- Pneumonia (infection of the lungs) caused by other bacteria.

- Other complications may be related to severe coughing, such as bloody noses, pneumothorax (air trapped inside the chest), or hernias.

- Other infections, such as middle-ear infections (otitis media), may occur.

- Although they are relatively uncommon, seizures and other complications involving the brain and nervous system can occur.

What puts your child at risk of pertussis?

- *The main risk factor for pertussis is not receiving proper childhood vaccinations.* Diphtheria, tetanus, pertussis (DTaP) vaccine is recommended for nearly all children. Your child should receive four doses of DTaP vaccine by age 18 months and another dose between 4 and 6 years.

- Vaccination programs for all children have reduced the number of cases of pertussis in the United States by 99%. Although a vaccinated child may still catch pertussis, the disease is likely to be much less severe.

- The *Bordetella* bacteria that cause pertussis spread easily from person to person. If your child is infected, everyone in your family and anyone with significant exposure to your child may need to take antibiotics to prevent infection.

- Pertussis most often occurs from summer to early fall.

How is pertussis diagnosed and treated?

- The diagnosis is suspected from the child's symptoms and confirmed by tests done on the mucous from the nose and throat. A complete blood count (CBC) can also help with the diagnosis.

- Infants with pertussis, especially those less than 3 months old, often need hospital treatment. Even if the baby seems OK between coughing attacks, pertussis can be dangerous because apnea (cessation of breathing) can occur.

- *Hospital care* is needed:

  - If your child's coughing attacks are severe.

  - If your child's skin begins to turn blue during attacks. This is called cyanosis, and it means your child is not getting enough oxygen. *This is an emergency!* Call 911 or another emergency number.

  - If your child cannot recover or remains exhausted after an attack. "Whooping" can actually be a good sign; it means that your child is strong enough to regain his or her breath after an attack.

  - If your child becomes unconscious (rather than just exhausted) after an attack.

  - In the hospital, your child may need extra oxygen to prevent complications related to inadequate oxygen levels. Rarely, if your child is having a lot of trouble breathing, mechanical ventilation (a breathing machine) may be needed.

- *Antibiotics.* If your child has definite or even possible pertussis, he or she will receive an antibiotic to kill the *Bordetella* bacteria. An antibiotic, usually erythromycin is given, although your doctor may choose a different medication. Additional antibiotics may be used if there is any chance that your child is developing pneumonia caused by other bacteria.

- *Isolation.* Your child needs to be isolated for 5 days after beginning antibiotic treatment to keep the infection from spreading to others. If your child is in the hospital, visits from family members may be limited. This is done to prevent any possibility of carrying the pertussis germ into or out of the hospital.

- *Family members may need treatment too.* Because the *Bordetella* bacteria spread so easily, you or other members of your family should also receive antibiotic treatment. Make sure you take the full amount of antibiotic prescribed. Additional vaccinations may be recommended for young children. If your child has been in close contact with other children or adults, especially at day care or school, they may also need treatment.

- *Home care.* If your child is well enough to be treated at home or to be discharged from the hospital, you will receive detailed instructions on home care, including keeping track of your child's coughing spells to make sure he or she is getting better. You should eliminate all smoking as well as any other sources of irritants in the air. Keep your home as quiet as possible, because excessive stimulation may trigger coughing spells.

When should I call your office?

When caring for your child with pertussis at home, call our office immediately if any of the following occurs:

- Your child's pertussis seems to be getting worse (coughing attacks become more frequent and severe) rather than better.

- Your child develops a new fever, or fast or noisy breathing. These may be signs of pneumonia.

- Your child develops any other new symptoms, such as earache.

The following situations are emergencies! Call 911 or another emergency number:

- Your child stops breathing.

- Your child seems to be having trouble recovering after a coughing attack, especially if his or her skin is turning blue.

- Your child becomes unconscious or confused after a coughing attack.

Pinworm Infection

Pinworms are tiny worms that can infect your child's intestinal tract. They may cause itching around the anus, especially at night. However, your child may have no symptoms at all.

What is pinworm infection?

Pinworm infection is infection with tiny worms. Pinworm infection is very common and spreads easily, especially among young children. The infection is not serious, but it can be uncomfortable. Simple treatments can get rid of the worms.

What does it look like?

- Pinworm infection may produce only mild symptoms or no symptoms at all.
- The main symptom is itching around the anus.
- Itching often occurs at night and may interfere with your child's sleep.
- In girls, itching may occur around the vagina.
- Your child may be irritable or restless.

What causes pinworm infection?

- Pinworms are common parasites. Their scientific name is *Enterobius vermicularis*; pinworm infection is sometimes called enterobiasis.
- Infection occurs when your child gets pinworm eggs into his or her mouth (ingestion).
- Pinworm infection spreads easily.

What are some possible complications of pinworm infection?

- Pinworm infection rarely causes any serious medical problems.
- Rarely, a small area of inflammation (granuloma) may occur around your child's anus.

What puts your child at risk of pinworm infection?

- Contact with other children infected with pinworms. This commonly occurs at school or day care centers.

- If one child in your home is infected, your other children may to become infected as well.
- Pinworms are most common in areas with warm climates.
- Infection is most likely to occur in places were children live, play, and sleep close together.

Can pinworm infection be prevented?

- Because pinworm infection is so common, it is very difficult to prevent.
- Try to keep children from putting unwashed hands into their mouths. Keep their nails short, because pinworm eggs get underneath the nails.
- Your child's treatment will include recommendations to avoid spreading the infection to others and to prevent your child from becoming infected with pinworms again.

How is pinworm infection diagnosed and treated?

Your doctor may have you do a "Scotch Tape test" at home. Early in the morning, before your child wakes up, press a piece of sticky tape on the area around your child's anus. The doctor will then look under the microscope to see if any eggs are stuck to the tape. He or she may provide you with a special paddle to use in performing this test.

- Your child will need treatment with worm-killing medications, which will be prescribed by the doctor.
- Your child should be given one dose of medication immediately. Depending on the medication, your child should take another dose in two weeks.
- While your child is being treated for pinworms, take steps to avoid spreading the infection or having your child's becoming infected again.
  - Have your child bathe each morning.
  - Wash underwear, pajamas, and sheets frequently.
  - Make sure your child washes his or her hands frequently. Keep fingernails short, and try to discourage your child from scratching around the anus.
  - Parents should also wash their hands frequently, especially after changing diapers.

When should I call your office?

Call our office if:

- Your child's symptoms of anal itching don't go away or come back after treatment for pinworm infection.

Pneumonia

Pneumonia is inflammation of the lungs usually caused by infection, most commonly with viruses or bacteria. Viral pneumonias usually clear up with supportive treatments; bacterial pneumonias are treated with antibiotics. Pneumonia is a major health problem for children worldwide, but in developed countries most pneumonias clear up without problems. Children with certain lung diseases or other health problems are at higher risk of pneumonia.

What is pneumonia?

Pneumonia is inflammation of the lungs usually caused by infection with viruses or bacteria. Most pneumonias resolve without problems. Pneumonia can be a serious illness. However, with the use of effective antibiotics for bacterial pneumonia, most children get better without complications.

There are many possible causes of pneumonia, and the most likely causes differ with age. In a younger child, it may be difficult to determine whether he or she really has pneumonia. The severity of pneumonia and the necessary treatment depend on many factors, including your child's age, his or her general health, and the cause of the pneumonia.

What does it look like?

The symptoms and severity of pneumonia in children vary widely. Some of the most common signs of pneumonia are:

- Cough.
- Fever, often high.
- Fast breathing.
- Difficulty breathing: you may see your child's chest caving in, ribs sticking out (retractions), belly going up and down, and nostrils flaring. *This is an emergency!* Take your child to the nearest emergency room immediately.
- Noisy breathing; you may hear "crackles" and wheezing as your child breathes.
- Chest pain may be present along with the other symptoms.
- If pneumonia is severe and your child is not getting enough oxygen in the lungs, he or she may become anxious, drowsy, or restless.
- Like other serious illnesses, pneumonia may cause dehydration. Symptoms include decreased urine and dryness inside the mouth.

What causes pneumonia?

Although bacteria and viruses are the most common causes, there are many other possible reasons for pneumonia. The most frequent causes differ by age group and time of year. To ensure effective treatment, your child may undergo tests to identify the specific bacteria or virus underlying his or her pneumonia.

The most common cause of pneumonia in young children is respiratory syncytial virus (RSV), a very common virus that also causes bronchiolitis (infection and inflammation of the very smallest breathing tubes).

What are some possible complications of pneumonia?

Most pneumonias, including bacterial pneumonias, resolve without a problem. Possible complications include:

- A collection of pus (abscess) may develop in the lungs. This often requires special treatment.
- Although this is very uncommon, severe pneumonia may lead to permanent changes in the lungs.

What puts your child at risk of pneumonia?

- Lung diseases, such as asthma, or cystic fibrosis.
- Breathing in foreign substances (aspiration), including food or acid from the stomach.
- Any nervous system problem that interferes with the normal ability to protect the airway.
- Any immune system problem that interferes with the ability to fight off germs.
- Other injuries, including trauma to the airway caused by general anesthesia for surgery.

Can pneumonia be prevented?

For children with specific diseases that place them at high risk of pneumonia, vaccines may help to lower the risk. A yearly influenza vaccination ("flu shot") is recommended for all children ages 6 months to 5 years as well as for children with asthma, diabetes, heart disease, or any other chronic disease.

All infants should receive the pneumococcal vaccine to prevent infection with *Streptococcus pneumoniae,* the most common cause of bacterial pneumonia in children. The usual recommendation for pneumococcal vaccine is four shots given by age 18 months.

All infants should also receive vaccinations to prevent a particularly dangerous type of pneumonia caused by *Haemophilus influenzae* type B (Hib) bacteria. The usual recommendation is four doses of Hib vaccine before age 18 months.

Pneumonia is most common in the fall or winter, when seasonal outbreaks of infection with respiratory viruses occur.

How is pneumonia diagnosed and treated?

- The diagnosis of pneumonia can be made based on what the doctor hears when listening to the chest with a stethoscope. Often a chest x-ray is needed to detect the pneumonia.

- Some tests on the blood or mucous may be done to help decide if the infection is caused by a virus or by bacteria.

- If bacterial pneumonia is suspected, your child may receive antibiotics. The specific antibiotic chosen may depend on the most likely bacterial cause.

- If the cause is suspected to be a virus and your child's pneumonia is mild, antibiotics will probably be unnecessary.

- Your child will be tested to make sure that enough oxygen is in his or her blood. This is usually done with a device called a pulse oximeter. It is usually placed on a finger and is not painful. Oxygen will be given if needed.

- If your child's pneumonia is not too severe, he or she can be treated at home, including taking oral antibiotics. Make sure your child drinks plenty of liquids to prevent dehydration.

- For infants and children with severe pneumonia, hospital treatment may be needed, possibly including intravenous (IV) antibiotics and fluids. Your child will be monitored closely for signs of worsening pneumonia or difficulty breathing.

- We may recommend a follow-up visit after a few weeks to make sure your child's pneumonia is getting better. Depending on the cause, it may take several weeks for the pneumonia to clear up completely.

- If your child's pneumonia does not clear up as rapidly or completely as it should, further tests may be recommended.

When should I call your office?

Call our office if:

- Your child's pneumonia symptoms (fever, cough, difficulty breathing, chest pain) do not seem to be getting better within 2 to 4 days.

- Your child's symptoms seem to be getting worse.

- Your child shows any signs of dehydration (dry mouth, not urinating).

- Your child seems to be having difficulty breathing: chest caving in, ribs sticking out (retractions), belly going up and down, and nostrils flaring. *This is an emergency!* Take your child to the emergency room immediately.

Rabies

Rabies is a deadly disease, spread by a bite from an infected animal. If your child has been bitten or scratched by a wild or stray animal, we may recommend rabies vaccination. Rabies shots are highly effective in preventing disease. Rabies vaccination is safe and has few side effects.

What is rabies?

Rabies is a deadly disease of the central nervous system (brain and spinal cord), caused by a virus. It is passed in saliva when an animal or human is bitten or scratched by an infected animal.

Because of pet vaccination programs, human rabies is rare in the United States and other developed countries. (However, it's still an important problem in some parts of the world.)

Rabies is very dangerous; if a person gets sick from a bite from a rabid animal, the chances of death are high. That's why rabies vaccination is frequently recommended after animal bites, especially from wild animals such as bats.

If your child is bitten or scratched by a wild or stray animal, call your doctor for advice immediately!

What causes rabies?

Rabies is caused by a virus that can affect many different kinds of animals. The most commonly infected animals in the United States are skunks, raccoons, foxes, and bats. Pet vaccination programs have greatly reduced the occurrence of rabies in dogs and cats. However, these kinds of animals may still be infected with rabies, especially if they are strays.

What does it look like?

Fortunately, human rabies is rare in the United States. When rabies does occur, it causes symptoms such as:

- Behavior changes or hallucinations.
- Spasms in the throat that make it very difficult to drink.
- Fear of water (hydrophobia).
- Possible paralysis of one or more limbs.

By the time any of these symptoms develop, the chances of death are high. Animals with rabies develop similar symptoms. If your child has been bitten by an animal, your doctor may ask how the animal was behaving. The average time from a bite or scratch to developing rabies is 4 to 6 weeks. However, the time can be as short as 5 days or as long as several months.

What puts your child at risk of rabies?

- Being bitten or scratched by an infected animal. Warn your children never to approach wild or stray animals.
- Traveling to certain foreign countries and exploring or playing around caves may increase the risk of being bitten or scratched by an infected animal.
- Contact with bats may cause rabies, even if your child is not bitten or scratched.

Can rabies be prevented?

- Make sure that all house pets receive all required rabies vaccinations. This includes not only dogs but also cats, ferrets, and other mammals.
- Make sure your child knows never to play with wild or stray dogs or cats. Rabies is more likely to spread from stray cats than from stray dogs.
- *If your child has been bitten or scratched by an infected animal, vaccination can prevent rabies from occurring.*

How is rabies treated?

Once rabies develops, the person who gets it is at high risk of death. That's why it's so important to get immediate medical care if your child has been bitten or scratched by an unknown animal.

Bite care. Any time your child is bitten by an animal, clean the area of the bite thoroughly.

- Scrub the area with soap and water.
- Rinse the area for at least 10 minutes. This may include rinsing with an antiseptic solution, such as Betadine (generic name: povidone-iodine).

Assessing rabies risk. Many factors affect your child's risk of developing rabies after a bite, including the type of animal, how it was behaving, and the rabies risk in your community.

- Tell your doctor as much as you can about the bite, including the animal's behavior.
- If the animal was acting strangely or very aggressively, there is a higher chance that it was infected with rabies.
- If the animal was a pet dog or cat that has been vaccinated, your child will not be at risk of rabies.
- If the animal was a stray dog or cat and it was captured, its behavior can be observed to tell whether it has rabies. If the animal was not captured, your doctor may recommend rabies vaccinations for your child, just to be safe.

This may depend on how often rabies is found in your area; the doctor may contact your local health department before deciding.

Rabies vaccination. If your doctor has any reason to believe that your child was bitten or scratched by an animal with rabies, rabies vaccinations will be recommended. It is very important to eliminate even the smallest chance that your child will develop this deadly disease.

- Treatment with rabies vaccine and rabies immune globulin (antibodies to rabies) should be given as soon as possible after the bite.

- Your child will be given one shot of vaccine and one shot of rabies immune globulin right away. These shots are given in the area of the bite.

- Over the next several weeks, your child will need four more shots. These shots are given in the arm. It is very important that your child receive all recommended shots.

- The risk of side effects is low. Vaccination is very effective in preventing rabies after an animal bite.

When should I call your office?

Call our office *any time* your child is bitten or scratched by a wild, stray, or unknown animal or has had contact with bats.

If your child is receiving rabies shots, call our office if any of the following occurs:

- Headache.

- Vomiting.

- Difficulty swallowing.

- Behavior changes.

- Muscle spasms.

- Fear of water.

Sexually Transmitted Diseases (STDs)

Sexually transmitted diseases (STDs) are a risk for anyone who is sexually active. They range from uncomfortable infections to life-threatening diseases like AIDS (acquired immunodeficiency syndrome). Many people with STDs don't even know it, making it easy to pass the disease on to their partners during sex. If you're sexually active, it's important to know about STDs and how to reduce your risk of getting them.

What are STDs?

STDs are a group of diseases with one thing in common: they are passed from one partner to another during sex. Anyone who is sexually active is at risk of getting an STD. However, STD rates are much higher for people who engage in certain high-risk behaviors, especially having a lot of sexual partners and not using a condom every time they have sex.

Fluid draining from the vagina or penis, pain when urinating, and sores on or around the genitals (vagina or penis) are often the first signs of an STD. However, many people have STDs without any symptoms. This includes people with dangerous infections like HIV (human immunodeficiency virus), the virus that causes AIDS (acquired immunodeficiency syndrome). Other STDs can cause lifelong medical problems, including infertility.

All STDs are preventable. Most, such as gonorrhea and syphilis, can be cured with medication. Others, like HIV/AIDS and genital herpes, cannot be cured but can still be treated and improved. If you have any questions or concerns about STDs, make sure to talk to your doctor.

What do they look like?

The symptoms of STDs vary a lot. Sometimes there are no symptoms at all. Other times, symptoms take a while to develop. During that time, you can still pass the disease on to your partner.

The main symptoms of STDs are:

- Fluid draining (discharge) from the vagina or penis. Females may notice an abnormal smell coming from the vagina.

- Pain when urinating. Although this can be a symptom of urinary tract infection, in teens it is often a sign of STDs.

- Males may notice swelling and pain in the area of the testicles or scrotum (*epididymitis*).

- Females may have itching or pain of the vagina or surrounding area (*vaginitis*).

- In both males and females, sores may develop on and around the genitals, including:

  - Ulcers (open sores) or blisters, which may be a sign of herpes simplex.

  - Warts (genital warts).

  - Tiny parasites (lice or "crabs").

- In females, additional symptoms such as fever and abdominal pain can be signs of pelvic inflammatory disease (PID). (See under "What are some possible complications of STDs?")

What causes STDs?

Bacteria. Several types of bacteria and other germs may cause infections in and around the genitals. More than one type of infection may be present at the same time. Some of these diseases are:

- Gonorrhea (produced by *Neisseria gonorrhoeae*), which can cause vaginal discharge, PID, and sometimes infection elsewhere in the body.

- Syphilis (caused by the spirochete *Treponema pallidum*), which is a highly contagious disease that can cause many complications if untreated.

- Infection with *Chlamydia*, which can cause vaginal discharge, PID, and other complications.

Viruses. Different viruses cause different diseases.

- Herpes simplex virus type 2. This virus causes outbreaks of painful genital sores. Herpes simplex type 1 usually causes cold sores of the mouth, but can also cause genital herpes.)

- HIV, which causes the life-threatening disease AIDS.

- *Hepatitis B virus*, which causes liver disease. This virus can be passed on both sexually and in contaminated blood.

- Human papillomaviruses (HPV), which cause warts on the genitals. In females, papillomavirus of the cervix (the opening of the uterus) may increase the long-term risk of cervical cancer.

Parasites.

- Lice ("crabs") may infest the area around the genitals, especially the pubic hair.

- *Trichomonas* causes vaginitis (with vaginal discharge) in females.

What are some possible complications of STDs?

- In females, bacterial infections like gonorrhea and chlamydial infections may cause a more serious infection deeper inside the reproductive system, including in the uterus (womb), ovaries, and ovarian tubes. This is called pelvic inflammatory disease (PID), and it may lead to an increased risk of infertility. Teenage girls are at highest risk of PID.

- Herpes simplex virus type 2 causes a lifelong infection, which may recur for a number of years. A pregnant woman with this type of herpes may pass the infection on to her baby.

- Hepatitis B virus can lead to liver disease. The virus may also be passed on from a pregnant woman to her infant.

- HIV can result in AIDS and destroys the immune system.

- Herpes, hepatitis B, and HIV can all be passed on from a pregnant woman to her infant. Other STDs can also cause serious complications in newborns.

- HPV can lead to cervical cancer.

What puts you at risk of STDs?

All sexually active people are at risk of STDs. The main risk factors are:

- Having a lot of sexual partners.
- Not using a condom every time you have sex.
- Having sex with gay or bisexual males.
- Using injected (IV) drugs.

Teens who start having sex at younger ages and those who use drugs or alcohol also seem to be at higher risk for STDs.

Can STDs be prevented?

- *Not having sex* is the best way to prevent STDs. There are many other ways to show affection and love for another person besides having sex. Never let anyone pressure you into having sex if you don't want to.

- *Limit partners*. The more sexual partners you have, the higher your risk of STDs.

- *Use condoms*. Using a condom every time you have sex reduces your risk of STDs, including HIV infection.

- *Know and talk to your partners*. Don't be shy about asking your partners whether they have any STDs. Remember that a person can look perfectly healthy and still have an STD.

How are STDs treated?

If you are diagnosed with an STD, it is essential to tell your partner(s). They will need medical examination and possible treatment too.

Treatment for STDs varies:

- Many STDs can be cured with antibiotics. These include gonorrhea, syphilis, and infections with *Chlamydia* and *Trichomonas*.

- Antibiotics may be given in a shot or pills. Make sure you finish your prescription completely; don't stop taking the medication just because your symptoms improve.

- *Pubic lice* can be eliminated with medications applied to the affected area.

- *Genital warts* can be treated with topical medications or frozen with liquid nitrogen. However, there is a risk that the warts will return after treatment.

- *Herpes* can be treated with antiviral medications, such as acyclovir. Your doctor can prescribe treatment when outbreaks occur and may recommend regular treatment to reduce the number of outbreaks.

  - To reduce the risk of spreading herpes infection, avoid having sex during outbreaks. However, it is sometimes difficult to tell because the virus can be present without sores.

  - Herpes infection is present for life, but symptoms become less common with time.

  - If you have herpes infection and become pregnant, there is a risk of infection for the infant. Be sure to mention this to your doctor.

- *PID* can be a serious infection, requiring more intensive treatment. This may include going to the hospital for intravenous (IV) antibiotics.

- *Hepatitis B virus* infection may resolve on its own. If not, treatment options are available.

- *HIV infection* is a lifelong problem. New treatments may reduce your risk of developing AIDS.

When should I call your office?

Call our office anytime you have questions or concerns regarding STDs, including how to prevent them.

During treatment for an STD, call our office if symptoms (for example, pain or fluid draining from the genitals) don't improve or if new symptoms develop.

Shingles (Herpes Zoster)

> Shingles is a disease that causes a blistering skin rash. It is produced by reactivation of the same herpes virus (varicella zoster) that causes chickenpox. Shingles is less common in children than in adults, and when it does occur in children it is usually mild. Shingles can be more serious in children whose immune systems aren't functioning normally.

What is shingles?

Shingles, also called *herpes zoster*, is a disease causing blisters on the skin in one particular part on the body. It is caused by the same virus that causes chickenpox, called varicella zoster virus. It is not the same as the virus causing the sexually transmitted disease genital herpes (that virus is called herpes simplex type 2).

After your child has chickenpox, the varicella zoster virus stays in his or her body for life. The virus lives in nerves. Shingles occurs when the virus becomes reactivated, causing a rash in the area served by that nerve. This is seen most commonly in adults and adolescents—it is much less common in healthy children under 10.

When it does occur, shingles in children is usually mild. However, it can be more frequent and severe in children with abnormal immune function or those infected with chickenpox before or shortly after birth.

What does it look like?

In healthy children, shingles is usually very mild:

- A blistering rash occurs in just one area of your child's body.

- The rash may be painful and itchy, and that area of the skin may be very sensitive. However, these symptoms occur less often in children than adults.

- New blisters may develop for a few days before the rash starts to fade. It usually clears up completely in a week or two.

Shingles can be more severe in children whose immune systems aren't functioning normally—for example, because of HIV infection or cancer treatment. These children may have a more painful rash, similar to that of adults. They may also develop more serious complications, which rarely or never occur in healthy children who have shingles.

What are some possible complications of shingles?

- In healthy children, serious complications are rare. There is a small risk that your child will have further outbreaks of shingles in the future.

- The rash may become infected with bacteria becoming crusty or oozing (impetigo).

- Adults with shingles sometimes develop a complication called postherpetic neuralgia, in which the skin remains overly sensitive to pain even after the rash has cleared up. However, this is rare in healthy children.

- If your child's immune system isn't functioning normally, he or she will be at higher risk of complications from shingles. The rash may become more frequent or widespread, or the virus may spread to other organs.

What puts your child at risk of shingles?

If your child's immune system isn't functioning normally, he or she will be at higher risk of shingles and of developing a more severe type of the disease.

Can shingles be prevented?

Varicella (chickenpox) vaccination is recommended for nearly all children. One dose is given after age 1 and again at age 4 to 6 years if your child hasn't already had chickenpox. (If your child has definitely had chickenpox, he or she doesn't need this vaccine.)

Having your child vaccinated against chickenpox will reduce his or her risk of shingles but will not eliminate it completely.

How is shingles treated?

- Your child may receive medications to help shingles clear up more quickly and to reduce the risk of complications. An antiviral drug such as acyclovir may be given for up to a week.

- However, because shingles is usually mild in children and the risk of complications is low, your doctor may decide that antiviral treatment is unnecessary.

- To avoid spreading the virus, keep blisters covered with bandages.

- Antiviral drugs will probably be prescribed if your child has severe shingles or is at high risk of complications.

When should I call your office?

Call our office if:

- Your child's skin rash hasn't cleared up in 1 week.

- Your child develops a red, crusty, or oozing rash.

- Your child's rash returns.

Sinusitis

Sinusitis is an infection of the sinuses, the air spaces behind the nose, below the eyes and the forehead. Sinusitis usually occurs after a cold. When sinusitis is caused by infection with bacteria, antibiotics can be helpful.

What is sinusitis?

Sinusitis is a common infection in children and adolescents, occurring after up to 2% of colds. The sinuses drain into the nose. Swelling in the nose can block the sinus openings and not allow drainage, resulting in sinus infection. When sinus infection is caused by bacteria, treatment with antibiotics is often recommended.

What does it look like?

- Bacterial sinusitis often develops after a cold. Symptoms such as runny or stuffy nose and cough may get worse after 5 to 7 days or fail to improve by 10 days.
- Cough is often present.
- Fever may develop after the first few days of a cold.
- Pus or thick, cloudy mucus may be coming from the nose.
- In teens and adults, sinusitis often causes headache or facial pain. These symptoms are less common in children.
- In children, sinusitis may occur in conjunction with middle-ear infection (otitis media).
- Other possible symptoms include bad breath, reduced sense of smell, or swelling of the face, especially around the eyes.

Symptoms can become severe, with a high fever and pus-like mucus coming from the nose. *If your child has these symptoms, call our office.*

What causes sinusitis?

The sinuses can become infected with the same viruses that cause the common cold. Viral infection of the sinuses usually causes no serious problems, as the infection clears up on its own.

However, the sinuses can become blocked during a cold, which increases the chances that infection with bacteria will occur. Bacterial sinusitis is less common than viral sinusitis but may require antibiotic treatment.

What are some possible complications of sinusitis?

Sinusitis may become a chronic problem, with symptoms such as a runny, stuffy nose and a cough lasting for several weeks or months.

- Although this is relatively uncommon, the infection can spread from the sinuses to other locations.
  - Although it is uncommon, infection can quickly spread to the area around the eyes (periorbital cellulitis) or even inside the eye socket (orbital cellulitis). *If your child develops swelling and redness of the skin around the eyes, eye pain, a change in vision, or difficulty moving his or her eyes, get medical care immediately.*
  - Rarely the infection can also spread to the bones of the skull, the inner lining of the skull, or even the brain itself.

What puts your child at risk of sinusitis?

- Colds, which are more common in the winter months and in children who attend day-care centers.
- Allergic rhinitis (hay fever) or asthma.
- Exposure to secondhand smoke at home.
- Repeated sinus infections may be related to allergies, problems with the immune system, or physical problems in the nose, such as a polyp.

Can sinusitis be prevented?

- The best way to prevent sinusitis is to try to avoid colds; having your child wash his or her hands frequently may be the best prevention.
- Getting a yearly influenza vaccination ("flu shot") may help to avoid sinusitis. However, sinusitis is more often related to colds than to the flu.

How is sinusitis treated?

- Antibiotics such as amoxicillin are the usual treatment for bacterial sinusitis. If your child is allergic to penicillin, other antibiotics can be used. Antibiotics are often given in the hope of helping your child feel better and preventing complications.
- Make sure your child takes the full dose of antibiotics prescribed; don't stop giving your child the medication just because he or she seems to be feeling better.

- Decongestants, nasal sprays, and other "over-the-counter" medications are often used for sinusitis but may not be very helpful. Don't use nasal decongestants for more than 3 to 5 days, as symptoms may get worse after treatment stops.

- Pain relievers (such as acetaminophen or ibuprofen) may help if your child is having headaches or facial pain.

- If the infection doesn't get better within a week, we may change your child's antibiotic treatment, order x-rays, or recommend a visit to an otolaryngologist (an ear, nose, and throat specialist).

- If your child's sinus infection is severe or if it seems to have spread, we may recommend putting him or her in the hospital, starting intravenous antibiotics, or seeing the otolaryngologist.

When should I call your office?

Call our office if:

- Your child's symptoms (for example, pus and fluid coming from the nose, headache, or facial pain) don't get better after 1 week.

- Your child's symptoms get worse (such as severe headache, vomiting, or high temperature).

- Your child's fever disappears and then returns.

If your child develops any of the following signs of spreading infection, get medical care immediately:

- Redness of the skin around the eyes.

- Outward displacement (bulging) of the eye, or double vision.

- Confusion; not acting like himself or herself.

- Eye pain, a change in vision, or difficulty moving the eyes.

- Severe or worsening headache.

- Neck stiffness.

Skin Abscesses

An abscess is a localized infection with a collection of pus. Abscesses may be called by other names, such as "boils" or "furuncles." They usually cause a painful, red swelling under the skin, which may occur anywhere on the body. Your doctor may perform a simple procedure to drain pus from the abscess. To help prevent abscesses, keep skin wounds clean and covered until they have healed.

What are abscesses?

An abscess is a localized collection of pus. It can occur anywhere in the body. An abscess of the skin is usually a minor problem that goes away with proper treatment. (Abscesses can also occur elsewhere in the body, including in the internal organs. This is a more serious problem, usually occurring as a complication of another disease or medical problem.)

The doctor may use a scalpel to drain away the infected fluid from inside the abscess. An antibiotic may be recommended to make sure the infection is completely eliminated. Even minor skin wounds can develop into abscesses without proper care.

What do they look like?

- An area of swelling on or under the skin. Abscesses are usually small at first outset but may gradually get bigger.

- Abscesses may occur anywhere on the body; the buttocks are a common location. The skin over the abscess may be inflamed (red, warm, and tender). Abscesses can be quite painful, depending on their size and location.

- Some abscesses may drain fluid on their own.

What causes abscesses?

- Abscesses are caused when a minor wound (such as a cut or scratch) becomes infected with bacteria (such as the common "staph" [Staphylococcus] bacteria).

- The infection becomes walled off or enclosed as the body attempts to fight off the germs. Abscesses may go unnoticed for some time, especially if they are located below the skin.

What puts your child at risk of abscesses?

Without proper wound care, any cut, scratch, or other wound may lead to an abscess.

Can abscesses be prevented?

- Wash all wounds thoroughly as soon as possible.

- Keep wounds covered with bandages until the skin closes over them.

- Teach children to keep their fingers away from wounds and scabs, since fingers may carry germs that lead to abscesses.

What are some complications of abscesses?

- The main complication is that the abscess will grow larger or spread to nearby areas.

How are abscesses treated?

Although most skin abscesses are not serious, they require medical care. Your doctor can provide proper treatment to relieve discomfort and prevent the infection from spreading.

- *Incision and drainage.* The doctor may perform a minor surgical procedure to drain infected fluid from the abscess. This "incision and drainage" procedure usually provides prompt pain relief. You will be given instructions on how to care for your child's wound after the procedure.

  - Usually, the doctor makes a small cut on the abscess to drain the pus. The cut may be packed with gauze to keep it open long enough for proper healing and to prevent the abscess from coming back.

- Some small abscesses may be treated with warm compresses and antibiotics, without incision and drainage.

- *Antibiotics.* Depending on your child's situation, the doctor may recommend antibiotics to kill any remaining bacteria. Make sure your child finishes the entire prescription, even if he or she is feeling better.

When should I call your office?

After treatment for an abscess, call our office if there is any sign that the infection is returning (recurrence of swelling, pain, warmth).

If your child develops fever, chills, or other signs of spreading infection, seek medical care as soon as possible.

Strep Throat and Scarlet Fever

Strep throat is caused by infection with the bacteria *Streptococcus*. In addition to sore throat, swollen glands, and other symptoms, some children develop a rash. When this rash is present, the infection is called *scarlet fever*. If your child has a strep infection, he or she will need antibiotics to treat it and to prevent rheumatic fever, which can be serious.

What are strep throat and scarlet fever?

Most sore throats are caused by virus, but strep throat is caused by the bacteria Group A Strepococcus. Treatment of this infection with antibiotics may help your child feel better and prevent rheumatic fever.

Some children with strep throat or strep infections elsewhere may develop a rash. When that occurs, the infection is called scarlet fever. The rash comes from toxins released by the strep bacteria. The infection is not more severe just because the rash is there.

Examining your child and performing some simple tests will tell your doctor whether or not your child has scarlet fever.

What does it look like?

- The first symptom of strep throat is usually a painful sore throat. Throat pain often develops rapidly, compared with the more gradual sore throat caused by infection with a virus (for example, sore throat with a cold).

- The throat and tonsils (glands at the back of the throat) look very red and swollen. You may see pus on the tonsils. The tongue may look very red and the area around the lips may look pale.

- Cough and runny nose are not commonly present or are mild.

- Other symptoms may include fever, headache, stomach pain, and swollen neck glands.

- Usually within a day or two, children develop a fine red rash. The rash feels rough, like sandpaper. It is sometimes described as looking like "sunburn with goose bumps."

- The rash may begin around the neck and then spread over the chest, back, and arms. It usually doesn't appear on the face. The bright red fades temporarily when you press on it. It may be most severe in the skin folds, such as the elbow crease, armpits, and groin.

- The area around the lips may look pale and the tongue very red.

- After a few days, the rash begins to fade. The skin usually begins to peel, as it often does after a sunburn.

What are some possible complications of scarlet fever?

Strep infection has some potentially serious complications. With proper treatment, most of these can be prevented. Complications include:

- Strep infection may cause an *abscess* (localized area of pus) in the throat.

- *Rheumatic fever.* This disease develops a few weeks after the original strep infection. It is felt to be caused by our immune system. It can be serious and can cause fever, heart inflammation, arthritis, and other symptoms. Your child can be left with heart problems called rheumatic disease. Rheumatic fever is uncommon now and can be prevented by treating the strep infection properly with antibiotics.

- *Acute glomerulonephritis.* This condition can also occur after a strep infection. It is an inflammation of the kidneys caused by our body's immune reaction to strep. The main symptom is blood-tinged urine (reddish in color). Though treating the strep infection does not prevent this disease, most children get completely better.

What puts your child at risk for strep throat?

Because strep infection is passed from person to person, the main risk factor is coming into contact with a person who has the strep bacteria. If anyone in your home or at your child's day-care center or school has strep infection, your child may be at risk. However, just because your child develops strep throat doesn't mean he or she will get scarlet fever.

Strep throat is uncommon in children under 2 years old. It becomes more common through early adolescence and less common during later adolescence and adulthood. Although your child may catch strep at any time of year, it occurs most commonly in winter and spring.

Can strep throat be prevented?

For most people, there is no practical way to prevent strep infection. The best way to protect your child is to have him or her avoid contact with people who have strep throat.

People who have had rheumatic fever may take antibiotics to prevent another episode of strep infection.

How are strep throat and scarlet fever diagnosed and treated?

- The doctor may be able to recognize scarlet fever just by examining your child and suspect a strep throat by the symptoms and exam.

- The doctor will probably perform some simple tests to identify strep throat using a swab sample taken from the back of your child's throat.

- A rapid antigen detection test can quickly tell whether your child has strep throat. Results are available within a half-hour. If the results don't show strep infection, your child may still need another test called a culture. The culture test is highly accurate but takes a day or two for the results to be known.

- If the doctor thinks your child has strep infection, he or she will prescribe an antibiotic, such as penicillin or amoxicillin. If your child is allergic to penicillin, other antibiotics are available. *To prevent rheumatic fever, it is very important that your child take the full dose of antibiotics prescribed,* even if he or she seems to be feeling better.

- Pain relievers such as acetaminophen or ibuprofen may relieve fever and sore throat pain. For older children, gargling with warm salt water may help the throat feel better. Anesthetic sprays and lozenges may also be helpful.

- Feeling sick and pain when swallowing will make it difficult for your child to eat and drink. Try feeding soft foods and give plenty of liquids for a few days. To prevent dehydration, make sure your child drinks enough liquids.

When should I call your office?

Call our office if:

- Your child's sore throat and other symptoms don't start to get better within 3 days after starting antibiotics.

- Your child's symptoms aren't completely better by 10 days.

- Your child's symptoms return after getting better. He or she may need further treatment, or an additional antibiotic.

- Your child has difficulty opening his or her mouth or is drooling.

Tetanus (Lockjaw)

> Tetanus is a serious disease causing uncontrollable muscle spasms. It is caused by bacteria, which are spread in bites and other wounds where the skin is broken. Fortunately, vaccines can prevent tetanus. If your child is not vaccinated, he or she is at increased risk of tetanus.

What is tetanus?

Tetanus is a disease producing spasms of the muscles. It is caused by a certain type of bacteria called *Clostridium tetani*. The tetanus bacteria have toxic (poisonous) effects on the nerves.

Tetanus bacteria are all around us, especially in the soil. Fortunately, the bacteria generally cause disease only when they get under the skin. Even a minor wound can cause tetanus, if the wound is contaminated by tetanus bacteria. That is why it is so important to keep your child's tetanus vaccinations up-to-date. If your child has a wound, we may recommend vaccination, depending on whether the wound is "clean" or "dirty" and on when your child last had a tetanus shot.

What does it look like?

Tetanus is a serious disease, causing uncontrollable muscle spasms.

- The usual first symptom is called trismus, or "lockjaw." The patient is unable to move his or her jaw because of muscle spasms. He or she may have difficulty chewing, swallowing, or moving the neck.

- Muscle spasms may spread downward throughout the body. The throat and chest muscles may become so stiff that the patient cannot breathe.

- Paralysis and spasms may occur, getting better gradually over time. Most patients survive, but they have a high risk of complications. Tetanus occurring in newborns carries a particularly high risk of death and permanent complications.

What causes tetanus?

Clostridium tetani bacteria are the only cause of tetanus. Tetanus is still a leading cause of death in some Asian and African countries.

What are some possible complications of tetanus?

- Death, especially in very young (and very old) patients.

- Pneumonia and other problems leading to difficulty breathing.

- Cuts, fractures, and other medical problems caused by severe spasms.

How can tetanus be prevented?

- *Immunizations.* Diphtheria, tetanus, pertussis (DTP) vaccine is recommended for nearly all children. Four doses are given in the first 18 months, another dose between 4 and 6 years, and another at 11 or 12 years. Regular "booster shots" are recommended every 10 years. The tetanus vaccine is very safe, with few or no side effects.

- Good wound care, especially for "dirty" wounds, may help to reduce the risk of tetanus.

- *If your child gets certain types of skin wounds,* good wound care and a possible tetanus booster vaccination are needed.

- If your child has a "clean" wound and you don't know if his or her tetanus shots are up-to-date, call our office.

Seek medical care immediately if your child has a "dirty" wound with obvious contamination, such as:

- Animal bites.

- Crush or puncture wounds.

- Obvious contamination of a wound with dirt, saliva, or feces.

- These "dirty" wounds need immediate and thorough cleaning to reduce the risk of tetanus as well as of other infections.

- If your child has a "dirty" wound and has had fewer than three tetanus shots, or if there is any doubt about his or her vaccination status, we may recommend additional treatment with tetanus immune globulin. This shot provides antibodies to fight the tetanus bacteria.

How is tetanus treated?

If your child develops any of the symptoms of tetanus, get medical care immediately.

- All patients who have tetanus need hospital treatment. A tetanus antitoxin must be given as soon as possible, along with antibodies to kill the tetanus bacteria.

- Muscle relaxants are given to treat muscle spasms. Because spasms can be triggered by even minor sounds, sights, and touch, the patient needs to be sedated and kept in a dark, quiet room. Recovery takes several weeks.

When should I call your office?

Be sure to call our office if your child has any type of deep or "dirty" skin wound, including animal bites or scratches.

Also call our office if your child has any significant wound and you are not sure whether his or her tetanus shots are up-to-date.

If you are pregnant and have any questions about your own tetanus vaccination status, mention this to your doctor.

Transient Synovitis of the Hip

> Transient synovitis of the hip is a common cause of pain and limping in children. The cause is unknown but may involve infection with a virus. Symptoms usually clear up in a few weeks. The doctor will monitor your child's recovery.

What is transient synovitis of the hip?

Transient synovitis of the hip is a condition causing sudden hip pain and limping in a young child. Usually, the child hasn't had any recent injury that could explain the pain. The condition is sometimes called "toxic synovitis."

The cause of transient synovitis of the hip isn't known for sure. Since it sometimes occurs shortly after a cold, infection with a virus may be the origin. In most cases, the condition is temporary and clears up in a few weeks.

What does it look like?

- Your child suddenly develops pain in one leg that causes him or her to limp.

- Your child may feel pain anywhere between the groin and the knee. Usually, there hasn't been a recent injury that could explain your child's pain.

- Most children have had a cold or mild respiratory infection a week or two before developing hip pain.

- Usually, no other symptoms are present. Your child may have a slight fever.

What causes transient synovitis of the hip?

The cause is unknown.

What are some possible complications?

Usually none. However, make sure your child gets follow-up medical care until the pain and limping are completely gone. It's important to make sure that your child's hip pain doesn't result from some other disease, such as arthritis.

What puts your child at risk of transient synovitis of the hip?

There are no known risk factors. Transient synovitis of the hip can occur at any age but is most common between ages 3 and 8.

How is transient synovitis of the hip diagnosed and treated?

- There are several possible causes of hip pain and limping in children. Your doctor may take an x-ray or recommend other tests to look for some of these less obvious causes. It is most important to be sure the symptoms are not caused by bacterial infection of the hip joint or nearby bones.

- Your child should take it easy and rest more for a few days, depending on how his or her hip feels. The doctor will want to know if the pain and limping are getting any better or worse.

- Use medications such as acetaminophen or ibuprofen to reduce pain.

When should I call your office?

Call our office if your child's hip pain isn't better after 1 week. We may recommend further tests to make sure your child doesn't have some other cause of hip pain or limping. Also call our office if your child develops any additional symptoms, such as:

- High fever.

- Severe hip pain or pain in other joints.

- Inability to put any weight on the painful leg at all.

- Swelling or redness around the hip.

Tuberculosis

Tuberculosis (TB) is a serious disease that is still a major threat to children and adults worldwide. Fortunately, active TB is now relatively uncommon in the United States, although it still occurs. A TB skin test sometimes shows inactive or latent TB infection. If this happens, your child may need treatment to eliminate the infection and prevent it from progressing to active TB.

What is tuberculosis?

Tuberculosis (TB) is a disease caused by infection with certain bacteria (called *Mycobacterium tuberculosis*). Throughout human history, TB has been a major source of illness. Although it is best known for causing serious infections of the lungs, TB infection can occur anywhere in the body.

Through effective prevention and treatment programs, active TB infection is now uncommon in the United States and other developed countries. However, TB still occurs in children as well as adults. It is a special risk for patients infected with HIV (human immunodeficiency virus, the virus that causes acquired immunodeficiency syndrome [AIDS]).

Skin testing for TB is performed in children with risk factors and in other situations. Some children without symptomatic active TB disease (no cough or other symptoms, and a normal chest x-ray) have a positive result on TB skin testing. This is called inactive or "latent" TB. If your child has latent TB, he or she will receive treatment to prevent active TB from developing.

What does it look like?

Active TB (disease with symptoms) is rare in otherwise healthy children. Cough is the most common symptom, although weight loss and fever may occur first. TB infection may progress rapidly or may remain latent for a long time. When infection spreads within the lungs, it causes definite symptoms, including cough, chest pain, and spitting up blood.

Latent TB (infection but no disease) is still uncommon but may occur. Your child will have no symptoms of TB; he or she will probably seem perfectly healthy. However, a TB skin test will show that he or she has been exposed to the bacteria that cause TB.

- Your doctor will perform a chest x-ray to find out whether your child has active TB disease. If so, effective treatments are available.

- If your child has no signs of active disease, your doctor may make the diagnosis of "latent" TB. In this case, your child will need a different kind of treatment to prevent active TB from developing.

What causes tuberculosis?

Infection with bacteria called *Mycobacterium* cause TB. The bacteria can spread easily if your child is in close contact with an infected person. The infection can be present for a long time before any symptoms develop.

What are some possible complications of tuberculosis?

TB is a potentially serious disease. Active or latent TB infection requires treatment to eliminate the infection.

Treatment prevents serious complications of TB, such as:

- Destruction of lung tissue.

- Bone infection.

- Lymph node infection.

- Meningitis (rare).

What puts your child at risk of tuberculosis?

- In the United States, TB is most likely to occur in children who were born in other countries. The TB infection rate is very high in certain parts of the world, especially in Africa, Asia, and Latin America.

- Most children are exposed to the TB bacteria at home by an infected family member. Less commonly, outbreaks of TB infection can occur in other settings.

- Infection with HIV is an important risk factor for TB. Children and adults with HIV infection are much more likely to develop active TB disease after being exposed to the TB bacteria. However, TB is usually curable even in patients with HIV/AIDS.

Can tuberculosis be prevented?

- Early identification and treatment of people with latent TB infection is the best way to prevent the infection from spreading and to prevent active TB.

- A vaccine for TB is used in some parts of the world, but it has some important limitations. Vaccination against TB is not recommended for most children in the United States.

How is tuberculosis diagnosed and treated?

- *Active TB* (disease) is rare among healthy children in the United States. If your child has a positive TB skin test, your doctor will ask about cough and other symptoms and perform a chest x-ray to see if active TB is present. If so, your child will receive medications to eliminate the infection. Treatment continues for a long time, usually 6 months. Your child will be closely monitored throughout treatment.

- *Latent TB* may be diagnosed if your child has a positive TB skin test but no cough or other symptoms and a normal chest x-ray. Your child still needs treatment to prevent the development of active TB disease.

  - Treatment for latent TB is usually with a medication called isoniazid (sometimes abbreviated "INH").

  - Your child must take INH for a long time, usually every day for 9 months.

  - Your doctor may recommend another medication instead of INH.

  - Side effects of INH are unusual in children. Your child will receive close medical follow-up to check for complications, such as liver or nervous system problems.

- *Drug-resistant TB* is an increasing problem. Some types of the bacteria that cause TB have become immune to the most commonly used medications. If your child's infection is with a drug-resistant type of bacteria, his or her treatment may have to be changed.

When should I call your office?

Whether your child has active or latent TB, he or she will receive close medical follow-up until treatment is complete.

During treatment, call our office if your child develops any of the following:

- Weight loss or loss of appetite.

- Fever.

- A bad cough with chest pain or spitting up blood.

- Abdominal pain or jaundice (yellow or orange color of the skin).

- Medication side effects, or if for any reason your child hasn't been taking prescribed medications.

Vulvovaginitis (Infection of the Vagina)

> Vulvovaginitis is inflammation (soreness, tenderness) of the vagina and surrounding area. These infections can cause itching, burning on urination, and fluid leaking from the vagina. After the doctor performs tests to find out the cause of the infection, treatment is generally effective.

What is vulvovaginitis?

Vulvovaginitis, sometimes called just vaginitis, is fairly common in girls. Several types of infection can cause itching and soreness of the vagina and the vulva (the tissue at the entrance to the vagina). Younger girls may develop "nonspecific" vaginitis related to hygiene problems.

Many other types of infections, including with bacteria and parasites, are possible. Some types of vaginitis result from irritation, with no infection at all. Yeast (candidal infection) is an uncommon cause of vaginal infection in girls before puberty.

Most causes of vaginitis clear up rapidly with treatment. To make sure your child receives proper treatment, the doctor may need to perform tests to identify of the cause of the infection.

What does it look like?

The most common symptoms of vulvovaginitis are:

- Itching and redness in and around the vagina.
- Fluid coming from the vagina (discharge).
- Pain when urinating.
- Irritation from certain soaps or poor hygiene that may cause itching and soreness but no discharge.

What causes vulvovaginitis?

- The main cause of vulvovaginitis in young girls is probably poor hygiene, leading to contamination with fecal (bowel movement or BM) material. Bacteria causing vulvovaginitis include *Streptococcus*, *Escherichia coli*, and *Staphylococcus*. Pinworm infection may also occur.
- The vaginal area is very sensitive in young girls and may be irritated by many different things. Possible causes include certain soaps or detergents and tight clothing or underwear.
- In young girls, sexually transmitted diseases (for example, gonorrhea or infection with the bacteria *Chlamydia* or the parasite *Trichomonas*) should lead to prompt evaluation for possible sexual abuse.

What are some possible complications of vulvovaginitis?

Usually none, but depending on risk factors for abuse, the doctor may check for sexually transmitted diseases.

What puts your child at risk of vulvovaginitis?

Infections and irritation of the vagina are common in young girls. For some girls, vaginitis is a frequently recurring problem. It usually clears up by the time your daughter reaches puberty.

Factors that increase the risk of vaginal infections include:

- Poor hygiene.
- Wearing tight clothing and underwear that does not allow for ventilation. In infants and toddlers, rubber pants or plastic-coated paper diapers may play a role.
- Using certain soaps and cosmetics, including douches and perfumed hygiene sprays.

Can vulvovaginitis be prevented?

- To reduce the risk of vulvovaginitis, avoid the risk factors listed above. Make sure your daughter changes her underpants every day. Cotton underpants provide the best ventilation.
- Teach your child how to keep her vaginal area clean. After bowel movements, girls should wipe backwards, away from the vagina.

How is vulvovaginitis treated?

Most causes of vulvovaginitis improve with simple treatments:

- Sitz baths: Have your daughter bathe sitting down in warm water, without soap or bubble bath.
- Make sure your child avoids things that may irritate the vaginal area, such as harsh soaps, perfumes, and tight clothes.
- Have your child practice good hygiene, and make sure she knows to wipe backwards after BMs, away from the vagina.

- If your daughter's vulvovaginitis seems more severe or doesn't go away, call your doctor's office. The doctor may perform a culture of the discharge from the vagina to find the exact cause of the infection. Proper antibiotic treatment can then be given to eliminate the infection.

When should I call your office?

Call our office if your daughter's symptoms (vaginal pain, itching, and discharge) do not get better with treatment or if they return after treatment.

West Nile Virus Infection

West Nile virus infection is a relatively new disease in the United States. The virus is spread by mosquito bites, so it generally occurs only in the summertime. Although West Nile virus can cause serious disease, it rarely does so in children. Steps to prevent mosquito bites will reduce your family's risk of infection.

What is West Nile virus?

In the last few years, outbreaks of West Nile virus have occurred each summer in the United States. The West Nile virus is one of a group of viruses called *arboviruses* that are passed on by mosquitoes or ticks. (Other diseases in this group include Western equine encephalitis, St. Louis encephalitis, and Colorado tick fever.)

West Nile virus can infect the central nervous system (brain and spinal cord) although that is uncommon. When that does happen, it usually involves older adults and is rare in children. When infection does involve the nervous system, it causes *encephalitis* (infection within the brain), *meningitis* (infection of tissue that covers the brain), or paralysis of certain muscles of the body.

Because West Nile virus is spread by mosquitoes, some commonsense measures to avoid mosquito bites can reduce your child's risk of disease. The same steps will also protect against other diseases spread by mosquitoes.

What does it look like?

- About 80% of people infected with West Nile virus have no symptoms.

- About 20% of people develop mild symptoms of West Nile virus. Symptoms start suddenly, including fever, headache and muscle aches, nausea and vomiting, a rash, and swollen lymph glands. The symptoms may last for as short a time as a few days, although some people don't get better for several weeks.

- Symptoms of encephalitis include confusion, headache, seizures, and behavior changes. Meningitis symptoms include headache, stiff neck, and vomiting. Paralysis means not being able to move certain muscle groups, like arms or legs. These are rare in children.

What causes West Nile virus infection?

- The virus is almost always spread by mosquito bites. The mosquitoes become infected after they bite infected birds.

- Very rarely, West Nile virus has been spread by blood transfusion. (Blood is now tested before transfusion, so this is no longer a risk.) Pregnant women who are infected may spread West Nile virus to their babies.

- West Nile virus *does not* spread between humans.

What are some possible complications of West Nile virus infection?

Although there is a small risk of death or permanent neurologic (brain) damage from severe West Nile virus disease, this occurs mainly in older adults, and is rare in children.

What puts your child at risk of West Nile virus infection?

- Mosquito bites! Taking steps to avoid mosquito bites will reduce your child's risk of infection with West Nile virus. (See "Can West Nile Virus infection be prevented?")

- Outbreaks occur in late summer to early fall.

- Cases of West Nile have occurred in most of the United States.

Can West Nile virus infection be prevented?

Taking steps to reduce exposure to mosquitoes and mosquito bites will reduce your family's risk of West Nile virus infection. Some of the steps you can take are:

- When outdoors, have your child use insect repellants containing the chemical "DEET."

- Keep your child's arms and legs covered; avoid bright-colored clothing.

- Use window screens to keep mosquitoes from getting indoors.

- Try to eliminate mosquito breeding areas. Cut back brush in areas where children play. Eliminate puddles, water buckets, and other possible sources of standing water where mosquitoes breed from your yard and garden.

How is West Nile virus infection treated?

- The diagnosis is proven by certain blood tests, usually testing for antibodies to the virus.

- There is no specific treatment for the infection.

- If the disease is mild, symptoms can usually be treated at home. Fever, aches, and other symptoms should get better in a week or so.

- Patients with more severe disease may need hospital care.

When should I call your office?

Call our office if anyone in your family develops symptoms of encephalitis, including:

- Severe headache.
- Changes in behavior or alertness.
- Stiff neck.
- Seizures.
- Vision changes.

Yeast Infections (*Candida* Vaginitis)

> Yeast infections of the vagina, particularly with *Candida* yeast, are a common problem in teenage girls. These infections cause pain and itching, sometimes with a white, creamy discharge from the vagina. Effective medications are available, but it's important to visit the doctor to make sure that yeast infection is the cause of the problem.

What are yeast infections?

Yeast infections are a fairly common problem in girls, beginning in puberty. Doctors estimate that three fourths of women will have a yeast infection some time during their lives. A family of yeasts called *Candida* is the most common cause of infection. These infections are sometimes called *Candida* vaginitis or "candidiasis."

Most yeast infections clear up rapidly with treatment with antifungal medications, some of which are available without a prescription. However, other vaginal infections can cause similar symptoms. To ensure proper treatment, the doctor may need to perform tests to be sure of the cause of the infection.

What do they look like?

The main symptoms of yeast infections are:

- Irritation of the vagina and surrounding tissues (vulva): burning or itching.

- Pain when urinating.

- Fluid draining (discharge) from the vagina. The fluid varies but often has a white, "cheesy" appearance.

- Pain during intercourse. Yeast infections are usually not spread to a partner through sex.

What causes yeast infections?

- Infection with *Candida* yeasts, especially *Candida albicans,* is the most common cause of yeast infection. It's normal to have small numbers of yeasts or fungi in the vagina. Symptoms of vaginitis only occur when the yeasts increase and grow out of control.

- Similar symptoms can be caused by other infections, such as bacterial vaginosis and infection with the parasite *Trichomonas.* To ensure proper diagnosis and treatment, have your child see your doctor.

What are some possible complications of yeast infections?

- Yeast infections usually clear up promptly with treatment but may come back. For some women, yeast infections are a frequently recurring problem.

What puts you at risk of yeast infections?

Yeast infections are a common problem for women and girls, beginning in the teen years. They are uncommon in younger girls, unless risk factors are present.
Risk factors for yeast infections include:

- Poor hygiene.

- Wearing tight clothing and underwear that does not allow for ventilation.

- Using certain soaps and cosmetics, including douches and perfumed hygiene sprays.

- Certain diseases, such as diabetes.

- Recent antibiotic treatment for a bacterial infection.

- Pregnancy.

- Using oral contraceptives (birth control pills).

Can yeast infections be prevented?

Avoid the risk factors listed above. Cotton underwear provides the best ventilation.

How are yeast infections diagnosed and treated?

- To determine whether a yeast infection is causing your child's symptoms, the doctor may look at a sample of her vaginal discharge under the microscope. If this yeast is present, effective antifungal (yeast killing) drugs are available to treat the infection.

- Some antifungal medications can be bought at the drugstore without a prescription. However, a doctor's visit is still a good idea to make sure the cause of the vaginitis is correctly identified. Your doctor may recommend a prescription-only antifungal drug.

- These medications may be given as creams or suppositories. A single-dose pill medication is available as well. Your doctor can recommend the best treatment for your situation.

- If your doctor gives you a prescription for antifungal drugs, make sure to finish the prescription, even if the symptoms have gotten better. Stopping treatment too early may allow the infection to come back.

When should I call your office?

Call our office if the symptoms (vaginal burning, itching, or discharge) do not get better with treatment or if they return after treatment.

Section XVII - Kidney and Urinary Tract

Bed-Wetting (Nocturnal Enuresis)

Bed-wetting can be a stressful problem for children and parents. Children generally don't wet the bed on purpose. Any child can have an occasional "accident," but medical attention may be needed if bed-wetting is a frequent problem. Behavioral and other types of treatments are available.

What's the medical definition of bed-wetting?

Bed-wetting is seen as a problem when a child who is old enough to have control over his/her bladder (urination) during the day and night wets the bed frequently for an extended period of time. A common definition is twice a week for about 3 months, or anytime bed-wetting is causing a significant problem in any area of your child's life (for example, causing embarrassment or teasing).

Generally, most children can stay dry both day and night after age 5. Bed-wetting becomes less common at older ages but can continue to occur into the teen years. The medical term for bed-wetting during sleep is *nocturnal enuresis*.

What are the types of bed-wetting?

- *Primary bed-wetting.* Bed-wetting has always been a problem.

- *Secondary bed-wetting.* Children who have been dry at night sometimes develop new problems with bed-wetting; the difficulty is often related to some stressful situation in your child's life.

- Some children wet themselves when they are awake (diurnal). This is a different condition and so the evaluation and treatment may be different.

What causes bed-wetting?

Many different factors can contribute to bed-wetting problems, including:

- *Genetics.* Bed-wetting runs in families.

- *Sleep problems.* Children who wet the bed may have a different type of sleep pattern the way the bladder works.

- *Differences in kidney function.* Minor differences in kidney function may interfere with your child's ability to know when he or she has to urinate.

- *Psychological issues.* Sometimes bed-wetting is related to stressful or traumatic experiences.

What are some possible complications of bed-wetting?

Besides embarrassment and family stress, there are few complications. By far, most children who wet the bed have no health-threatening disease or physical abnormality.

What affects your child's risk of bed-wetting?

- If you or anyone else in your family had problems with bed-wetting, your child may be at higher risk.

- Constipation probably increases bed-wetting.

- Bed-wetting is more common in boys than girls, especially at younger ages.

- At age five, 7% of boys and 3% of girls wet the bed. Even in the teen years, bed-wetting is a problem for 1% of boys (but very few girls).

How is bed-wetting treated?

Assessment. Your doctor will ask detailed questions about the bed-wetting behavior. If the problem is simply nighttime bed-wetting, a urine test (urinalysis) may be done. This is mainly to check for infection or diabetes.

Treatment options. Your doctor may recommend one or more of the following treatments:

- Home "do's and don'ts" (behavioral treatment):

  - *Do* try to get your child's cooperation in dealing with the problem.

  - *Do* have your child urinate before going to bed.

  - *Do* make a chart of dry nights, or help your child do so. Offer small rewards for each dry night. Increase the rewards once your child stays dry for several nights in a row.

  - *Don't* wake your child repeatedly to take him or her to the bathroom.

  - *Don't* punish or embarrass your child. Rewards are much more effective than punishment.

- Night-time alarm. A simple "bell-and-pad" alarm system is commonly used. This type of device is a useful addition to the "do's and dont's" listed above and can be very effective. However, the child must be willing to use it.

- The alarm is set off by urine. The goal is to get your child to wake up and go to the bathroom or to clean up the bed.

- After using this device for at least 3 to 4 weeks, your child will be better able to recognize the urge to urinate. For most children, bed-wetting stops after use of this device. Sometimes, however, the problem returns, and the device is needed again.

- Medications may be tried if other treatments don't help. However, medications are less effective than the nighttime alarm device. The problem may return after your child stops taking the medication. Two main medications are used:

- Desmopressin, which decreases the amount of urine produced.

- Imipramine (Tofranil), an antidepressant drug, may be helpful. However, it can have serious side effects, especially if your child takes an overdose.

- Psychotherapy (counseling) is sometimes helpful, especially for children who start wetting the bed after some traumatic or stressful event.

When should I call your office?

Call our office if problems with bed-wetting continue, or if they return after your child gets better.

Glomerulonephritis

Glomerulonephritis is a disease caused by inflammation in the kidneys. There are many possible causes. The first symptom is usually blood in the urine. Sometimes, glomerulonephritis is a short-term problem with no permanent kidney damage. At other times, it is an early sign of chronic (long-lasting) kidney disease. If your child has glomerulonephritis, we will probably recommend a visit to a specialist (a pediatric nephrologist) for further tests and treatment.

What is glomerulonephritis?

Glomerulonephritis is a condition caused by inflammation of the glomeruli, tiny structures that do the filtering work of the kidneys. It has many possible causes, ranging from an immune reaction, infections elsewhere in the body, autoimmune diseases (in which the immune system attacks the body's own tissues), and genetic disorders.

Tests may be needed to determine the cause of your child's glomerulonephritis. Your doctor will probably recommend visits to a kidney specialist (pediatric nephrologist) for further testing and treatment. In many children, glomerulonephritis clears up without treatment. Others are at risk of kidney complications later in life, and some may develop progressive kidney disease.

What does it look like?

Your child may have some or all of the following symptoms:

- Blood in the urine. This is the main symptom of glomerulonephritis, no matter what the cause. The medical term for blood in the urine is *hematuria.*

  - The urine usually appears brown, like cola, and sometimes is rust-colored. (Bright red blood in urine is rare.)

  - Sometimes the urine looks normal, but blood or red blood cells are found on testing or seen under the microscope.

  - Blood may be present for a few days or several weeks.

- Protein in the urine may be detected on a urine test (urinalysis).

- There may be a decreased amount of urine, even if your child is drinking enough liquids. (Kidney function may be reduced.)

- High blood pressure; this may cause headache or seizures if very elevated.

- Pain in the abdomen or side, usually not severe.

- Swelling (edema) of tissues beneath the skin, most often in the feet and lower legs.

- Glomerulonephritis sometimes occurs as a complication of other chronic diseases, such as lupus erythematosus or sickle cell disease.

What causes glomerulonephritis?

Many different diseases may lead to glomerulonephritis. A number of these involve some type of immune reaction:

- Immune reaction to infections—often with group A streptococci (the bacteria that cause strep throat)—is one of the most common causes.

- Other immune system abnormalities.

- Certain genetic diseases.

- Rheumatic diseases and vasculitis (blood vessel inflammation) can lead to an immune reaction, causing inflammation in various organs, including the kidneys.

What are some possible complications of glomerulonephritis?

- Glomerulonephritis may be a temporary problem that goes away with or without treatment. (For example, nearly all children with glomerulonephritis after strep throat recover within a few weeks.)

- For glomerulonephritis from some other causes, most children recover completely but may be at increased risk of kidney disease as adults.

- Glomerulonephritis sometimes leads to progressive kidney disease (continuing damage to kidneys).

Can glomerulonephritis be prevented?

Regardless of the cause of glomerulonephritis, evaluation and appropriate treatment are needed to reduce the risk of kidney damage.

How is glomerulonephritis treated?

Treatment depends on the cause. A kidney specialist (pediatric nephrologist) can perform tests to find out what is causing your child's glomerulonephritis and recommend appropriate treatments.

If symptoms are severe, your child may need hospital treatment: for example, if kidney function is very reduced, if not enough urine is being produced, or if blood pressure is greatly increased.

Treatments may include:

- Giving the right amount and type of fluids until kidney function improves.

- Medications to reduce high blood pressure, if present.

- Steroids or other drugs for some types of glomerulone-phritis.

When should I call your office?

Your doctor (or the kidney specialist) will give you a list of specific things to watch out for, depending on the cause of your child's glomerulonephritis.

Call our office or go the emergency room if your child develops:

- Blood in the urine.

- Decreased urination.

- Headaches.

- Edema.

Hemolytic-Uremic Syndrome

Hemolytic-uremic syndrome (HUS) is one of the most common causes of sudden kidney failure in children. It most often results from gastrointestinal infection with a certain type of bacteria called *Escherichia coli* 0157:H7. This is a serious condition that requires aggressive medical treatment. The chances of full recovery are good, but some children with HUS are at risk of kidney problems later in life.

What is hemolytic-uremic syndrome?

Hemolytic-uremic syndrome is a serious kidney disease usually occurring in children under age 4. Most of the time it results from eating foods contaminated with a type of *Escherichia (E.) coli* bacteria. Other causes are also possible. The disease causes damage to the kidney and blood vessels, resulting in sudden kidney failure and blood abnormalities, including anemia (low blood hemoglobin levels).

Children with HUS need immediate and intensive medical care, often including dialysis to replace lost kidney function. With aggressive treatment, most children survive. Some of these children may be left with severe kidney damage (end-stage renal disease), which requires continued dialysis or even a kidney transplant. In the years after recovering from HUS, your child will need close medical follow-up, as the risk of kidney-related complications is high.

What does it look like?

- Most cases of HUS begin with acute diarrhea, usually caused by eating contaminated food. The diarrhea is often bloody. Other symptoms may include fever, vomiting, and abdominal pain.

- Occasionally, the illness may start with an upper respiratory infection (a cold).

- Kidney and other problems develop within 5 to 10 days after the start of the infection, with symptoms including:

  - Pale skin (from anemia).

  - Fussiness.

  - Weakness, lack of energy.

  - Decreased urination, that is, not going to the bathroom or wetting diapers. This may be caused by dehydration or kidney damage. *If your child doesn't urinate for 12 hours, go to the emergency room immediately.*

- Dehydration: symptoms include dryness inside the mouth, decreased tears when crying, sunken eyes or "soft spot" (fontanelle) on the top of the head.

- Small red spots (called petechiae) on the limbs.

What causes hemolytic-uremic syndrome?

Most often, HUS occurs as a complication of infection with a specific type of bacteria called *E. coli* 0157:H7. The bacteria are usually spread from contaminated food.

- This specific *E. coli* bacteria can be found in the intestines of cattle and other domesticated animals. This is one reason to make sure meat is cooked well enough before eating it.

- Other bacteria and viruses can cause HUS, but these are less common.

Kidney problems aren't caused by the infection itself. Instead, they result from a toxic substance produced by the bacteria during the infection. This substance, called "Shiga toxin," damages the blood vessels of the kidneys. The result is abnormal clotting and other types of damage to the blood cells.

What are some possible complications of hemolytic-uremic syndrome?

HUS is a serious illness. In the past, most children with HUS died. Today, with aggressive medical care, 90% survive.

The main complication is kidney damage. Severe kidney damage (end-stage renal disease) occurs in about 9% of children who survive the initial illness. Later in life, other kidney-related complications can occur.

Children with HUS are at risk of a number of other complications, including problems with the heart, brain and nervous system, and gastrointestinal system.

Can hemolytic-uremic syndrome be prevented?

- Make sure meat is cooked well enough before eating, especially beef.

- If your child develops bloody diarrhea, see your doctor. In general, your child should not be treated with antibiotics before the cause of this symptom is known for sure. If the cause is infection with *E. coli* 0157:H7, antibiotics could increase the chance of developing HUS.

How is hemolytic-uremic syndrome treated?

Children with HUS need immediate hospitalization and aggressive medical care. This phase of your child's care will probably be directed by a kidney specialist (pediatric nephrologist) and blood specialist (hematologist). Treatment may include:

- *Proper fluids and electrolytes* (sugars, salts, and other chemicals the body needs), often given through a vein (intravenously or IV).

- *Dialysis*. Your child will probably receive some type of dialysis treatment to make up for lost kidney function, including the ability to produce enough urine and filter wastes and toxins.

  - Your child may undergo *hemodialysis,* in which waste products are removed by filtering your child's blood through a special dialysis machine.

  - However, many children with kidney failure undergo a different procedure called *peritoneal dialysis.* Special fluids are placed in your child's abdomen to absorb waste products. The fluids are then removed from your child's body, taking the waste products with them.

- Treatments to reduce high blood pressure.

- Treatments to ensure proper nutrition.

- Treatments for less common complications, such as seizures and strokes.

- There are other potential treatments whose value is less clear or that are used in unusual circumstances. Your doctor will explain these treatments, if they are needed.

Although HUS is a serious illness, most children recover without lasting problems. It may take a while for your child to recover completely.

There is a chance that your child will be left with reduced kidney function or permanent kidney damage after HUS. Even if kidney function returns to normal, your child will need long-term medical follow-up because of an increased risk of kidney problems later in life.

When should I call your office?

Call our office if you have any questions about treatment for HUS or about long-term follow-up after your child has recovered.

Henoch-Schönlein Purpura

Henoch-Schönlein purpura (HSP) is a condition most commonly causing a skin rash with arthritis. It results from inflammation of blood vessels (vasculitis). Other organs may also be involved, including the kidneys and gastrointestinal tract. The cause of HSP is unknown—it usually occurs after a cold. Most children with HSP recover completely, but it's important to watch for complications related to the kidneys and gastrointestinal system.

What is Henoch-Schönlein purpura?

Henoch-Schönlein purpura (HSP) is a vasculitis (inflammation of the blood vessels), usually involving the immune system. The most common symptom is a rash, mainly on the legs, buttocks, and abdomen. Arthritis (joint pain and swelling), abdominal pain, and other symptoms can occur as well. Another name for HSP is *anaphylactoid purpura.* ("Purpura" means a rash caused by bleeding under the skin.)

Most children with HSP recover without complications, although complete recovery may take several weeks. However, problems may result from vasculitis involving other organs, especially the kidneys and intestines. Some of these complications are serious, so your child should be watched closely while he or she is recovering.

What does it look like?

- Usually, the illness starts with an upper respiratory infection (cold). Other symptoms may occur suddenly or gradually.
- The main symptom is a *rash:*
  - The rash begins as pink spots that often look and feel like hives or welts. The bumps gradually change from red to purple to brown before they finally fade.
  - The rash usually appears on the lower half of the body, especially the legs, buttocks, and lower abdomen.
  - The rash usually appears in "crops," which last 3 to 10 days. After clearing, the rash may reappear. It may take a few days to a few months between crops.
  - Swelling (edema) may occur in several areas of the body, including the buttocks, face, or hands and feet. Swelling of the scrotum (the sac containing the testicles), if it occurs, can be very painful.
- *Arthritis* (joint pain and swelling) occurs in most children with HSP:
  - Pain occurs mainly in the knees and elbows but usually clears up within a few days.
- Abdominal pain.

- Blood in the urine *(hematuria).* The urine usually appears brown, like cola, but sometimes rust-colored.
- Other possible symptoms include:
  - Diarrhea, sometimes with blood.
  - Low-grade fever.
  - Fatigue (low energy).

What causes Henoch-Schönlein purpura?

The cause of HSP is unknown. Genetic and immune system factors may play a role.

What are some possible complications of Henoch-Schönlein purpura?

The two main complications of HSP are disease involving the kidneys and gastrointestinal tract:

- *Glomerulonephritis,* which involves inflammation of the kidneys.
  - Occurs in one fourth to one half of children with HSP.
  - In most cases, the kidney involvement clears up without causing major problems. Your child will be followed up closely until this occurs.
- *Gastrointestinal involvement.*
  - There is a risk of serious complications related to blockage of the intestines, called intussusception.
  - *If your child has bloody or dark red bowel movements, get medical help immediately.*
- Other types of organ involvement are possible but rare, such as seizures and other nervous system problems or testicular torsion (twisting of the testicles).

What puts your child at risk of Henoch-Schönlein purpura?

- Most common in children ages 2 to 8.
- Usually occurs during the winter.
- Twice as common in boys as girls.

How is Henoch-Schönlein purpura treated?

Most cases of HSP clear up without any specific treatment. There is little that can be done to make the disease resolve more quickly. It usually takes 3 to 10 days to clear up.

Simple treatments can help to reduce the symptoms of HSP:

- To avoid dehydration, make sure your child gets enough liquids.

- Give acetaminophen to reduce pain.

- Avoid hard physical activity.

- If the scrotum is painful or swollen, keep it elevated and apply an ice pack.

  - If your child develops severe pain in the scrotum, call our office immediately.

- *Kidney involvement.* If your child has glomerulonephritis, we may recommend evaluation by a kidney doctor (pediatric nephrologist). This specialist can perform tests to measure your child's kidney function and recommend appropriate treatments. For example, medications may be given to control high blood pressure.

- *Intestinal obstruction* is a potentially serious complication that requires immediate treatment in the hospital. If symptoms are severe, steroids are often helpful and may prevent obstruction.

- *Other complications* (such as seizures or blood-clotting problems), although very uncommon, may also require evaluation and possible treatment.

When should I call your office?

Call our office if your child's rash and other symptoms come back after going away, if they get worse instead of better, or if brown or rust-colored urine is present.

Call our office immediately if your child develops any of the following signs of serious complications:

- Bloody bowel movements.

- Severe pain in the abdomen.

- Coughing up or vomiting blood.

- Severe pain in the scrotum.

- Seizures.

Kidney Stones (Urolithiasis)

You may think of kidney stones as something that happens only in adults, but children can get them too. Most children with kidney stones (but not all) have some type of underlying disease, for example, a kidney problem or metabolic disorder. Tests are usually performed to see if your child has one of these underlying diseases. Many stones pass by themselves, but others require treatment.

What are kidney stones?

Kidney stones are collections of crystallized material that form into stones somewhere in the urinary tract. (The urinary tract includes the *kidneys,* which filter urine; *ureters,* tubes that bring urine to the bladder; the *bladder,* which holds urine and expels it through the urethra; and the *urethra,* through which urine flows out of the body.)

The stones may be made up of several different substances, most commonly calcium. Many factors can cause or increase the risk of stones, such as having too much calcium in the urine or infections or surgery of the urinary tract. In some cases, kidney stones run in families.

If your child has a kidney stone, your doctor will likely recommend tests to see if he or she has any condition responsible for the stone. Some stones pass on their own (go out with your child's urine). If not, other treatment options are available. With proper treatment and follow-up, most children with kidney stones have no complications.

What do they look like?

Symptoms of kidney stones vary, but may include:

- Blood in the urine. Sometimes the blood is visible, but other times it is detected on urine tests. In the latter case, the stone may not be causing any symptoms.

- Depending on where the stone is located, pain may occur on your child's side, or in the lower abdomen or genital area. This pain is sometimes called *renal colic.* Pain may come and go.

- Difficulty urinating, depending on stone location. Your child may feel like he or she has to urinate but be unable to do so. This may be a sign that your child is passing a kidney stone.

- Your child may pass urine with small amounts of gravel-like material. This is a sign that your child is passing a stone.

What causes kidney stones?

Many causes are possible:

- *Metabolic abnormalities* are the most common cause of kidney stones in children. This refers to problems with a person's metabolism that lead to abnormal amounts of minerals (like calcium), hormones, enzymes, and other chemicals.

  - The most frequent cause is higher than normal levels of calcium in the urine (hypercalciuria). This can result from increased absorption of calcium from the intestines or problems with absorption of calcium by the kidneys.

  - High levels of oxalate. It can be found in what we eat such as spinach and vitamin C. More oxalate is absorbed into our bodies with certain intestinal diseases. Our bodies can also make too much of it.

  - Several other metabolic abnormalities are possible but less common.

- *Kidney and urinary tract problems* may increase the risk of kidney stones. Repeated urinary tract infections with certain bacteria and certain types of surgery on the urinary system are special risk factors for stone formation.

- Many other diseases are associated with kidney stones, including cystic fibrosis (a genetic disease resulting in lung and digestion problems).

- Taking certain drugs can also increase the risk, including steroids and the diuretic furosemide (Lasix).

- In some cases, no apparent cause of kidney stones is found. These cases are called *idiopathic.* The diagnosis of idiopathic kidney stones is made only after tests to make sure your child doesn't have other known causes.

What are some possible complications of kidney stones?

Treatment reduces the risk of complications related to kidney stones. Possible complications include:

- Urinary tract infections.

- Kidney damage.

- Other complications may be related to the underlying disease that is responsible for the kidney stones.

What puts your child at risk of kidney stones?

Risk factors depend on the cause. General risk factors for kidney stones include:

- Dietary factors, especially very high calcium intake, a lot of foods containing oxalate, or very high doses of vitamin C.

- The risk is higher in boys than in girls.

- If you or others in your family have had kidney stones, your child may be at higher risk.

- Kidney stones are less common in African-American families.

- A long period of immobilization or bed rest increases the risk of kidney stones by increasing the amount of calcium in the urine.

Can kidney stones be prevented?

Depending on the cause of kidney stones, some preventive measures can be recommended:

- Make sure your child drinks plenty of liquids.

- Diet changes may be recommended for oxalate stones.

How are kidney stones treated?

Treatment for kidney stones depends on your child's specific situation. Factors to consider include:

- The size of the stone.

- Where it is located.

- What it is made of.

- Whether it is causing any blockage or infection.

We will recommend a visit to a doctor specializing in the diagnosis and treatment of urinary problems (a pediatric urologist) or a kidney specialist (a nephrologist). Treatment options include:

- *Letting the stone pass.* Many small stones eventually pass on their own (go out with your child's urine). This may be less likely to happen in young children. Passing a stone can be quite painful.

- *Endoscopy.* A simple procedure may be performed to temporarily widen (dilate) part of the urinary system to allow the stone to pass more easily. An endoscope is an instrument placed through the urethra, into the urinary tract. It allows the doctor to see the problem and perform certain procedures.

- *Lithotripsy.* A procedure called lithotripsy uses lasers or sound waves to break up stones, allowing them to pass.

- Surgery is rarely needed to remove kidney stones.

- *Treating the cause.* Other treatments may be recommended, depending on the problem causing your child's kidney stone.

- *Drinking fluids.* Because stones are caused by overly high levels of certain substances in the urine, drinking plenty of fluids will help to prevent further stones.

- *Diet changes.* If high calcium levels are the cause of your child's kidney stone, your doctor may recommend reducing the amount of dairy products in his or her diet. This has to be done carefully to make sure your child's body is getting enough calcium.

- *Medications* may be recommended, depending on what is causing your child's kidney stones. For example, a drug called allopurinol can help to prevent stones made of uric acid.

When should I call your office?

Call our office if your child has:

- Pain when urinating.

- Blood is seen in the urine.

Posterior Urethral Valves

Posterior urethral valves are a relatively common birth defect in boys. The urethra is the tube that carries urine from the bladder to be passed out of the body. In this condition, abnormal valves in the urethra block the flow of urine. This results in enlargement of the bladder and other complications, some of which can be severe.

What are posterior urethral valves?

Posterior urethral valves are a congenital (present at birth) condition in which abnormal tissue develops in the urethra. The abnormality blocks the flow of urine passing from the body. The problem may be recognized before birth on ultrasound scans.

Depending on how severe the blockage is and how long before it is recognized, posterior urethral valves can lead to serious kidney damage, along with other complications. Surgery can be performed to remove the abnormal valves. Your child will need close medical follow-up to assess kidney function once the diagnosis is made.

What does it look like?

Many boys with posterior urethral valves have their condition recognized before birth. The abnormality can be detected on routine ultrasound scans performed during pregnancy. The scan shows enlargement of the fetal bladder and kidneys.

If your son's posterior urethral valves are not diagnosed before birth, you may notice symptoms such as:

- Poor urinary stream or difficulty urinating.

- Urinary tract infections.

- Problems with toilet training or bed-wetting.

What causes posterior urethral valves?

The cause of the abnormal tissue is unknown. Posterior urethral valves are not a genetic condition—your other children are not at increased risk of this or other abnormalities.

What are some possible complications of posterior urethral valves?

The extent of damage to the bladder, kidneys, and other parts of the urinary system depends on how severe the blockage is and how long it has been present.

- Kidney damage may remain after treatment in about 30% of boys with posterior urethral valves.

- Backward flow of urine (from the bladder, through the ureters, up to the kidneys) may occur. This is called *vesicoureteral reflux,* and it is seen in about 50% of patients.

- Even after successful treatment for posterior urethral valves, your son may need long-term medical follow-up to manage problems such as not being able to control urination (incontinence) or frequent urinary tract infections.

What increases your child's risk of posterior urethral valves?

Posterior urethral valves are a relatively common congenital condition, affecting about 1 in 8000 newborn boys. Girls do not develop this condition.

Can posterior urethral valves be prevented?

There is no way to prevent posterior urethral valves. Prompt diagnosis and treatment reduce the risk and seriousness of complications.

How are posterior urethral valves diagnosed and treated?

Diagnosis. Once the problem is suspected, it is usually diagnosed by a procedure called a *voiding cystourethrogram* (VCUG).

- The VCUG is done to take x-ray pictures of your child's urinary tract. A thin tube (catheter) is placed into the urethra (opening of the penis) and gently pushed to the opening of the bladder. Dye is put into the bladder through the catheter.

- X-ray pictures are taken as your child urinates. This allows the doctor to see the abnormal valves or any other problems of the bladder or urethra.

- Once posterior urethral valves are recognized, a doctor specializing in the treatment of urinary or kidney diseases (a urologist or nephrologist) will probably manage your child's care.

- A catheter may be placed to restore normal urine flow. This simply means placing a tube in the bladder to let urine flow out freely.

- Additional tests are performed to find out how well your child's kidneys are functioning and to assess the rest of the urinary system.

Treatment of the abnormal valves is fairly simple. Usually this is done through a procedure called *endoscopy.*

- The endoscope is an instrument like a telescope that is placed into your son's urethra. This allows the doctor to see and remove the abnormal tissue.

- Your son will be under anesthesia for the endoscopy procedure. It has a very high success rate with few complications and a short recovery time.

Follow-up care is essential to assess and manage any remaining problems with the kidneys or urinary function.

- Follow-up care may be needed if your son has any lasting kidney damage.

- Antibiotics may be recommended to prevent urinary tract infections. This is particularly true if vesicoureteral reflux (backward flow of urine to the kidney) is present. Yearly follow-up examinations will probably be recommended to monitor your child's kidney function and growth.

- Excessive urination, sometimes called *polyuria,* can be a problem. It can quickly lead to dehydration if your son develops some other illness causing fluid loss, such as vomiting or diarrhea.

- Incontinence (difficulty controlling urination) can be a problem after treatment of posterior urethral valves. Further evaluation and treatment may be needed. Follow-up treatment plays an important role in preventing future kidney damage.

When should I call your office?

Call our office if any of the following problems occur, before, during, or after treatment for posterior urethral valves:

- Slow growth or weight gain.

- Little or no urination.

- Signs of urinary tract infection: frequent urination, pain and pressure or a burning feeling, abnormal-smelling urine, fever.

- Signs of dehydration: dryness inside the mouth, no tears when crying, sunken eyes or "soft spot" (fontanelle) on top of the head.

Urinary Tract Infections

Urinary tract infections are a relatively common problem in children, especially girls. Some children have repeated urinary tract infections. Prompt treatment is needed to prevent complications, especially spreading of the infection to the kidneys.

What are urinary tract infections?

Urinary tract infections (UTIs) are infections of the bladder (called *cystitis*), kidney (called *pyelonephritis*), or both. They are usually caused by bacteria and occasionally by a virus. The infections are often caused by spread of bacteria from fecal (bowel movement) material.

Symptoms of UTIs include frequent urination, pain when urinating, and fever. These infections almost always need treatment to get rid of the bacteria and to reduce the risk of complications, which can sometimes cause permanent kidney damage.

What do they look like?

The main symptoms of UTIs include:

- Pain and/or a burning feeling when urinating. Your child may also feel pain in the pelvic area, abdomen, back, or side.
- Frequent urination. Your child may suddenly and urgently have to go to the bathroom and be unable to control his or her urination. Wetting "accidents" in a toilet-trained child are a common sign of UTIs.
- Abnormal-smelling urine.
- Fever, which is often present with kidney infections but usually not with bladder infections.
- In babies, fever may be the only symptom. (However, some babies also have a poor appetite or vomiting.)
- Nausea and vomiting and sometimes mild diarrhea.

What causes urinary tract infections?

- Germs (bacteria) growing anywhere within the urinary system. The bacteria usually come from contamination with fecal (bowel movement) matter. (Bacteria that are normal and harmless in the intestine can cause infection if they get into the urinary system.)
- Occasionally a virus called an adenovirus can cause an infection of the bladder. These infections usually produce blood in the urine.

What are some possible complications of urinary tract infections?

Without proper treatment, UTIs may lead to kidney damage. That's why it is so important to call our office as soon as possible whenever your child develops symptoms of a UTI.

What increases your child's risk of urinary tract infections?

- The risk is higher in girls than boys, especially after the first year. Three to five percent of girls have at least one UTI compared to 1% of boys.
- Children with one UTI are at higher of repeated UTIs.
- The risk is higher in boys who have not been circumcised.
- Other factors that may increase the risk of UTIs include:
  - Constipation.
  - Poor hygiene.
  - Urine-withholding behaviors: rushing to the bathroom, waiting till the last minute to urinate.
- UTIs are a frequent symptom of many different problems with the urinary system, including:
  - Vesicoureteral reflux (backward flow of urine from the bladder to the kidney).
  - Urinary tract obstruction (blockage).
  - Neuropathic bladder (problems with nerve supply to the bladder).
  - Any problem requiring placement of a tube (catheter) to drain urine.

Can urinary tract infections be prevented?

- To reduce the chance of UTIs, avoid the risk factors listed above.
- Teach girls how to keep the vaginal area clean. After bowel movements, your daughter should wipe backwards, away from the vagina.
- If your child has had previous problems with the urinary system, proper medical follow-up can help to reduce the frequency of UTIs.

How are urinary tract infections diagnosed and treated?

Diagnosis. Diagnosis is based on your child's symptoms, evaluation of a urine sample (urinalysis), and urine cultures.

- Urinalysis is an evaluation of the urine for signs of infection, such as pus cells. Children with UTIs usually have white blood cells (pus) in the urine.

  - The urine culture test is the only way to make sure that a UTI is present. It's important to make sure the urine sample used for this test isn't contaminated by germs from the skin or elsewhere. Older children can simply urinate into a cup. For infants, a small tube (catheter) can be placed into the urethra (the tube where urine flows out) to get a urine sample.

  - If bacteria are present in the urine, they will grow in the culture from the urine sample. It takes about a day before the culture results are known. This provides information on the type of bacteria present and what antibiotics will work to treat them.

- The doctor may recommend starting antibiotic treatment before the culture results are known. Antibiotic treatment can always be changed or stopped later, if needed.

- *Antibiotics.* Your child will get a prescription for antibiotics to kill the bacteria causing the infection.

  - Very ill children, especially babies, may need treatment in the hospital. In this case, antibiotics are often given through a vein or intravenously (IV). Your child will also receive fluids and other treatments until he or she starts getting better.

  - Otherwise, your child can recover at home while taking antibiotics. Antibiotics may be given in shot or pill form. Make sure your child finishes his or her antibiotic prescription, even if the symptoms have gotten better. Stopping treatment too early may allow the infection to come back.

  - Antibiotic treatment may continue for about 7 to 14 days. Kidney infections (pyelonephritis) need longer treatment than bladder infections (cystitis).

- *Follow-up.* The doctor will need to see your child again to make sure that the UTI is completely gone.

  - If your child does not seem better within a few days, another culture or tests may be performed.

  - Especially in infants and young children, special tests may be done to examine the kidneys and bladder. The goal is to check whether your child has any urinary system problems that may have contributed to the UTI. If such a problem is discovered, appropriate treatments can be recommended.

Call our office any time your child has symptoms of a possible UTI. 🛈

🛈 When should I call your office?

During treatment for UTI, call our office if your child's symptoms aren't getting better, if the symptoms get worse, or if new symptoms develop.

After treatment, call our office any time your child has symptoms of a possible UTI: 🛈

- Frequent urination.

- Loss of control over urination.

- Pain when urinating.

- Fever in babies, without typical symptoms of a cold or other illness.

Vesicoureteral Reflux

Vesicoureteral reflux is "backwards flow" of urine. When your child urinates, some of the urine in the bladder flows back toward the kidneys instead of out of the body. It is most often a congenital (present since birth) condition. Kidney damage may occur if the reflux is severe or there are frequent or severe kidney infections. Antibiotics may be used to prevent infection. Vesicoureteral reflux often resolves with time. Surgery can be performed if needed.

What is vesicoureteral reflux?

Vesicoureteral reflux (VUR) most commonly results from a birth defect involving the urinary system. Normally, urine flows from the kidney, through tubes called the ureters, into the bladder, and through the urethra out of your child's body. VUR occurs when some urine from the bladder flows back up the ureters, toward the kidney, when your child urinates. This happens because the ureters aren't properly connected to the bladder. The condition is most commonly present since birth (congenital).

The backward flow of urine can lead to kidney damage. This risk depends on how severe the reflux is. Urinary tract infections are often the first sign of VUR. In other children, VUR is detected during tests for problems with urination or suspected kidney disease.

Prompt recognition and treatment can prevent or reduce the damage caused by VUR. Most children are treated with antibiotics to prevent infections until the abnormality causing urine reflux clears up. Most mild cases resolve with time. In certain situations, surgery may be done to fix the reflux problem.

What does it look like?

VUR is most often recognized as part of the evaluation for a urinary tract infection in an infant or young child. Children most commonly evaluated for VUR include:

- Girls younger than 3 to 5 years old who have their first urinary tract infection.
- A school-aged girl who has had more than one urinary tract infection.
- Any boy with a urinary tract infection.
- In children 2 years or older, symptoms of urinary tract infection include:
  - Pain with urination.
  - More frequent urination.
  - Sometimes fever, nausea and vomiting, or diarrhea.

- Abdominal, side, or back pain.
- In infants or toddlers, symptoms may include:
  - Just fever.
  - Sometimes vomiting or decreased appetite.
  - Abnormal-smelling urine.

VUR itself causes no symptoms. Sometimes, VUR is diagnosed during tests for other problems, such as difficulty urinating or frequent urination.

What are some possible complications of vesicoureteral reflux?

- Damage to the kidneys. Over time, VUR, usually associated with infections of the kidneys, can, if severe enough, cause scarring and damage to the kidneys.

What increases your child's risk of vesicoureteral reflux?

- VUR affects about 1% of children.
- VUR runs in families:
- The risk of VUR is much higher for children with various other kidney or urinary tract diseases, especially those causing blockage of urine flow.

Can vesicoureteral reflux be prevented?

Prompt diagnosis and treatment may prevent complications.

How is vesicoureteral reflux diagnosed?

A test called a *voiding cystourethrogram* (VCUG) is performed to find out whether your child has VUR and, if so, how severe it is.

- The test is performed by placing a small tube called a catheter into your child's bladder. Catheter placement does not harm your child, although he or she may find it upsetting. If needed, a mild sedative may be given to relax your child.
- Usually, a small amount of dye is placed into your child's bladder, along with enough liquid to fill the bladder. Then x-rays are taken while your child is urinating. These x-ray pictures can be used to tell whether VUR is present and how severe it is.

Your child will probably also have an *ultrasound test* of the urinary system, to see whether there is any damage to the kidneys. This test uses sound waves to produce pictures of the urinary tract. It can give information on other abnormalities, and about how VUR and infections have affected the kidneys.

How is vesicoureteral reflux treated?

Treatment depends on the cause and severity of VUR. Your doctor may recommend a visit to a kidney specialist (a nephrologist) or a doctor specializing in the treatment of urinary tract diseases (a urologist).

- *Antibiotics.* For some cases of reflux, antibiotics are given to prevent urinary tract infections until the reflux clears up.

  - Your child should take the antibiotics every day. By preventing infections, antibiotics help to prevent damage to the kidneys.

  - Your child will undergo regular follow-up tests to see whether the VUR has resolved. This usually occurs by age 6 or 7.

- *Surgery.* In some situations, the urologist may recommend surgery to correct the abnormality causing your child's VUR:

  - If the VUR is very severe, if reflux is worsening despite antibiotics, or if repeated infections have caused kidney damage, surgery may be recommended immediately.

  - Surgery for VUR is highly effective, with success rates of 95% or higher. Even for children in the most severe category of VUR, the success rate is around 80%.

  - Although surgery is highly effective in curing VUR, it is very important to be alert for any signs of continued problems with urination or urinary tract infections.

- *VUR as a complication.* The situation may be different if your child has VUR occurring as a complication of other urinary tract diseases. In this case, the specialist directing your child's care (a urologist or nephrologist) can advise you of the best treatment options for your child.

When should I call your office?

Call our office if your child has any symptoms of urinary tract infection (frequent urination, pain, fever, nausea and vomiting).

Section XVIII ▪ Musculoskeletal— Orthopedic

Bowlegs and Knock-Knees

You may notice that your child's knees are pointed outward (bowlegs) or inward (knock-knees). Babies and young children often look bowlegged or knock-kneed. However, this is usually normal, and the child outgrows it.

What are bowlegs and knock-knees?

Bowlegs (genu varum) means simply that the legs bow outward, and knock-knees (genu valgum) that they are turned inward at the knees. Parents are often concerned that their toddler looks bowlegged as he or she is learning to walk. Later in childhood, children may develop a knock-kneed appearance. Both of these are normal stages of development that children usually outgrow.

Rarely, bowlegs is a sign of the disease rickets (usually vitamin D deficiency) or other medical problems requiring treatment. Serious medical problems causing knock-knees are even less common.

What do they look like?

Bowlegs. When your child is standing or walking, the knees are far apart and the legs bow outward and then turn inward at the foot. This is normal in babies and toddlers, up to about 2 years old.

Knock-knees. The knees are close together and the lower legs are farther apart when your child is standing or walking. This is normal at around 3 or 4 years of age. It usually resolves by about age 7.

What causes bowlegs and knock-knees?

Bowlegs and knock-knees are most often normal stages in your child's skeletal development. In most children, the legs, knees, and feet are normally aligned by school age or soon after.

Sometimes, the angle of bowlegs or knock-knees is more severe, or the problem doesn't go away as the child grows.

- *Bowlegs* may result from some other conditions that need treatment:

- *Rickets* is a disease usually caused by inadequate levels of vitamin D, which bones need to grow normally. Although not as common as it once was, rickets can still occur. It is a special risk for breast-fed babies who do not receive vitamin D, usually in the form of vitamin supplements.

- *Blount's disease* is a condition in which the top of the lower leg bone does not develop normally. The cause is unknown, but if your child has this disease, the problem of bowlegs may get worse as he or she grows.

- *Knock-knees* are less commonly caused by conditions requiring treatment, unless they are related to a serious injury (such as a broken leg) or cerebral palsy.

How are bowlegs and knock-knees treated?

For most children, bowlegs and knock-knees are a normal part of their development and do not need treatment. Bowlegs are common up to about age 2, and knock-knees until around ages 5 to 8.

- If your child has bowlegs caused by rickets, he or she will require vitamin D treatment and sometimes other treatment. Bowlegs and other bone problems will improve with treatment.

- If your child has Blount's disease, he or she will be referred to an orthopedic doctor (a specialist in bone-related problems) for further evaluation and treatment.

When should I call your office?

Call our office if you are concerned that your child may have bowlegs or knock-knees, especially if:

- The legs look severely affected.

- The condition continues past the normal age for bowlegs (about 2 to 3 years) or knock-knees (about 7 years), or if it is severe.

- The condition interferes with your child's walking, playing, or other activities.

- Your child develops any symptoms, such as pain or aching after activity.

Flatfoot (Pes Planus)

Men with flatfoot were once ineligible for military service because doctors thought they wouldn't be able to march! Now we know that flatfoot causes little or no problem for most adults or children. Babies' and toddlers' feet may look "flat," but this appearance usually goes away as your child grows.

What is flatfoot?

Flatfoot simply means that the normal arch of the foot is missing, or "flat." Most children with the "flexible" type of flatfoot have no pain and no problems walking or running. The arch is present when your child is not putting weight on the foot. Usually, flexible flatfoot does not need treatment.

Other, less common so-called "rigid" types of flatfoot can cause pain and interfere with activity. The arch is absent even when your child is not putting weight on the foot. Rigid flatfoot often occurs in children with other medical problems that interfere with normal development of the foot bones or with diseases that affect muscles (such as cerebral palsy).

What does it look like?

- The foot appears flat on the floor when your child is standing or walking. Depending on severity, the arch may be reduced but is still present. In severe flatfoot, the inside part of the foot may bulge out where the arch would normally be.

- With flexible flatfoot, the arch appears normal when your child isn't putting any weight on the foot, or when he or she stands on tiptoe. The foot usually does not feel painful.

- Your child's foot moves normally. If your child's foot motion is reduced, this may be a sign of the less common rigid type of flatfoot.

- Rigid flatfoot may be painful, especially if your child is active.

What causes flatfoot?

- Flatfoot is usually congenital (present from birth). Your child may simply have loose ligaments (the tough connective tissue that holds the joints together).

- Babies' and toddlers' feet may look flat because of the normal loose ligaments and fat in the area. For most children, the normal foot arch develops by age 6.

What are some possible complications of flatfoot?

- Most children with flatfoot have no symptoms and no complications.

- If foot pain develops, it can usually be easily treated using arch supports inserted into the shoes.

What puts your child at risk of flatfoot?

If you or other family members have flatfoot, your child may be more likely to have it.

Can flatfoot be prevented?

Since flatfoot is usually congenital, there is no way to prevent it.

How is flatfoot treated?

- Most children with the flexible type of flatfoot need no treatment. There is no type of exercise, special shoe, shoe insert, or other treatment that can change the shape of the foot.

- For babies and toddlers, flatfoot is normal. The normal foot arch usually develops by age 6.

- If your child is having foot pain or other symptoms or is having problems wearing shoes, arch supports may be helpful.

- Your doctor may take x-rays to make sure there are no bone abnormalities.

- Inexpensive arch supports are available at drugstores. Custom-made arch supports are more expensive and often not needed.

- If your child has one of the rigid types of flatfoot, a visit to a bone and joint specialist (an orthopedic surgeon) may be recommended for further evaluation and treatment.

When should I call your office?

Call our office if your child develops foot pain, trouble wearing shoes, or other symptoms related to flatfoot.

Fractures

Fracture of even a small bone can be a serious injury. In children, fractures involving the "growth plate" at the end of a bone are a special problem. This is the place where new bone grows, and treatment of these fractures is needed to avoid complications.

What are fractures?

A fracture is a break in a bone. Commonly fractured bones in children include the arm, wrist, and finger bones; the collar bone; and the bones of the leg, ankle, and toes.

Because of differences in the developing skeleton, fractures in children are different from those in adults. Young children with fractures can develop certain complications that don't occur in older children and adults. Fractures also heal more quickly in children than in adults.

What do they look like?

The symptoms of fractures depend on how and where the injury occurred. Common symptoms include:

- Pain—sometimes severe, but not always.
- Bruising.
- Swelling and tenderness.
- Your child may be unable or refuse to use the limb that is injured.

Even for doctors, it can be difficult to tell the difference between a bone fracture, a muscle strain or sprain, or a bruise. X-rays may be needed to tell when a fracture is present.

What causes fractures?

The accident or injury causing the fracture is usually obvious, but not always. Arm and wrist fractures often result from falling onto the outstretched hand. Finger or toe fractures usually result from a direct blow.

Of course, fractures can also result from car crashes and other major accidents. They may also result from child abuse.

What are some possible complications of fractures?

- *Growth plate fractures.* When children get fractures, it is important to find out whether the fracture includes the growing end of the bone, or "growth plate." If so, the growth plate must be in the proper position as the fracture heals. Otherwise, complications related to abnormal

bone growth may occur. For example, the limb with the fracture may end up being shorter than the opposite limb.

- For some fractures, surgery may be needed to make sure the growth plate is in the proper position.
- Growth plate injuries are not a risk for teenagers after they have stopped growing: around 14 to 16 years for girls, 16 to 18 years for boys.

- *Open fractures.* These are fractures in which the bone is showing. Infection is possible.
- *Nonunion.* The fracture may not heal properly, and the two ends of the broken bone are not united.
- *Malunion.* After healing, the ends of the broken bone may not be properly lined up, resulting in abnormal appearance or function.
- *Compartment syndrome.* Excessive swelling or pressure related to a fracture can interfere with the blood supply to a part of the body.
- Seek medical attention immediately if your child develops any change in color, numbness or tingling, coldness, or extreme pain or swelling of the toes or fingers.

What increases your child's risk of fractures?

- Anything that reduces the amount of bone mass can increase the risk of fractures: for example, radiation treatments for cancer.
- More severe fractures have a higher risk of complications related to abnormal bone healing.

How are fractures treated?

Because their bones are still growing, children's fractures usually heal rapidly. Treatment depends on:

- Which bone is fractured.
- How severe the fracture is.
- Whether the fracture involves a joint.
- Whether the fracture involves a growth plate.

The main goals are to have the bone heal properly and to restore normal function of the injured limb. The broken piece or pieces of bone must be lined up properly for normal healing to occur.

- *Broken finger or toe bones* may be treated in the doctor's office. For finger fractures, a splint may be applied. Broken toes may be "buddy-taped" to the neighboring toe. Your child should reduce his or her activity level for 4 to 6 weeks while the fracture heals.

- For other types of fractures, your child may be sent to see a bone and joint specialist (an orthopedic surgeon).

- *Reduction.* Bones with fractures in which the broken bone is not lined up properly need to be straightened. This is called reduction. A *closed reduction* means the doctor puts pressure on the bones to move them into the proper position without any surgery. Some fractures are so bad that surgery is needed to straighten the bone. This is called an *open reduction.*

- *Casting.* A cast is placed on the fractured area to keep the fragments in place while the bone is healing. X-rays can "see" through the cast, so these may be used to monitor your child's fracture as it heals.

  - The cast will need to be in place for several weeks for complete healing to occur.

  - Keep an eye on the fingers and toes beyond the point of the fracture. Excessive swelling or pressure underneath the cast can cause problems.

- Be careful not to let your child's cast get wet. Seal the cast in a plastic bag for bathing.

- Itching under a cast can be a problem. Make sure your child doesn't stick anything under the cast to scratch.

- *Pain.* All fractures are painful. Medications such as acetaminophen, ibuprofen, or narcotics, if necessary, can help to control your child's pain during the initial healing process.

When should I call your office?

Call your orthopedic surgeon's office or our office if:

- Your child has continued pain after a fracture that does not respond to medications.

- Your child's cast or splint falls off or becomes damaged.

- Get medical attention immediately if your child develops any change in color, numbness or tingling, coldness, or extreme pain or swelling of the toes or fingers.

Ganglion Cyst

A ganglion cyst is a lump that develops on your child's hand or wrist or occasionally the foot. These cysts are usually harmless and often go away on their own. If the cyst becomes large or causes lasting pain, minor surgery can be done to remove it.

What is a ganglion cyst?

A ganglion cyst is a small pouch of tissue that forms in the wrist or hand and fills with joint fluid (synovial fluid). Ganglion cysts are most commonly found on the top of the wrist or back of the hand but may occur on the underside of the wrist or on the fingers. The cyst may get bigger when your child moves the joint.

What does it look like?

- A round, firm lump on the wrist or hand. The cyst may appear suddenly or gradually.
- The cyst may get bigger with exercise, smaller at rest.
- If it is large, the cyst may cause some pain or numbness or interfere with normal movement.

What causes ganglion cysts?

A small opening forms in the capsule surround the joint.

What are some possible complications of ganglion cysts?

Ganglion cysts are usually harmless. Occasionally, they may press on nerves, causing numbness or weakness.

What puts your child at risk of ganglion cysts?

- Ganglion cysts are more common in teens than in younger children.
- They are more common in girls than in boys.

How are ganglion cysts treated?

Ganglion cysts often go away on their own. Treatment may be recommended if the cyst is causing symptoms (such as pain or numbness) or is interfering with normal joint movement.

- Aspiration: a needle is placed to draw the fluid out of the cyst. This treatment can be repeated if the cyst comes back.
- Surgery: a minor surgical procedure can be performed to remove the cyst. Surgery is usually successful in eliminating the cyst completely and permanently.

When should I call your office?

Call our office if:

- Your child has a ganglion cyst causing symptoms such as pain or numbness or if the cyst interferes with normal joint movement.
- Your child has a ganglion cyst that comes back after treatment.

Growing Pains

"Growing pains" are a common experience for preschool and school-aged children. They are episodes of pain in your child's legs. No one knows for sure what causes growing pains; they may just be muscle spasms that occur after an active day's playing. Although they can be quite painful, brief episodes of growing pains in the legs are normal and harmless.

What are growing pains?

Growing pains are episodes of pain in your child's legs. They are most common in preschool and preteen children. Although the pain is real, the cause of growing pains in children is unknown. One explanation is that the pains may result from muscle contractions or spasms, usually at the end of a day of active playing.

What do they look like?

- Pains often occur at night or when your child is resting.
- Pain usually occurs in the lower legs.
- Pain does *not* occur in the joints (hips or ankles).
- Rubbing the legs lessens the pain.

What are some possible complications of growing pains?

None. Unless there is another explanation for your child's leg pain, the pains will go away completely with no harmful effects.

What puts your child at risk of growing pains?

Growing pains are a very common, even normal, experience for children.

Can growing pains be prevented?

Since the cause is unknown, there is no clear way to prevent growing pains. Stretching the muscles before exercise or activity may be helpful.

How are growing pains treated?

- Rubbing your child's legs may make the pain lessen.
- Pain medications (acetaminophen or ibuprofen) may be helpful.

When should I call your office?

Occasional episodes of growing pains are harmless and can be safely treated at home.
Call our office if:

- Your child has leg pain after an accident or injury.
- Your child has pain in the leg joints, not just the muscles.
- Your child has severe leg pain or tenderness.

Legg-Calvé-Perthes Disease

Legg-Calvé-Perthes disease is a hip disease that occurs in growing children. Your child may start limping but feel little or no pain. Especially in young children, Legg-Calvé-Perthes disease may heal on its own with no treatment needed. However, some children need treatment to prevent or correct hip deformities.

What is Legg-Calvé-Perthes disease?

Legg-Calvé-Perthes disease affects the "ball" of the hip joint at the top of the thigh bone (femur) in growing children. For some reason, the blood supply to this part of the bone (the ball) becomes interrupted. Part of the bone dies, resulting in pain and limping. Treatment depends on your child's age and the severity of his or her symptoms.

What does it look like?

- Your child starts limping. Limping usually develops gradually over time. It tends to get worse when your child is active.
- Most children do not have much pain. When present, pain is in the front of the thigh, anywhere between the hip and the knee.
- Hip motion may be limited.
- Sometimes, both hips are involved.

What causes Legg-Calvé-Perthes disease?

The blood supply to the ball of the hip joint becomes reduced. The cause is unknown.

Whatever the cause, the reduced blood supply causes some of the bone to die. It may be only a small area, or the entire ball may be affected. The bone stops growing until new blood vessels can develop. Treatment may be needed to keep the ball in its proper position in the hip socket, so that the new bone grows in the proper shape.

What are some possible complications of Legg-Calvé-Perthes disease?

If the bone does not regrow in the proper way, various types of hip deformities may develop.

Children with Legg-Calvé-Perthes disease have a higher risk of arthritis of the hip in adulthood. This risk is greater if your child is older when Legg-Calvé-Perthes disease develops, or if the hip joint is not normal after the bone heals.

What puts your child at risk of Legg-Calvé-Perthes disease?

Although the cause is unknown, certain risk factors for this hip disease have been noticed:

- Legg-Calvé-Perthes disease most commonly occurs around 6 to 7 years but can occur at any age between 2 and 12 years.
- Legg-Calvé-Perthes disease is more likely to be found in boys than in girls. However, the problem may appear at an earlier age and tends to be more severe in girls.

Can Legg-Calvé-Perthes disease be prevented?

- Since the cause is unknown, there is no known way to prevent Legg-Calvé-Perthes disease.
- Once the condition is present, early treatment is important to reduce the risk of hip deformity.

How is Legg-Calvé-Perthes disease treated?

Depending on your child's age and the severity of Legg-Calvé-Perthes disease, options range from close observation with no or occasional treatment to bracing or to surgery. Your child will probably be sent to a bone and joint specialist (an orthopedic surgeon) for further evaluation.

- *No treatment.* Especially if your child is under 6 years old, he or she may receive no specific treatment at first. Frequent medical follow-up, including doctor visits and x-rays, may be recommended.
- *Temporary treatment.* Depending on his or her symptoms, bed rest or stretching exercises may be recommended as your child's hip heals. During the healing process, your child may have episodes of pain and reduced motion.

More definitive treatments may be needed to make sure the damaged bone heals properly and to prevent arthritis from developing. These treatments are more likely to be needed if your child is older, overweight, or has loss of hip motion.

- *Bracing.* A brace, or sometimes a cast, may be recommended. The goal is to keep the ball of the joint inside the hip socket. This ensures that the healing bone will take on the proper shape to fit inside the hip joint. Your child may have to wear the cast or brace for a year or longer, until the hip bone begins to heal.

- *Surgery.* Sometimes surgery rather than bracing is recommended. If your child's Legg-Calvé-Perthes disease does not heal properly, surgery may be needed to correct the hip deformity.

When should I call your office?

Call your orthopedic surgeon's office or our office if your child develops new or severe pain, limping, or loss of hip motion during treatment for Legg-Calvé-Perthes disease.

Nursemaid's Elbow
(Pulled Elbow)

> Nursemaid's elbow is a partial dislocation of one of the forearm bones at the elbow. It is a common injury in toddlers, often caused by an adult's pulling or swinging the child by the arms. Usually, nursemaid's elbow is easily treated by the doctor's putting the dislocated bone back in place.

What is nursemaid's elbow?

Nursemaid's elbow is a partial dislocation of the "radial head," which is one of the bones of the elbow. Because this bone is not fully developed in toddlers, it is easy for one of the elbow ligaments to slip over the end of the bone.

Nursemaid's elbow is not a serious injury, and it is relatively easy to correct. Because the joint is so flexible in young children, the ligament slips back into place easily. However, the injury can easily happen again, so you must be careful to avoid pulling or tugging on your child's arm.

What does it look like?

- Your child has pain and difficulty moving his or her arm.
- Often, he or she starts crying immediately after being lifted or pulled by the arm.
- Your child refuses to move the arm or to let you move it. He or she usually holds the arm in a bent position in front of the body, as if it were in a sling.
- Your child may otherwise be happy and playful—he or she just refuses to move the injured arm.

What causes nursemaid's elbow?

- Pulling or jerking on your toddler's arm, for example, pulling your child up a step or swinging him or her by the arms.
- In about one half of children with nursemaid's elbow, the exact cause of the injury is unknown.
- Nursemaid's elbow most often occurs in toddlers ages 1 to 3 years. It rarely happens after age 5 because the skeleton has matured.
- If your child has had this type of elbow injury in the past, it is not uncommon for it to happen again.

What are some possible complications of nursemaid's elbow?

As long as the injury is recognized and treated properly, complications are rare.

Can nursemaid's elbow be prevented?

Yes. Do not pull on your baby's or toddler's arms.

- Don't pull him or her by the outstretched arms up a step or curb or out of a car seat.
- Don't swing your child by the arms.
- Don't jerk on your child's arms, especially when you are angry. (Nursemaid's elbow is sometimes called "temper tantrum elbow" because the injury sometimes happens when the child is having a tantrum.)

The proper way to lift an infant or toddler is under the armpits or by the upper arms, never by the hand or wrist.

How is nursemaid's elbow treated?

- The doctor can usually move the elbow joint back into proper position. This can be done in the office or emergency room, usually with no need for anesthetic.
- *Do not* try to move the elbow yourself.
- It may take more than one try before the elbow moves back into place.
- You may hear a "pop" or "click" as the elbow moves back into place.
- Your child will likely be upset and cry while the doctor is manipulating the elbow. Crying usually stops not long after the elbow position is returned to normal.
- Your child will probably be able to use the arm soon after treatment. However, this may take a while if he or she is afraid to move the arm.

When should I call your office?

Call our office if your child develops new or repeated symptoms of nursemaid's elbow (refusal to move the arm, crying after being pulled or jerked by the arm).

Osgood-Schlatter Disease

Osgood-Schlatter disease is a condition causing pain just under the kneecap, not in the knee joint. It occurs most commonly in children who play sports, mainly in the preteen and teen years. The pain usually goes away by the time your child is done growing. We may recommend that your child temporarily reduce sports activity.

What is Osgood-Schlatter disease?

Osgood-Schlatter disease is a problem caused by irritation of the growing bony bump (tibial tubercle) just below the knee, where one of the powerful knee tendons is attached to the bone. The most common cause of irritation is your child's participation in frequent sports or other activities. Osgood-Schlatter disease is a common cause of knee pain in children and teens.

What does it look like?

- The main symptom of Osgood-Schlatter disease is pain just below the knee. The bony bump under the knee may be tender and swollen.

- Pain usually starts after your child has been playing sports or other activities. Once he or she rests for a while, the pain goes away. Pain may be present in one or both knees.

- Osgood-Schlatter disease is most common in children in their early teens who play sports involving sprinting and jumping, such as football, basketball, soccer, gymnastics, or ballet.

- Girls are most likely to have Osgood-Schlatter disease between 8 and 14 years and boys between 10 and 15 years. The problem is more common in boys, but this may change as more girls play sports.

What causes Osgood-Schlatter disease?

The condition is felt to be caused by irritation and tiny fractures (very small breaks) in the bony bump (called "tibial tubercle") below the knee. A tendon from the knee attaches at the bump and pulls on the bone (which can cause the problem) when the child is active. This type of damage most often occurs in active children, especially those who frequently play organized sports.

What are some possible complications of Osgood-Schlatter disease?

- For most children, Osgood-Schlatter disease causes no lasting problems: the pain goes away by the time your child is done growing.

- Surgery is rarely needed but may be considered if problems with Osgood-Schlatter continue.

How is Osgood-Schlatter disease treated?

- Rest or reduced activity is the main treatment for knee pain caused by Osgood-Schlatter disease. Your child may have to reduce playing sports and other activities that aggravate the knee pain, such as playing basketball or climbing stairs.

- If the pain is mild, reduced activity may be the only treatment needed.

- For more severe pain, give your child pain relievers or anti-inflammatory drugs (such as ibuprofen) or ice packs.

- A program of stretching the leg muscles and strengthening the quadriceps muscles (the muscles of the front of the thigh) may be recommended.

- Wearing a pad under the knee may help keep the area from becoming irritated.

- If knee pain becomes more severe and persistent, your child may have to stop playing sports for a while. Rarely, a knee immobilizer or cast may be used. After several weeks, your child can gradually resume sports activities.

- Even if your child's Osgood-Schlatter disease is mild, it may take a year or longer for knee pain to go away completely.

When should I call your office?

Call our office if:

- Your child continues to have significant knee pain despite treatment.

- Your child develops severe pain or swelling of the knee.

- Your child starts limping.

Patellofemoral Pain Syndrome

Patellofemoral pain syndrome, sometimes called "runner's knee," is the most common cause of chronic knee pain. It is an "overuse" syndrome, caused by too much activity of the knee, especially in sports involving running and jumping. Simple treatments are usually effective, such as reducing sports activity and using exercises to strengthen the leg muscles.

What is patellofemoral pain syndrome?

Patellofemoral pain syndrome is pain involving the kneecap, or patella. It most often occurs in teenage athletes but can happen in younger children as well. Although patellofemoral pain syndrome is not a serious condition, physical activity may have to be decreased and exercises done to strengthen the leg muscles before their knee pain goes away.

What does it look like?

- Pain in the front part of the knee in the area around the kneecap.

- Pain develops gradually, with no apparent injury.

- Pain is usually worse in one knee than the other.

- Pain is worse when going up stairs, after squatting or running, or after sitting for a long time.

- Occasional swelling can occur.

What causes patellofemoral pain syndrome?

- Patellofemoral pain syndrome is most often caused by too much physical activity. It may occur in runners, basketball players, and volleyball players. No particular injury causes the pain. Instead, pain develops gradually, over time.

- Weakness of the upper leg muscles—especially the front of the thigh (quadriceps)—seems to play a role in this type of pain. That's why strengthening of these muscles is an important part of treatment.

What are some possible complications of patellofemoral pain syndrome?

Proper treatment and rehabilitation are needed to protect the knee against future injury, especially in athletes.

Although patellofemoral pain syndrome is the most common cause of knee pain, there are many other possible reasons for knee pain in young athletes, such as joint dislocation or arthritis. Your child needs medical evaluation to make sure the cause of the pain is identified and treated.

What puts your child at risk of patellofemoral pain syndrome?

This kind of knee pain is most common in teenage athletes involved in running or jumping sports.

How is patellofemoral pain syndrome treated?

Treatment may include:

- *Reduced physical activity.* It may be necessary to reduce or temporarily stop the activity causing your child's knee pain.

- *Medications.* Pain relievers such as ibuprofen or other nonsteroidal anti-inflammatory drugs (NSAIDs) may help.

- *Exercises.* Exercises to strengthen the quadriceps muscles (front of the thigh) may be useful.

- *Bracing.* A brace or sleeve may be used to support the knee joint and surrounding area.

- *Rehabilitation.* The doctor may recommend that your child undergo a formal rehabilitation or a physical therapy program if symptoms persist or are severe.

When should I call your office?

Call our office if:

- Your child has continued knee pain despite reduced activity and other treatments for patellofemoral pain syndrome.

- Your child starts limping.

- Your child develops other knee symptoms, such as "locking" or "giving out."

- Your child develops severe swelling or pain in the knee.

Scoliosis

> Scoliosis is an abnormal curvature of the spine. It is most common in girls during puberty. Depending on the degree of your child's scoliosis, evaluation and treatment by a bone and joint specialist may be needed.

What is scoliosis?

Scoliosis is a curve that develops in the spine as your child grows. It occurs most commonly in teenage girls as they go through puberty. Many causes are possible, but usually no particular cause is found (that is, it is "idiopathic"). Scoliosis may range from mild, requiring no treatment, to severe, requiring bracing or surgery. If your child's scoliosis is more than mild, your doctor will probably recommend that you visit a bone and joint specialist (an orthopedic surgeon).

What does it look like?

The curve is most noticeable from the back as your child bends forward—the ribs on one side of the back look higher than on the other side. You may also see that the spine is not straight and a side-to-side curve is present.

- The curve may first be noticed on a routine school screening program.

- Your child's shoulders may be at different heights. One hip may seem higher than the other.

- Back pain may indicate more severe scoliosis or the presence of additional spinal problems. Children with idiopathic scoliosis usually don't have significant back pain.

- Symptoms involving the nervous system, such as weakness, increased muscle tightness, or trouble controlling urination, often means scoliosis is not the only problem. A complete medical evaluation would be needed.

- X-rays may be taken to diagnose your child's scoliosis and see how much of a curve is present.

What causes scoliosis?

There are many possible causes of scoliosis, but the most common type is idiopathic. This simply means that no particular cause can be identified. Idiopathic scoliosis most often develops in adolescents, age 11 or older. It is less common in children between 4 and 10 years old, and even rarer in babies and toddlers. Idiopathic scoliosis seems to run in families.

Several other causes of scoliosis are possible. For most of these, other abnormalities are present as well:

- *Congenital scoliosis.* Abnormal spinal curve is already present at birth or develops soon afterward.

- *Neuromuscular scoliosis.* Abnormal spinal curve can occur as a complication of various diseases affecting the nerves and muscles (for example, cerebral palsy, spinal cord tumors or injuries, or polio).

- *Other genetic conditions.* Scoliosis can occur in children with some uncommon genetic diseases (such as neurofibromatosis or Marfan's syndrome).

- *Unequal leg length.* If your child's legs are different lengths, this may look like scoliosis. Careful evaluation may be needed to determine whether scoliosis is really present.

What are some possible complications of scoliosis?

- The main complication is that the abnormal spinal curve will get worse over time.

- Very severe scoliosis can result in difficulties with the spinal joints or in heart and lung problems. These serious complications occur mostly in children with neuromuscular causes of scoliosis.

What puts your child at risk of scoliosis?

- If you or others in your child's family have had scoliosis, your child may be at greater risk.

- Girls are at higher risk of having scoliosis than are boys. Girls are also more likely to have worsening scoliosis requiring treatment.

- Although scoliosis is less common in children under 11, it can be more difficult to treat in younger children.

- Scoliosis is a possible complication of various diseases or genetic disorders (such as cerebral palsy and spinal cord tumors or injuries, neurofibromatosis, or Marfan's syndrome).

Can scoliosis be prevented?

There is no known way to prevent scoliosis, especially the idiopathic form. Treatment may help to prevent scoliosis from getting worse.

How is scoliosis treated?

Treatment for scoliosis depends on the severity of the abnormal spinal curve and the chance that it will get worse over time.

- *Observation.* Most children with scoliosis do not need treatment because they have only a mild spinal curve. If your child's scoliosis is more severe, he or she will probably be sent for evaluation by an orthopedic surgeon.

- *Bracing.* If your child has more severe scoliosis or has a high likelihood of worsening spinal curve, a brace may be recommended. Braces are useful only if your child is not yet finished growing. Bracing doesn't return the spinal curve to normal but may help keep it from getting worse.

- *Surgery.* If your child's scoliosis is quite severe, or if it gets worse despite bracing, surgery may be recommended. Surgery is the only treatment that can actually reduce the spinal curve. Although surgery is sometimes needed for children with severe idiopathic scoliosis, most children who undergo surgery have other causes of scoliosis.

- Other treatments for scoliosis—including exercise, physical therapy, electrical stimulation, and chiropractic treatment—have not been proven to be effective.

When should I call your office?

Call our office if:

- Your child has any other symptoms related to scoliosis, especially back pain.

- Your child has any neurologic symptoms, such as weakness, increased muscle tightness, or trouble controlling urination.

Slipped Capital Femoral Epiphysis (SCFE)

Slipped capital femoral epiphysis (SCFE—often pronounced "skiffy") is a common hip problem in teenagers. The top of the immature thigh bone (the femur) slips partially off the ball of the joint. If your child has SCFE, he or she may need surgery to stabilize the bone.

What is slipped capital femoral epiphysis (SCFE)?

In SCFE, the ball of the joint (the capital femoral epiphysis) slips so that it no longer sits in the correct position on top of the thigh bone. The ball remains in the hip socket. The severity of your child's symptoms depends on how severe the slip is.

Because it affects growing bone, SCFE almost always occurs in young adolescents. It is more common in boys than girls and often occurs in teens who are overweight. Treatment is needed to restore the normal joint and prevent complications of the hip.

What does it look like?

In most teens with SCFE, the slip is *stable:* although the ball has started to slip off the top of the joint, it is still well attached. Your child with stable SCFE may have:

- Mild discomfort at first.
- Hip pain that increases as the slip gets worse. Sometimes knee pain is the main symptom.
- The child can walk on the leg, although usually with a limp.
- Limited hip motion.

In other children, the slip is *unstable*: the ball is no longer firmly attached to the top of the thigh bone. In unstable SCFE:

- The slip usually occurs suddenly.
- Pain is severe; your child may suddenly collapse.
- Your child may be unable to walk or to put any weight on the leg, even if it is supported.
- Hip motion may be very limited and painful.

What causes SCFE?

- The exact cause of SCFE is unknown. Hormones may play a role, because SCFE often occurs in children with growth disorders or other hormonal diseases. Children who develop SCFE before puberty (age 10 or younger) may be more likely to have hormonal diseases, especially hypothyroidism (low thyroid hormone levels).
- Being overweight is probably a contributing factor.
- Trauma or sports injuries sometimes lead to SCFE. However, there is often no obvious injury.

What are some possible complications of SCFE?

Serious complications of SCFE are possible:

- Osteonecrosis (sometimes called avascular necrosis): If the blood supply to the ball of the hip joint is reduced, the bone may die.
- Chondrolysis: Loss of the cartilage of the hip joint.

If complications occur, or if pinning to repair the damaged bone is unsuccessful, more surgery may be needed.

What puts your child at risk of SCFE?

- It usually occurs in the early teens: 13 to 14 years in boys, 11 to 12 years in girls.
- The risk is higher in boys than in girls.
- The risk is higher in African Americans than in whites.
- Being overweight is a major risk factor: most teens with SCFE are obese.
- SCFE may run in families.
- Hypothyroidism (low function of the thyroid gland).
- The risk is higher in children with certain medical problems, including kidney disease or treatment for cancer.

How is SCFE treated?

- X-rays are performed to confirm that your child has SCFE and to see how severe it is.
- If SCFE is present, it is important to keep weight off the affected hip as much as possible. Your child should start walking with crutches immediately. A visit to a bone and joint specialist (an orthopedic surgeon) will be recommended by your doctor as soon as possible.
- The most common treatment for SCFE is to place one or two pins through the bone to repair the slip.

When should I call your office?

- Call our office if your child develops hip pain, especially if it is severe.

- Call your orthopedic surgeon if your child has increased pain after a procedure to treat SCFE.

Sprains and Strains

Sprains and strains are common injuries in active children. A sprain is an injury to the ligaments in and around joints. A strain is an overstretched or "pulled" muscle. Any time your child has an injury causing a lot of tenderness, swelling, or difficulty moving a limb or joint, you should seek medical advice.

What are sprains and strains?

Sprains are common athletic injuries in children. The ankle is the most commonly sprained joint, but wrist, finger, and knee sprains may occur as well. Sometimes it's difficult to tell a sprain from a fracture. You should always seek medical attention if your child has more than a mild sprain.

Strains, sometimes called "pulled muscles," are also very common. Strains happen away from the joint. The upper leg is a common site for strains, as are the chest, groin, and shoulders.

What do they look like?

- *Ankle or knee sprains.* Ankle and knee sprains are common sports injuries. Ankle sprains most often result from a fall with the foot turned inward. Knee sprains may result from various causes, such as a direct hit or jumping and landing off-balance. The joint is painful, especially when your child tries to move it. If there is a lot of pain or swelling around the injury or if your child cannot walk on the injured leg, seek medical attention.

- *Wrist or finger sprains.* Sprains of the wrist and hand joints may also occur. For example, your child's finger may get jammed in a ball game. If your child has significant pain or swelling, get medical attention.

- *Muscle strains.* Strains can occur in almost any muscle. Strains of the thigh muscles are common, especially in active or athletic children. Muscle strains may be seen when the muscle is overstretched during sports or other activities, from a direct hit, or for other reasons. Symptoms include pain, tenderness, and occasionally swelling.

What are some possible complications of sprains and strains?

The major concern is that a bone fracture may be present in addition to the damaged joint ligaments, especially with sprains. That's why it's important to seek medical evaluation if your child has more than a mild sprain, with swelling, bruising, moderate to severe pain, limping, or inability to use the injured limb or joint normally.

With any type of sprain or strain, there is a chance of reinjuring the joint or muscle. This is especially true in young athletes who don't give their injuries the time and rest they need to heal.

What puts your child at risk of strains and sprains?

- Strains and sprains usually occur in older children, especially athletes. Because young children's ligaments are so flexible, they have relatively few joint sprains.

- Not stretching before and after physical activity puts your child at risk for strains and sprains.

Can strains and sprains be prevented?

- Stretching before and after physical activity is often recommended to reduce the risk of muscle strains and sprains.

- If your child has had a significant joint sprain, he or she may be at risk of injuring the joint again. Strengthening exercises and other recommended rehabilitation techniques may help to reduce this risk.

How are strains and sprains treated?

For *mild muscle strains or sprains,* the usual recommended treatment is rest, ice, compression, and elevation. To remember these steps, just think of the word "RICE":

- *Rest.* Use the injured area as little as possible for the first day or two after the injury. Passive movement, which does not produce pain, will keep the joint from becoming stiff. Try to keep your child off an injured leg, especially if the knee or ankle is injured.

- *Ice.* Put an ice pack on the injured area. This will help to control swelling and pain. Don't put the ice directly on your child's skin because the cold may cause skin damage. Instead, put the ice in a plastic bag and wrap it in a cloth. For muscle strains, heat (for example, a heating pad) is sometimes recommended instead of or in addition to cold.

- *Compression.* Wrapping the injured area in an elastic bandage may help to reduce swelling.

- *Elevation.* If possible, have your child raise the injured muscle or joint while he or she is resting.

Medications such as acetaminophen or ibuprofen may help to control pain. In mild strains and sprains, the injured joint or muscle should start to feel better in a day or two.

For more *severe muscle strains and sprains,* other treatments may be required. If the ligament or muscle is completely torn, it may need to be repaired by surgery.

When should I call your office?

Call our office if:

- Your child has a joint or muscle injury producing swelling, significant pain, or difficulty moving the joint.

- Your child is limping or is unable to move the injured joint without pain.

- Your child's sprain or strain doesn't seem to get better after a day or two of "RICE" or other home treatments.

Tendinitis and Tennis Elbow

> Tendinitis means inflammation of a tendon, the part of a muscle that attaches to bone. Tendinitis is not common in young children but can occur in older children and teens, especially athletes. "Tennis elbow" is one common type of tendinitis.

What is tendinitis?

Tendinitis is inflammation (pain and swelling) of the tendons attaching muscle to bone around a joint. Tendinitis usually results from overuse, that is, performing the same motion over and over again. Tendinitis of the elbow is sometimes called "tennis elbow," although it can result from other activities as well.

What does it look like?

- Pain and some swelling near a joint, such as the elbow, shoulder, back of the ankle (Achilles' tendon), back of the thigh (hamstrings), or even a finger joint.

- Weakness or difficulty moving the joint, especially when performing repetitive motions.

- In tennis elbow, the bony point on the outside of the elbow may become inflamed (epicondylitis).

What causes tendinitis?

Tendinitis is an overuse injury, most often caused by performing the same motion over and over again. Tendon damage builds up until it becomes difficult or painful to perform that particular motion. In tennis and other sports, the injury may result from incorrect technique. Many other activities may also cause tendinitis, such as:

- Golf (elbow tendinitis).

- Baseball or other throwing sports (shoulder or elbow tendinitis).

- Running (Achilles' tendinitis).

- Basketball or other jumping sports (knee tendinitis).

What are some possible complications of tendinitis?

- Usually, tennis elbow and other forms of tendinitis clear up with simple treatments, especially rest and the use of anti-inflammatory medications (such as ibuprofen).

- Rarely, tendinitis leads to a tear of the muscle or tendon, requiring surgery.

What puts your child at risk of tendinitis?

Tendinitis most often occurs in older children and teens who play sports or participate in other rigorous activities. In tennis and other sports, tendinitis may result from incorrect technique. Tendinitis is rare in younger children.

Can tendinitis be prevented?

Learning and following correct technique—for example, the proper tennis stroke—may help to prevent tendinitis or keep it from recurring.

How is tendinitis treated?

- *Rest.* Have your child take a break from the sport or other activity that is causing pain. It is especially important to stop any repeated motions that are irritating the tendon.

- *Medications.* A few days of treatment with anti-inflammatory medications such as ibuprofen may help to reduce pain and inflammation.

- *Rehabilitation.* Depending on the cause and location of the tendinitis, specific exercises or other rehabilitation such as splinting may be recommended

Usually, tendinitis improves after a few weeks of rest and simple treatments. If pain and inflammation continue, other therapy may be needed. We may recommend a visit to an orthopedic surgeon (a specialist in treating bone and joint problems).

When should I call your office?

Call our office if your child's tendinitis symptoms (pain, swelling, or tenderness) don't improve within a few weeks or if your child's pain or swelling becomes severe.

■ Torticollis ■

Torticollis, or twisted neck, is relatively common in children. There are many possible causes, most related to spasm of the neck muscles. Not all causes of torticollis are serious. However, any problem with abnormal position or movement of the neck needs to be evaluated by a doctor.

What is torticollis?

Torticollis is a symptom related to turning or bending of the neck. Many different causes are possible. In newborns, torticollis usually results from injury during labor and delivery or the infant's position in the womb. Less often, it is caused by birth defects. In older children, torticollis may result from injuries to the neck muscles, common infections, or other causes.

What does it look like?

- Abnormal twisting of the neck. Usually, your child's head is tipped toward one side, with the chin pointing in the other direction.

- Painful spasms of the neck muscles may occur.

- Other symptoms may be present, depending on the cause. For example, there may be a tender lymph node (gland) if the cause is infection.

What causes torticollis?

There are many possible causes of torticollis. In most children, the problem is only temporary or can be managed with simple treatments. Less often, torticollis is a more serious problem. If your child has torticollis or any problem moving his or her neck, it's important to get medical evaluation to find out what's causing the problem.

In newborns, torticollis most often results from causes related to the muscles in the neck and shoulder area. It may be caused by injuries to the neck muscles during a difficult delivery. At other times, it's simply the way the infant was positioned in the womb. Less commonly, different types of birth defects may cause torticollis in a newborn.

In older children, possible causes of torticollis include:

- Injury to the neck muscles. Sometimes the trauma is minor, such as sleeping in an awkward position. Much less often, the vertebrae in the neck may become dislocated or fractured because of trauma.

- Infections or inflammation in the neck. The lymph nodes in the neck may become infected or inflamed, interfering with normal neck motion. Less commonly, torticollis may be caused by a deeper infection such as an abscess in an area of the throat. Arthritis or other bone diseases are also possible causes.

- Even less frequently, torticollis may result from injury or diseases of the nervous system.

What are some possible complications of torticollis?

- For most common causes of torticollis, there are few complications.

- Rarely, if torticollis persists in a newborn, surgery may be needed.

What puts your child at risk of torticollis?

In newborns, large size, difficult delivery, and abnormal position during birth may increase the risk of torticollis.

Can torticollis be prevented?

Torticollis is usually an unexpected, unpreventable problem. Identifying and treating the cause may prevent complications related to abnormal movement and positioning of the neck.

How is torticollis treated?

Usually, the doctor can tell what caused your child's torticollis by examining him or her and asking some questions. If the cause is not clear, x-rays and other tests may be required.

Treatment for torticollis depends on the cause:

- *For newborns* with torticollis, gentle motion of the head and neck is recommended to stretch the muscles. Often, a physical therapist is involved. To avoid injury, this should be done only as recommended by a doctor.

- *For older children* with torticollis related to infection or inflammation, treatment may include:

  - Antibiotics for the specific infection.

  - Rest.

  - Anti-inflammatory medications (such as ibuprofen).

  - Passive motion to keep the muscles from getting stiff. However, the motion should not be painful, and you should never use force to move the neck.

- If the cause is related to trauma (even sleeping position) treatments may include:

  - Muscle relaxants such as Valium (generic name: diazepam).

  - Passive motion.

  - A soft collar or brace to support the neck.

- For other causes of torticollis, it is essential to obtain and follow medical advice.

When should I call your office?

- Call our office any time your child has an abnormal position or movement of the neck.

- If your child's torticollis is related to infection or trauma, call our office if there is no improvement within a few days.

- Call our office if symptoms get worse or if your child develops any neurologic problems (such as numbness or weakness in the arms and hands).

Section XIX ▪ Nervous System

Bell's Palsy

Bell's palsy is a relatively common condition that causes weakness or temporary inability to move the muscles on one side of the face. Your child's mouth may droop on one side. If he or she has trouble closing the eye on the affected side, steps may be needed to protect it against drying out. Bell's palsy almost always clears up within a week or two, with no treatment needed.

What is Bell's palsy?

Bell's palsy is weakness of the muscles on one side of the face. The weakness is caused by damage to the facial nerve, which controls the muscles of the face. "Palsy" means paralysis, but this type of paralysis is almost always temporary.

Bell's palsy usually follows a recent infection with a virus. In 95% of cases, the muscle weakness clears up within a week or two. Usually no treatment is needed. Eye drops or sometimes an eye patch may be necessary to keep the eye from getting too dry.

What does it look like?

- Fairly sudden loss of movement on one side of your child's face. The loss of movement may be total but is more often partial.

- The entire half of the face is affected, from forehead to mouth. Your child's mouth may droop on one side. He or she may be unable to close one eye; because of this, tears may flow constantly from the eye.

- The facial feeling is normal; the face does not feel numb.

- Bell's palsy can occur at any age. It most often begins about 2 weeks after infection with some type of virus. The most common infection is with herpes simplex virus, which causes cold sores. However, the virus may not have caused any illness at the time.

- Your child may have loss of taste on one side of the tongue (this occurs in about one half of cases).

What causes Bell's palsy?

The cause isn't certain. Some type of immune reaction to recent infection with a virus (most often herpes simplex, the virus that causes cold sores) is probably involved. By the time Bell's palsy occurs, the infection is no longer present.

What are some possible complications of Bell's palsy?

- If your child can't close his or her eye completely, there is a chance that the eye (cornea) could be injured from drying out too much.

- A small minority of patients (5%) are left with permanent weakness of the facial muscles.

- Otherwise, there are few complications.

What increases your child's risk of Bell's palsy?

- There are no specific risk factors besides recent infection with a virus. Bell's palsy can occur at any age, from infancy to the teen years (adulthood as well).

- For newborns, the risk of Bell's palsy is higher if the delivery was difficult—especially if forceps had to be used to assist the birth. In this case, the cause of the palsy is trauma (pressure) caused by the forceps.

Can Bell's palsy be prevented?

There is no practical way to prevent Bell's palsy.

How is Bell's palsy treated?

- Usually, no treatment is needed. The condition clears up on its own within a week or two.

- Some doctors may prescribe oral steroids for this condition. They may also include an antiviral drug to treat the herpes simplex virus, since it is commonly associated with Bell's palsy.

- If your child cannot close his or her eyes or blink normally, steps may be needed to keep the eye from drying out. The doctor may prescribe special eye drops to protect the eye, especially at night. The eye also may be patched or taped shut.

- If tears are dripping from the eye, make sure your child has tissues to dry them! Keep your child from rubbing the eye as much as possible.

- Call our office if full facial motion has not returned within a few weeks. Additional tests may be needed if the condition continues for a longer time.

When should I call your office?

Call our office if your child doesn't recover full motion of the facial muscles within a few weeks.

Cerebral Palsy

Cerebral palsy is the term for a group of conditions that cause abnormal development or damage to parts of the brain that control muscle functions and movement, such as strength or walking. It is usually present at birth. Children with cerebral palsy have a lack of muscle control and other disabilities that are generally present for life. However, the disabilities are not always severe and generally do not get worse. A team approach to health care is best for children with cerebral palsy.

What is cerebral palsy?

- Cerebral palsy (CP) is a term used to describe damage to the brain that has occurred early in its development due to a number of causes. The damage usually occurs before birth but sometimes occurs during birth. Recognized causes include premature birth, infections, metabolic or hormonal diseases, genetic diseases, and bleeding or clotting within the brain. Pinpointing the cause is an important goal of your child's diagnosis.

- The motor disorders (affecting strength and body movement) and other disabilities resulting from CP vary a lot. Some children with CP have normal intelligence with relatively minor muscle and movement problems. Others need a wheelchair or have reduced intelligence or other medical problems.

- Depending on your child's needs, several professionals will be involved in his or her care.

- While it is true that CP can be caused by lack of oxygen during a difficult labor and delivery, this is not the case in most children.

What does it look like?

The main abnormalities caused by cerebral palsy are poor muscle strength and control over movement of various parts of the body (motor function). Generally, the damage to your child's brain remains the same over time—it doesn't get any worse as your child grows.

Several types of motor disorder are possible, depending on the exact brain injury. Some children have mild or minimal muscle problems, while others have severe disabilities.

- *Spastic hemiplegia.* Some children with CP have weakness in the muscles on one side of the body. Your child will use one hand much more often than the other. Walking is delayed and is better on one side. Uncontrolled tightness of the muscles (spasticity) is common. About one third of children with spastic hemiplegia develop epilepsy, and about one fourth have reduced intelligence.

- *Spastic diplegia.* Children with this type have decreased movement and increased muscle tightness more in the legs than arms. The legs may be very weak and reduced in size, while the upper body develops more normally. Intelligence is usually normal; the risk of epilepsy is low.

- *Spastic quadriplegia.* The most severe type is weakness in the muscles of both arms and legs. Children with this form of CP have high rates of mental retardation and epilepsy. Many other problems are possible, such as difficulty swallowing and severe tightening of muscles, leading to permanent deformity.

- *Athetoid cerebral palsy.* This is a less common pattern in which the muscles are initially weak and floppy, rather than too tight. With time, the limbs become rigid and tight, with abnormal positioning. Feeding and speech problems are common. Intelligence is often normal, and the risk of seizures is low.

Every child with CP is different! Your child may have a mix of these patterns. Careful diagnosis is needed to determine the extent and cause of your child's disabilities.

What are some possible complications of cerebral palsy?

Complications vary a lot, depending on your child's situation. For example, muscle tightness can lead to permanent deformity (contractures). Contractures cause limited movement around the joints, for example, inability to straighten the arm or leg completely. Swallowing problems can lead to pneumonia. Many other complications are possible.

The original damage caused by CP doesn't change much over time. However, muscle tightness may cause contractures, which further limit movement. Good physical therapy can reduce this risk.

How is cerebral palsy diagnosed?

Diagnosis is a key first step in managing CP. Often the abnormalities are not seen at birth but become apparent as your baby develops. Your child will undergo a complete evaluation to assess the extent of his or her disabilities and to make sure that CP is the correct diagnosis.

- Magnetic resonance imaging (MRI) scans or other imaging tests that show a picture of the brain will be performed to determine the extent and location of the injury to your child's brain.

- Other tests may be recommended, depending on your child's situation. Genetic testing is especially important if a genetic (inherited) cause of CP is suspected.

How is cerebral palsy treated?

Unfortunately, there is no cure for CP. The brain damage causing your child's disability is permanent.

However, many treatments and other kinds of help are available for children with CP. The results are best when a team of health professionals from different fields is involved in your child's care. The team may include doctors from various specialties (an orthopedic surgeon, a neurologist), physical therapists, occupational therapists, and others.

You'll receive training in special ways of caring for your child with CP that limit the impact of his or her muscle disorder. Some of the different treatments are:

- Stretching exercises, directed by a physical therapist, to help prevent permanent muscle deformities (contractures).

- Assistive devices or aids that may be used to help your child get around, such as braces, walkers, or a wheelchair.

- Surgery is sometimes recommended to loosen tight muscles, particularly around the hip or Achilles' tendon.

- Medications may help to reduce muscle tightness.

- Other types of devices may be used to improve communication skills. Many children with CP can benefit from special education and other educational services. A psychologist or other mental health professional can be helpful as well.

Your child will receive close follow-up to prevent and/or treat some of the medical problems that can occur in CP.

When should I call your office?

Call our office if you have any questions about caring for your child with CP. Our office can help to put you in touch with appropriate specialists or community resources.

Where can I get more information about cerebral palsy?

Here are a few contacts to get you started in learning what your family needs to know about living with CP:

- The National Institute of Neurological Disorders and Stroke. Information and publications are available on the Internet at *www.ninds.nih/gov.*

- United Cerebral Palsy. On the Internet at *www.ucp.org* or call (1-800) 872-5827.

- March of Dimes Birth Defects Foundation. On the Internet at *www.marchofdimes.com* or call 1-888-MODIMES (663-4637).

Guillain-Barré Syndrome

Guillain-Barré syndrome is a nervous system disease caused by an abnormal immune system response to infection. A week or two after a minor illness, your child develops muscle weakness or paralysis that gradually gets worse. In severe cases, the paralysis may lead to difficulty breathing. Guillain-Barré syndrome usually requires at least some time in the hospital for observation and supportive care. Most patients recover completely, but this may take weeks to months.

What is Guillain-Barré syndrome?

Guillain-Barré syndrome is a nervous system disease caused by our own immune system attacking certain nerves in the body. The exact cause of this reaction is unknown, but it usually follows a relatively minor illness caused by infection with a virus. Guillain-Barré syndrome can occur at any age. Most children recover without further problems.

What does it look like?

Most cases of Guillain-Barré syndrome start with sudden weakness of the lower leg muscles. Over the following days, the weakness spreads gradually upward. Abnormal sensations (tingling, numbness) may be present as well.

The symptoms most often occur a week or two after a relatively minor illness, for example, acute diarrhea (gastroenteritis) or a cold.

Over a period of days to weeks, the muscle weakness continues to spread upward, through the body to the arms. The weakness may worsen, to the point where your child cannot move the muscles at all (paralysis).

In more severe cases, weakness or paralysis continues to spread upward to the muscles of the throat, tongue, jaw, and face ("bulbar" muscles). This paralysis is particularly serious because it can interfere with your child's ability to eat, drink, and prevent choking. The paralysis can also lead to problems with breathing and heart rate. Close monitoring and support in the hospital may be needed so that your child can survive this period.

Fortunately, Guillain-Barré syndrome usually resolves on its own. On average, the weakness and paralysis start to clear up after 2 to 3 weeks. Return of function starts at the top of the body and gradually spreads downward.

Most patients recover completely, although it may take months before full muscle strength returns. Some patients are left with some degree of muscle weakness or abnormal sensation. There is a small risk of another attack of Guillain-Barré syndrome in the future.

What are some possible complications of Guillain-Barré syndrome?

The most serious complication is difficulty breathing. This can become severe enough to require a respirator (ventilator) to help your child breathe. This type of paralysis occurs in about one half of patients with Guillain-Barré syndrome, and it can develop very quickly.

What increases your child's risk of Guillain-Barré syndrome?

- Fortunately, Guillain-Barré syndrome is uncommon, affecting about 1 in 100,000 people.

- Besides a recent infection, there are few known risk factors. It is unknown why some people develop Guillain-Barré syndrome while others do not.

- About 7% of survivors of Guillain-Barré syndrome have future attacks. The repeat attacks are usually not as severe as the initial one.

Can Guillain-Barré syndrome be prevented?

There is no known way to prevent Guillain-Barré syndrome.

How is Guillain-Barré syndrome treated?

Guillain-Barré syndrome requires prompt recognition and hospital treatment. Because paralysis can develop quickly, all patients need hospital care and monitoring, at least at first. Your child's care will likely involve a specialist in nervous system diseases (a neurologist).

- *Supportive care.* The main goal of treatment is to provide your child with supportive care until he or she recovers. Depending on the severity of the weakness/paralysis, this may include:

  - Intravenous (IV) fluids if he or she cannot drink normally.

  - Constant nursing care to prevent complications of muscle weakness/paralysis such as breathing or eating problems or bed sores.

  - Special machines used to monitor heart, lung, and other critical body functions. If your child has trouble breathing on his or her own, mechanical ventilation may be needed. A ventilator is a machine that helps your child breathe. Mechanical ventilation will be continued until your child is strong enough to breathe on his or her own again.

- *Other treatments*. If your child's weakness and paralysis are spreading rapidly, certain treatments may be given with the intent of reducing the duration and severity of the attack:

  - Intravenous immune globulin (IVIG). The most common treatment, IVIG, is a solution of antibodies that affect the immune system. These antibodies seem to reduce inflammation and swelling of the affected nerves.

  - Plasmapheresis. Used less commonly, plasmapheresis is a way of filtering the blood to remove antibodies and other substances that may be causing Guillain-Barré syndrome.

- The length of time your child spends in the hospital depends on the severity of the attack. Usually, once muscle function has started to return, he or she will be sent home to continue recovering.

Having a child develop Guillain-Barré syndrome is a stressful event for your family. Counseling and other mental health services may be helpful.

When should I call your office?

Your child will receive close medical monitoring and follow-up. He or she will probably stay in the hospital until recovery is well under way.

During recovery and afterward, call our office if your child develops any possible sign of a repeat attack of Guillain-Barré syndrome, such as sudden muscle weakness or abnormal sensation, especially in the lower legs.

Headaches (Tension and Migraine Types)

Headaches are common in children. Migraine headaches are seen fairly often in younger children and teens, whereas tension-type headaches are more likely to occur after puberty and in the teen years. Various treatments are available for migraines, including drugs to help prevent them from occurring. Headaches often occur during nonserious infections. Occasionally headaches occur with serious conditions, such as infections involving the brain, injury or bleeding in the brain from trauma or other causes, brain tumors, or high blood pressure.

What do they look like?

Headaches are a common medical problem, particularly with infections such as the flu, sinusitis, and strep throat. *If headaches are severe or occur with repeated vomiting, confusion, or unusual sleepiness, you should contact your doctor right away.* Children or teens with repeated headaches should be evaluated by their health care provider to be sure there is not a more serious cause.

Migraines are a common cause of repeated headaches in children and teens.

- Pain may be severe and at times, disabling. Migraines can last anywhere from an hour to a few days.

- Pain is often described as "pounding" and occurs on one or both sides of the head. Often nausea and/or vomiting is present. Lights often bother your child's eyes; loud sounds are also disturbing.

- Some people may get an *aura*—this is another symptom that may come before the headache. An aura can be a warning sign that a headache is coming. Sometimes an aura occurs during the headache. The most common auras are visual (involving the eyes), such as seeing bright, flashing lights; others include tingling in the face or hands and other symptoms.

- Your child often prefers to be in a dark, quiet room once the headache comes on.

- A number of other unusual and uncommon types of migraines may occur. Most children with migraines have a relative or family member who also has these types of headaches.

Tension-type headaches are more common in children after puberty and among teenagers. They often occur during times of tension or emotional stress/anxiety.

- Tension-type headaches last anywhere between a half hour and a week. Pain is most commonly described as "pressing" or "tightening." It usually occurs on the front part of the head and is not very severe.

- Since the symptoms of tension-type headaches aren't as specific as those of migraines, it is especially important to be sure there is not another cause of the headaches.

Toddlers and infants can develop headaches too, but they can't tell you that their head hurts. Instead they may fuss or repeatedly rub their head or eyes.

How are headaches diagnosed?

- The diagnosis of migraine headaches is usually made by the presence of typical symptoms and a normal physical examination. If the symptoms aren't clear or if the nervous system examination is not normal, other tests may be needed.

- The most common tests are special imaging of the brain such as an MRI (magnetic resonance imaging) or a CT scan (computed axial tomography). These tests show the structures in the brain and any abnormalities, such as a tumor or swelling.

- Most headaches occurring with a cold, the flu, or other infections with fever are not serious. However, it's important to call or see your health care provider if the headaches have unusual features. A complete history and physical examination help determine if other, more serious causes of headache are present:

  - Infections involving the brain (such as meningitis).

  - Blood clots in the brain from trauma (such as a fall or child abuse, the latter caused for instance by shaking a baby).

  - Brain tumors and high blood pressure.

How are headaches treated?

Some basic steps can help make headaches less frequent and severe:

- Reduce stress for your child as much as possible. Counseling may be helpful if stress continues to be a problem.

- Be sure your child gets enough sleep.

- Don't allow your child to skip meals, particularly breakfast.

- Have your child lie down in a quiet, dark room, especially with a migraine.

- Have your child avoid caffeine.

Medications:

- Simple pain relievers like ibuprofen (Advil) or acetaminophen (Tylenol) can reduce headache pain.

- If headache is accompanied by a lot of nausea or vomiting, your doctor may prescribe an anti-emetic drug like Phenergan (generic name: promethazine) that helps prevent these symptoms. This drug may be taken either orally or rectally. If your child knows a migraine is coming on, give him or her the medicine as soon as possible.

- A number of prescription medications can help stop a migraine if the simple pain medicines are not working well enough. Some newer medications, such as Imitrex (generic name: sumatriptan) are available for teenagers and adults. They are not used as often in children because they have not been studied long enough in that age group.

- If your child's migraine headaches are unusually severe or frequent, we may recommend using medications for prophylaxis (prevention). This means taking a medication daily to try to prevent headaches from occurring. A number of medicines are used for this purpose, including beta-blockers (propranolol), tricyclic antidepressants (amitriptyline), antihistamines/antiserotonins (cyproheptadine), and anticonvulsants (topiramate).

- Certain types of alternative treatments are sometimes helpful, such as breathing and relaxation exercises or biofeedback

If your child has a severe headache that does not respond to the usual treatments, call our office or take your child to the emergency room.

When should I call your office?

Call our office if:

- There is a change in the type of your child's headaches.

- Headaches become more frequent or more severe.

- Headaches continue despite treatment.

Call our office or go to the emergency room if your child has any of the following:

- Sudden, very severe headache.

- Headache with behavior changes or seizures.

- Persistent vomiting that has not occurred with past headaches.

Hydrocephalus

Hydrocephalus is a condition in which excess fluid builds up within the brain. Hydrocephalus is not a single disease—rather, it results from problems with the normal cerebrospinal fluid flowing within and around the brain and spinal cord. Excess fluid can cause increased pressure within the brain. This can damage the brain, leading to developmental disabilities, reduced intelligence, and other complications. Prompt diagnosis and treatment are essential to lessen the impact of hydrocephalus.

What is hydrocephalus?

Hydrocephalus ("hydro" = water, "cephalus" = head) is excessive buildup of cerebrospinal fluid (CSF) within the skull. The CSF is a normally clear fluid that carries important chemicals to the brain, removes wastes, and helps cushion the brain.

Hydrocephalus has many possible causes. Often it is a congenital condition (present from birth), but it can develop in older children and adults as well. Any condition that interferes with the normal flow of CSF can cause hydrocephalus.

The excess fluid causes the normal spaces (ventricles) within the brain to become too large. In infants, the first sign of hydrocephalus is usually enlargement or too rapid growth of the head. This happens because a baby's growing skull can still easily increase in size. Since the skull cannot expand in older children, the first symptoms of excessive pressure in these children may include vomiting, vision changes, or balance problems.

Treatment to remove the excess CSF must begin as soon as possible. This is usually done by placing a device called a shunt, which drains the fluid from the brain. These shunts carry a risk of infection and other complications. Children with hydrocephalus may develop mental and physical disabilities. These risks are related to the cause and severity of the disease.

What does it look like?

In infants:

- The first sign of hydrocephalus is that the baby's head is growing faster than normal and may appear big. The doctor often discovers this when the head is measured at well baby visits.

- The "soft spot" (fontanelle) on top of your baby's head may be wide or bulging. The forehead may be wider than normal.

- Your baby's normal development, such as rolling over or crawling, may be slow.

- Many other symptoms are possible, including vomiting, sleepiness, and fussiness.

In older children:

- Enlargement of the head cannot occur.

- Symptoms are more general, including mood changes, extreme tiredness, poor appetite, and vomiting.

- Headaches.

- Over time, personality changes, falling grades, doing poorly at school.

- Balance problems, loss of control over leg muscles.

Symptoms of hydrocephalus vary a lot, depending on cause, severity, and other factors. Your child may have some, all, or none of these symptoms.

What causes hydrocephalus?

Anything that interferes with the normal cycle of cerebrospinal fluid:

- Some patients have blockage of the normal flow of CSF within the brain. This is called "obstructive" hydrocephalus and is most often caused by a defect or abnormality that the baby was born with (congenital).

- Other patients have problems with the normal absorption of CSF within the brain. This is called "non-obstructive" hydrocephalus. It is most commonly caused by bleeding inside the brain (intraventricular hemorrhage) in a premature infant.

- Others causes result from later illness or injury, such as meningitis, head injury, or brain tumors.

What are some possible complications of hydrocephalus?

- Children with hydrocephalus often have some degree of mental and physical disability. These symptoms are affected by the cause and severity of the hydrocephalus, other birth defects or injuries, and how quickly treatment is started to relieve pressure on the brain.

- The shunts used to treat hydrocephalus carry a risk of infection and other serious complications. Patients with shunts need close medical follow-up.

What puts your child at risk of hydrocephalus?

- Hydrocephalus is relatively common; it may affect 1 out of 500 infants at birth.

- Some of the abnormalities that cause hydrocephalus are genetic (inherited) disorders.

- Premature infants are at higher risk, especially those with bleeding inside the brain (intraventricular hemorrhage).

- Hydrocephalus may occur after other diseases involving the brain and nervous system, such as meningitis, head injuries, or brain tumors.

How is hydrocephalus diagnosed?

- In infants, hydrocephalus is usually recognized by the abnormal enlargement of the baby's head. Infants with hydrocephalus may be diagnosed before birth by routine ultrasound scans.

- In older children, because the head cannot expand, hydrocephalus may be more difficult to recognize. However, it may be suspected based on your child's symptoms and what the doctor finds on physical examination.

- Once the problem is suspected, the doctor will recommend tests, such as ultrasound, magnetic resonance imaging (MRI), or computed tomography (CT), that can take pictures of the brain. These tests will confirm the excess fluid buildup in your child's brain. They will also help to determine the cause and severity of your child's hydrocephalus.

How is hydrocephalus treated?

Shunt placement. The main treatment is placement of a device called a *shunt*. An operation is required to place the shunt system.

- The shunt is basically a long tube with one end placed in the space inside the brain where fluid is building up (called the *ventricle).* The other end of the tube is placed in the abdominal space (called the *peritoneum).* This device is called a "ventriculoperitoneal (VP) shunt."

- The VP shunt works by draining excess fluid from the brain into the abdomen, where it is harmlessly absorbed. When working properly, shunts are very effective in reducing the pressure on your child's brain.

- Shunts are complex devices that are prone to several types of problems. They may break down or become blocked, interrupting fluid drainage. Another potentially serious problem is infection, causing symptoms of fever, sore neck, and redness of the skin over the shunt. *All of these problems are emergencies requiring immediate medical attention.*

Follow-up care. Hydrocephalus is a serious and complex medical condition. Your child will need close medical follow-up. A surgeon specializing in the brain (a neurosurgeon) will be the doctor in charge of placing and taking care of the VP shunt. Our office will play an important role in providing follow-up care and in deciding when you need to see the neurosurgeon.

- Many children with hydrocephalus need special education or other special services to address their mental and/or physical disabilities. Early intervention should start as soon as your child's disability is diagnosed.

- Having a child with hydrocephalus can be very stressful for your family. Counseling, support groups, and other forms of therapy may be helpful.

- With close medical follow-up and other necessary services or support, many children with hydrocephalus go on to live normal, active lives.

When should I call your office?

Learning to recognize the warning signs of shunt problems and complications is an important part of caring for a child with hydrocephalus. Get medical attention immediately if your child develops any of the following:

- Rapid head enlargement (in an infant), vomiting, sleepiness, behavior changes.

- Severe headache or new headache.

- Signs of shunt infection: fever, sore neck or shoulders, redness of the skin over the shunt.

- Any change in vision.

- Any neurologic abnormality (for example, weakness or loss of muscle control, loss of bladder control).

Where can I get more information?

The National Institute of Neurological Disorders and Stroke. Information and publications are available on the Internet at *www.ninds.nih/gov.*

Muscular Dystrophy

Muscular dystrophy is the term for several inherited diseases that gradually damage muscle tissue. Each of these diseases is caused by a different gene abnormality and therefore cause different symptoms. Some are present at birth, whereas others do not appear until childhood or even adulthood. Unfortunately, there is no cure for muscular dystrophy. Treatment can help to manage some of the complications.

What is muscular dystrophy?

Several different diseases may be called "muscular dystrophy." However, they are actually unrelated diseases, caused by different gene abnormalities. The one thing they have in common is that they all cause gradual destruction of muscle tissue.

Some muscular dystrophies are already apparent at birth. Others don't appear until adolescence or even young adulthood. These diseases vary in how quickly they develop, the severity of the disability, and the expected change of survival. There is no cure for any form of muscular dystrophy. Treatments can help to maximize your child's functioning and quality of life and may help to slow the course of the disease.

What does it look like?

There are many different muscular dystrophies. Each is caused by a specific abnormal gene, and each has specific symptoms. The three most common muscular dystrophies are Duchenne, Becker, and myotonic muscular dystrophy.

- *Duchenne muscular dystrophy.* Muscle weakness first appears in early childhood, usually by age 6. An abnormal walking pattern (gait) is often the first sign.

  - This muscular dystrophy occurs only in boys, but the abnormal gene is carried by females ("X-linked").

  - Intelligence is reduced, but most patients are not severely mentally handicapped.

  - Walking becomes increasingly difficult. Even with treatment, most patients lose the ability to walk by age 12.

  - Muscle weakness spreads and worsens. Weakness of the muscles used in breathing and swallowing makes it increasingly difficult to keep the airways clear. Limitations on how well the limbs can straighten, called contractures, occur. Contractures limit movement of the limbs and can cause abnormal curving of the spine (scoliosis).

  - Weakness of the heart muscle develops (cardiomyopathy). This may further reduce your child's activity level.

- *Becker's muscular dystrophy.* Similar to Duchenne muscular dystrophy, but it develops later and is usually less severe.

  - Also occurs only in boys: first symptoms usually appear in the late teens or early adulthood.

  - Fewer learning problems than in Duchenne muscular dystrophy.

  - The pattern of increasing muscle weakness is similar to that in Duchenne muscular dystrophy but slower to develop. However, the same types of disabilities eventually appear. Many patients die before age 40.

- *Myotonic muscular dystrophy* (sometimes called Steinert's disease) affects various types of muscle. Other problems may include diseases of the heart, thyroid gland, and eyes (cataracts).

  - Muscle weakness usually develops around age 5. Affected infants may have a typical facial appearance. A severe newborn form can rapidly cause death.

  - The first sign is "myotonic" muscle contractions. This means that the muscles are very slow to relax after being used. The muscles of the fingers and face are affected first, other muscles later on. Speech may be affected because of weakening of the tongue and facial muscles.

  - About half of patients have reduced intelligence but are usually not severely mentally handicapped. The rest have normal intelligence.

  - Muscle weakness spreads very slowly; most patients can still walk even in late adulthood.

Many other types of muscular dystrophy are possible, each with its own pattern of onset and severity. Some types develop early and progress rapidly. Other forms develop later in life, develop slowly, and have little or no impact on life expectancy. Testing is an important first step to determine what type of muscular dystrophy your child has.

What causes muscular dystrophy?

Each form of muscular dystrophy is caused by a specific genetic (inherited) abnormality. The gene defects are already present at birth, even if muscle weakness and other symptoms don't develop until later.

What are some possible complications of muscular dystrophy?`

All forms of muscular dystrophy cause progressive breakdown and destruction of muscle fibers. Some forms involve other parts of the body. The exact complications caused by this muscle degeneration depend on which form your child has.

What increases your child's risk of muscular dystrophy?

- Duchenne muscular dystrophy occurs in about 1 in 3600 newborn boys. Myotonic muscular dystrophy affects about 1 in 30,000 infants.

- The genes for muscular dystrophy run in families. Some, like the gene abnormalities that cause Duchenne and Becker muscular dystrophies, are "X-linked." This means that the gene is carried by females but the disease appears only in males. *Genetic counseling* can help you to understand this risk.

How is muscular dystrophy diagnosed?

- Your child will probably be referred to a *geneticist* (a specialist in inherited diseases) or a *neurologist* (a specialist in diseases of the nervous system). Besides performing tests to diagnose the disease, they will explain the risk of it occurring in children you or other family members may have in the future.

- *Genetic testing.* Some form of genetic testing is needed to identify the gene abnormality causing your child's disease. The same tests may be performed on the parents and other family members. This will help to determine where the abnormal gene came from and to identify family members who might pass it on to future children.

- *Muscle biopsy.* A sample of your child's muscle tissue may be obtained for examination under the microscope.

How is muscular dystrophy treated?

Unfortunately, there is no cure for muscular dystrophy. However, treatments are available to help keep your child functioning as well as possible and to prevent and manage complications.

Treatments for muscular dystrophy depend on your child's specific medical problems. Physical therapy may help to keep muscles working as long as possible. Braces and other aids may be used to assist your child's mobility. Surgery is sometimes recommended to help preserve or improve your child's functioning. If the heart is involved, medications may be needed.

Regular medical follow-up is needed to preserve your child's heart and lung function as much as possible. Close attention to issues like diet and immunizations can help to preserve your child's health.

Mental health care and support are also important. Depression can be a problem, especially for adolescents with muscular dystrophy. Having a child with such a serious disease can be overwhelming for parents. Several national and local organizations are available to provide information and support for children with muscular dystrophy and their families.

Where can I get more information about muscular dystrophy?

Here are a few contacts to get you started in learning what your family needs to know about living with muscular dystrophy:

- The National Institute of Neurological Disorders and Stroke. Information and publications are available on the Internet at *www.ninds.nih/gov.*

- The Muscular Dystrophy Association. On the Internet at *www.mdausa.org* or call 1-800-FIGHT-MD (1-800-344-4863).

Tics and Tourette's Syndrome

Tics are repeated, involuntary muscle movements. Common examples are frequent eye blinking or twitching of the mouth; many other types are possible. Some habits (such as thumb sucking or hair twirling) are similar to tics but don't develop as suddenly. Some tics need to be evaluated to be sure they are not really seizures. One possible diagnosis is Tourette's syndrome, a complicated type of tic disorder that is usually lifelong.

What are tics?

Tics are involuntary, uncontrolled, and repeated muscle movements or actions that are repeated in some way. There are three main types of tics:

- *Transient tic disorder.* The most common type, which usually goes away on its own. More common in boys, transient tic disorder usually resolves in about a year. Common types of tics in this disorder include eye blinking, facial movements, and throat clearing.

- *Chronic motor tics.* These types of tics generally do not go away. They can involve up to three different types of muscle groups; for example, eye blinking combined with other types of facial movements. (The word "motor" means that muscles are involved.)

- *Tourette's syndrome.* A lifelong disorder that is usually inherited (genetic). It can involve many types of motor tics (eye blinking, facial movements) and vocal tics (different kinds of sounds, such as grunting).

Stressful situations can increase tics, so parents should not respond negatively when they occur. As children get older, they may learn some control, especially in public. Some tics may require testing to make sure they are not really seizures.

What do they look like?

- Practically any type of movement that occurs frequently can be a tic. In addition to the examples above, tics may consist of squinting, wrinkling of the nose, or twitching around the mouth.

- Some tics are sounds, such as grunting.

- Your child may seem unaware of the tic and may have trouble stopping the tic even if you tell him or her to, but he or she may be able to control it for a short time.

- Many childhood tics are a temporary problem that goes away after a few weeks or months. Others, such as those related to Tourette's syndrome, are lifelong.

What causes tics?

- The cause of common, temporary childhood tics is unknown. They may be at least partly genetic (inherited). Stress doesn't cause tics, but sometimes it seems to make them worse.

- Occasionally, tics can be unmasked by certain medications but are not caused by them. Stimulant medications used to treat attention deficit–hyperactivity disorder (ADHD) do not cause tics. (However, some children with tics also have ADHD.)

- Occasionally, tics may be related to or may flare up after an infection with *Streptococcus* bacteria (for example, strep throat).

What are some possible complications of tics?

Tics can be an embarrassing problem for your child. Teasing and other social problems may occur.

What puts your child at risk of tics?

- Tics are a common, usually temporary problem.

- They are more common in boys than girls.

- They most commonly occur between ages 4 and 7 years.

- Tourette's syndrome may run in families.

How are tics treated?

- Usually, no treatment is necessary. Most childhood tics go away on their own, usually within a few weeks or months.

- Try not to pay too much attention to your child's tics or other habits. Calling attention to or commenting on the tic creates stress, which may make the tic worse.

- Don't scold or punish your child for the tics. Even if your child can consciously control the tic for a time, he or she isn't "doing it on purpose."

- Try to reduce stress in your child's life. If there is any stressful situation that may be contributing to the tic, discuss it with your doctor. Also, be sure to tell the doctor if the tic is causing embarrassment or teasing for your child, or if other social problems are present.

- If tics are causing a lot of interference with your child's home or school life, mental health counseling or behavioral management may be helpful. Biofeedback may also improve the situation in some cases.

- In some children, certain medications usually used for psychiatric conditions can be helpful, for example, risperidone or haloperidol. These drugs have a number of side effects and so are only prescribed if really needed.

- If your child is believed to have Tourette's syndrome, we will probably recommend a visit to a specialist in the treatment of nervous system diseases (a neurologist) or mental health disorders (a psychiatrist).

- Most of the time, unless Tourette's syndrome is present, tics eventually clear up on their own.

When should I call your office?

Call our office if:

- Your child's tic doesn't improve or go away within a few months.

- The tic seems to be getting worse, especially if muscles in different areas of the body are involved.

- Your child is having social problems, problems at school or at home, or other issues that you think might be contributing to or resulting from the tic.

Section XX ▪ Newborn

Ambiguous Genitalia and Intersex Conditions

> Some infants are born with "ambiguous genitalia." This means that the visible genitals—penis and testicles or vagina and clitoris—aren't clearly either male or female. There are many possible causes of these conditions. Expert testing is needed to determine the diagnosis, sexual identity, and best treatment for your baby.

What are ambiguous genitalia?

Ambiguous genitalia are one of many different conditions in which the outer genitals don't clearly appear male or female. They are sometimes called "intersex" conditions.

Most babies with ambiguous genitalia have the genes of either a male or female, but with some additional characteristics of the opposite sex. Special tests, including genetic testing, are needed to determine your infant's exact diagnosis and to decide on the best management. Infants with some intersex conditions may also have other medical problems that need treatment.

For parents, it's upsetting to be told their newborn has ambiguous genitalia. Expert medical diagnosis and treatment and sensitive follow-up care can help to provide your baby with the best chance of a happy, healthy life.

What do they look like?

There are many causes and possible appearances of ambiguous genitalia. For many children with intersex conditions, the external genitals are not clearly male or clearly female. Infants with complete "androgen insensitivity"—in which male hormones don't have the normal effect—look like females but are actually males.

- The genitals may look either like a small penis or an enlarged clitoris. The vagina may appear closed, resembling a scrotum (the sac containing the male testicles), or the scrotum may show some separation, resembling a vagina. Some infants have elements of both male and female genitals. Many variations are possible.

- The internal sex organs may not match the appearance of the external genitalia. For example, a baby who seems to have a penis may have ovaries, while a baby with undescended testes (male testicles that have not dropped to their normal position in the scrotum) may seem to have a vagina.

- Many infants with ambiguous genitalia are otherwise healthy, with no other medical problems. Babies with some genetic conditions have other associated abnormalities.

What causes ambiguous genitalia?

Most cases are related to genetic (inherited) defects affecting the hormones involved in determining the appearance of the genitals (sexual characteristics). Initial examination and testing focus on finding the underlying cause of your infant's condition.

It's important to understand that, in every infant, the male and female genitals start out the same during early development of the baby in the womb. The development of the genitals is affected by genes and by many substances the body produces (such as hormones). That's why so many different conditions can end up causing ambiguous genitalia: they interfere with the normal processes that determine whether the genitals will turn out to be male or female.

Some of the main causes of ambiguous genitalia are:

- *Congenital adrenal hyperplasia.* This is related to several different genetic defects that affect enzymes involved in making hormones in the adrenal gland. (The adrenal gland is a small organ near the kidney that produces a number of different hormones, including those affecting development of the genitals.) Congenital adrenal hyperplasia may cause girls to develop male characteristics or boys to develop female sexual characteristics in childhood. Some forms can cause severe illness.

- *Androgen insensitivity syndromes.* Babies with this condition are genetically male (have male sex chromosomes). However, they have a defect that doesn't allow male hormones to properly affect the development of the genitals. Some male babies with androgen insensitivity look female, but others have more features that make them look male.

- *Sex chromosome abnormalities.* These are various genetic abnormalities in which the baby doesn't have the normal sex chromosomes of either a male (XY) or a female (XX). These include the rare condition in which the infant is a "true hermaphrodite," with both ovarian (female) and testicular (male) tissue.

- *Problems during pregnancy.* Some conditions in the mother during pregnancy can lead to problems in sexual development of the baby. These may include hormone-producing tumors or certain medications.

Many other causes are possible. Babies with ambiguous genitalia don't always fall into clear categories. Expert testing and diagnosis/identification will seek to provide the best possible information on the cause of your baby's condition.

What are some possible complications of ambiguous genitalia?

Many infants with ambiguous genitalia or intersex conditions are otherwise healthy. Others have additional medical problems that need treatment. For example, some forms of congenital adrenal hyperplasia can lead to problems with electrolyte balance and blood pressure.

- Some causes are associated with other birth defects.

- Many children with conditions causing ambiguous genitalia are unable to have children as adults. However, this is not always the case.

What puts your child at risk of ambiguous genitalia?

- Many of the genetic diseases that cause ambiguous genitalia run in families. You may carry the genes for these abnormalities without being aware of it. In many cases, however, there is no previous family history of genetic disease.

- There are some rare conditions arising during pregnancy—such as hormone-producing tumors or certain medications—that can cause ambiguous genitalia.

Can ambiguous genitalia be prevented?

Genetic counseling can help you to understand the risk of passing one of these intersex conditions on to future children. Otherwise, there is no practical way to prevent these conditions or to diagnose them before birth.

How are ambiguous genitalia diagnosed?

Examination, testing, and diagnosis are the essential first steps in determining the cause of your child's condition, finding out whether there are any accompanying medical problems, and deciding on the most appropriate treatment.

These evaluations are performed by experts in diagnosing these complex conditions, for example, a geneticist (a specialist in genetic diseases) or an endocrinologist (a specialist in gland and hormone diseases).

The results of some key tests will have a major impact on your child's diagnosis and treatment, including:

- Genetic tests. These will determine which, if any, genetic abnormality your child has. Parents and other family members may be tested as well.

- Hormone levels and other blood tests.

- Ultrasound or other tests to assess your child's genitals and internal organs of reproduction. It is especially important to determine whether ovaries or testicles are present.

How are ambiguous genitalia treated?

Your child's treatment will depend on the results of a full evaluation:

- *Hormone treatments* may be needed immediately. This is especially important for some infants with congenital adrenal hyperplasia.

- *Counseling* is an important part of treatment. The families of children with ambiguous genitalia need detailed information about their child's condition and emotional support to deal with the stress of this difficult time.

- *Sex assignment* is a difficult and sensitive issue. Although not always, sometimes a decision needs to be made as to whether the child is to be raised as a boy or a girl. Most experts feel it is important to make this decision as soon as possible after birth. Sex assignment can affect surgical issues.

- *Surgery* on the ambiguous genitalia is often required. In many situations, it is easier for the surgeon to create a functioning vagina than a functioning penis. As a result, many children with intersex conditions are raised as girls. This is obviously a difficult and emotional decision to make. Input and advice from various medical and mental health professionals can provide parents with information to help sort through all these issues.

- *Follow-up* is needed to monitor your child's growth and development. Further medical treatment may be needed as your child grows, especially around the time of puberty. Emotional and social support are important as well. With expert medical care and support, many children with intersex conditions grow up to lead normal lives.

When should I call your office?

Going through the diagnosis of an intersex condition is a very stressful time for your family. Call our office if you need help finding support or expert information regarding your child's condition.

Our office will continue to oversee your child's general health care. Call our office if you have any questions or concerns about your child's general health.

Apnea of the Newborn (Interrupted Breathing)

> Apnea is interruption of breathing for a certain amount of time or when accompanied by a change in skin color. Apnea is a common problem in premature babies; it may result from a wide range of medical problems or may occur on its own. Evaluation and testing are essential. Home monitoring may be recommended for apnea of any cause. As long as there are no other medical problems, most infants with apnea eventually outgrow the condition.

What is apnea of the newborn?

In newborns, apnea is defined as a pause in breathing for 20 seconds or longer, or with a change in skin color or a drop in heart rate. Apnea is common in premature infants. When no specific cause is found, it is termed "apnea of prematurity."

Many other diseases and medical problems can cause apnea in newborns. A search is needed to identify the cause. Some infants with episodes of apnea may receive a monitor for use at home to detect apneic events. Your doctor will tell you what action to take if your baby's apnea monitor sounds an alarm.

Some babies, including full-term infants, have "periodic breathing"—this is *not* apnea. It consists of a few pauses in breathing, usually lasting a few seconds. There may be a series of pauses, followed by normal breathing.

What does it look like?

- Infants with apnea have periods of not breathing, generally while sleeping.

- Apnea is most common in premature infants.

- The pauses in breathing are relatively long—over 20 seconds.

- Apnea can also be present if pauses in breathing are accompanied by other abnormalities:

  - Blue color of the skin, called *cyanosis,* usually starting around the lips.

  - Slowing of heart rate, called *bradycardia.*

- Periodic breathing can occur in premature or full-term infants. This is *not* apnea! Your baby's breathing stops for a few seconds. There may be a series of pauses, followed by periods of normal breathing. There is no color change and no slowing of the heart rate. This breathing pattern usually clears up when your baby is a little older.

What causes apnea of the newborn?

- *Apnea of prematurity* is a common problem in premature infants. The cause is unknown. These babies have no other disease that is causing apnea. It may be related to immaturity of the parts of the brain that control breathing.

- The more premature the baby, the more frequent episodes of apnea may be. Apnea usually starts between the 2nd and 7th days of life.

- Apnea in full-term babies is unusual. Testing is needed to identify the cause.

- Other causes of apnea are possible. These include problems with the brain or heart, infections, low blood sugar levels or electrolyte problems, and abnormalities of the central nervous system. For some babies, apnea is related to gastroesophageal reflux disease (GERD) or abnormal "spitting up."

What are some possible complications of apnea of the newborn?

Frequent episodes of apnea can result in your baby's not getting enough oxygen, which could be harmful to the brain.

What puts your newborn at risk of apnea?

Prematurity and the medical problems associated with it are the main risk factors for apnea in newborns.

- *Apnea developing beyond the first 2 weeks after birth in a premature infant, or at any time in a full-term infant, may be particularly serious. Immediate medical evaluation is needed.*

How is apnea of the newborn diagnosed?

In premature infants, apnea is commonly noticed by doctors or nurses or sometimes by parents. If the nature of the apnea is unclear, a sleep study (*polysomnography)* is done.

This test measures how long the episodes of apnea last and other information about the episodes, such as the amount of oxygen in the baby's blood.

How is apnea of the newborn treated?

- *Home monitoring* may be recommended if your baby is still having episodes of apnea by the time he or she goes home from the hospital. The home monitor is a device used to monitor your baby's breathing during sleep. An alarm goes off if breathing is interrupted. Unfortunately, alarms sometimes go off accidentally, when no apnea has occurred.

  - In most cases, gently touching or stroking your baby's body will arouse him or her enough to breathe.

  - You will be taught how to perform cardiopulmonary resuscitation (CPR) in case your baby doesn't start breathing again. This involves giving breaths to the baby and helping the heart to pump blood.

- *Medications* may be given if apnea is considered severe. These drugs stimulate your infant to breathe. Two commonly used drugs are caffeine and theophylline.

- *Nasal continuous positive airway pressure (nCPAP)* may be used for severe apnea. This is a device that helps your baby breathe by gently blowing a steady supply of air into the nostrils. (It is not the same as mechanical ventilation, in which a machine called a ventilator is used to take over the work of breathing for your baby.)

- Other medical problems causing apnea (such as brain injury, infection, or heart problems) are treated if present.

- Most babies with apnea of prematurity outgrow the problem after a few weeks—by the time they have reached their original due date. Home monitoring may continue for a month or two after that.

When should I call your office?

Most babies with apnea no longer need medications or monitoring after leaving the hospital.

If your baby is sent home with a monitor, you'll be trained in how to use it and how to respond to alarms.

- *If your baby has apnea with cyanosis (blue color of the skin) or slowed heart rate (bradycardia), call our office or go to the emergency department immediately.*

Baby's First Weeks— Newborn Care

Healthy babies can usually go home from the hospital 2 days after birth. New parents have a lot of questions about caring for their newborn. This handout answers basic questions about caring for a newborn infant in the first few weeks. If you have questions about caring for your baby or any concerns about his or her health, call our office.

How do I care for a newborn baby?

That's the question asked by every new parent. Even when it's not their first baby, parents may need a "refresher course" when a new baby comes along.

The newborn period is a special time when your baby adjusts to life outside the womb. Newborns sleep a lot and have to eat frequently. They may cry frequently and need a lot of attention.

A newborn infant can place a lot of demands on the parents, especially a mother who's recovering from labor and delivery. This handout answers some "Frequently Asked Questions" for the parents of newborns.

What are the basics of newborn care?

Bringing baby home. You must take care of some important safety steps before taking your newborn home:

- *Car seat.* You must have an approved car seat to drive your baby home from the hospital. Infants under 1 year old must ride in a rear-facing car seat, properly installed in the back seat.
- *Home safety/childproofing.* Make sure your home has working smoke detectors (check batteries). Ask your doctor for advice on childproofing your home.
- *No smoking!* Avoid smoking around your baby and discourage others from smoking inside your home.

  Feeding.

- *Breast versus bottle.* Breast milk is the recommended diet for your newborn. Mothers will receive breast-feeding instruction after delivery. If you choose not to breast-feed or there are medical reasons why you can't, infant formula is an acceptable alternative to breast-feeding.
- *Avoid giving your baby supplemental bottles,* at least until breast-feeding and milk production are well established. Breast-fed babies need additional vitamin D, found in multivitamin supplements. Additional iron and fluoride may be recommended as well.
- *How often?* Healthy infants want to feed frequently during the first week—every 2 to 4 hours. Breast-fed infants may need to be fed more often than bottle-fed infants. Breast-feeding stimulates the breasts to make more milk. It's normal for the baby to lose a little weight during the first week. Your baby should be gaining weight by the end of the second week. In general, until your baby has gained enough weight, he or she should be breast-feeding at least eight times per 24 hours.
- *How much?* If you're breast-feeding, it can be difficult to tell how much milk your baby is getting. Generally, if your newborn is satisfied after nursing, sleeps between feedings, and gains weight, he or she is getting enough milk. After the first few days, diapers should be wet every 4 hours or so.

  Sleeping.

- *How much? How often?* Generally, newborns sleep most of the day for the first few months.
  - They generally sleep for 1 to 4 hours at a time, followed by 1 to 2 hours of awake time. Most babies settle into a nightly sleep routine by 2 to 3 months.
  - Most babies do not sleep 5 to 6 hours through the night until they are at least 3 months old. Until that time, your baby will probably wake up at least once during the night to be fed (2 a.m. feeding).
- "Back to sleep."
  - *Place babies on their backs to sleep!* This is the most important thing you can do to reduce your infant's risk of sudden infant death syndrome.
  - Your baby should sleep in a crib with a firm mattress. The mattress should be covered by a fitted sheet. Don't use a top sheet, pillows, or blankets. Dress your baby in sleepwear that is appropriate for the temperature.
- *Bathing.* Babies don't need to be bathed every day—once every few days is fine. Give only sponge baths for the first couple of weeks, until the umbilical cord stump falls off. (Your doctor will give you instructions on caring for the umbilical cord.)
  - When you start giving your baby tub baths, use a basin or special "baby tub" with no more than 2 inches of water. Use only mild soap, if any.
  - Support your baby's head during the bath.
  - *Never leave your baby alone in the bath, even for a few seconds!*

- *Crying.* Some newborns cry a lot. Although crying sometimes means your baby needs feeding or a diaper change, at other times it's difficult to tell why he or she is crying. Hold and comfort your baby, gently rocking, singing, or talking to him or her. Call our office if you find it difficult to comfort your baby.

- *Illnesses.* If your baby seems sick or warm, take his or her temperature. The best way to take a newborn's temperature is to use a rectal thermometer. If the temperature is 100.4°F (38°C) or higher, call our office.

- *Urine and stools.* After the first few days, diapers should be wet every 3 to 4 hours or so. Your baby will probably pass the first dark green "meconium" stool within the first 48 hours after birth, usually in the hospital. After that, your baby's stools (bowel movements) will be green or yellow and soft. This varies; in breast-fed babies, stools may be looser (more liquid).

- If your baby goes for more than 6 hours without wetting the diaper, this may be a sign of dehydration, which can develop very quickly in babies. If stools are very watery and frequent (diarrhea), this may be a sign of illness, especially if your baby has a fever. (However, it's normal for babies to pass stool every time they feed.)

- *Emotions/postpartum depression.* It's normal for new mothers to feel tired and "stressed out." As much as possible, keep in touch with your sources of support (family, friends). Some new mothers may develop postpartum depression in the weeks and months following the birth of a new baby.

  - *If you feel down or unhappy or are having trouble handling the demands of caring for a new baby, call your doctor's office.*

- *Taking baby out.* Your baby must be in an approved car seat every time he or she goes in the car. It is fine to take your baby out for walks in a stroller. Dress your baby appropriately for the weather; there is no need to "overdress" your baby on warm days. On sunny days, keep the baby's skin covered, since babies get sunburned easily.

- A parent (or other responsible caregiver) needs to be present at all times. It's fine to leave your baby in another room, as long as you can hear him or her if she cries.

- *Skin rashes.* There are several types of skin rashes that are common and harmless in newborns. Just to be sure, ask your doctor if your newborn develops a rash.

- *Doctor's office visits.* The doctor will want to see your infant for several "well-baby" visits. The first visit will probably be 2 or 3 days after your baby goes home, with another visit at 1 or 2 weeks. (Your doctor may recommend a different office visit schedule.)

  - At these visits, the doctor will check to make sure your baby is doing all right, give recommended immunizations (vaccinations), and answer any questions about infant care. Between office visits, it's a good idea to write down any questions you want to ask your doctor.

When should I call your office?

Call our office if you have questions or concerns about caring for your baby.

Between well-baby visits, call our office immediately if any of the following occur:

- Vomiting (not just simple spitting-up).

- Diarrhea.

- Dehydration (caused by vomiting or diarrhea).

  - Baby going over 6 hours without wetting the diaper. (With highly absorbent disposable diapers, this may be hard to judge. It may help to place a cotton ball on the penis or vagina.)

  - Reduced wetness inside the mouth.

  - Irritability or extreme tiredness.

  - In very severe cases, sunken eyes or "soft spot" (fontanelle).

- If you're not sure your baby is getting enough breast milk or formula.

- Your baby is running a fever—temperature 100.4°F (38°C) or higher, measured by a rectal thermometer. Even without a fever, call if your baby is irritable or refusing to eat.

- Umbilical cord problems, especially redness of the skin around the cord, active bleeding, fluid coming from the cord stump, or very foul odor.

- Excessive crying.

- Depression in the mother—feeling overwhelmed.

- Jaundice: yellow or orange color of the baby's skin.

Circumcision

Circumcision is a simple surgical operation to remove the foreskin, a piece of skin that covers the tip of the penis in boy babies. There's no official recommendation to routinely have male newborns circumcised. Circumcision may reduce the risk of certain medical problems later in life, but there is also a small risk of complications from the surgery. The final decision depends on your family's preferences.

What is circumcision?

In newborn boys, the skin of the penis goes a little bit past the "tip" (glans) of the penis. This piece of skin is called the foreskin. Circumcision is a simple operation to remove the foreskin.

Sometimes there are medical reasons why circumcision should or should not be done. Research has shown that circumcision reduces the risk of certain medical problems later on in life. On the other hand, there is a small risk of complications from the procedure. For most parents, the decision as to whether or not to have their son circumcised depends on cultural, religious, or personal reasons.

How is circumcision done?

Circumcision is usually done a day or two after your baby is born. The procedure is fairly simple and doesn't take very long. There are different methods of circumcision, but all involve removing (cutting) the foreskin.

Your baby will be awake for the procedure. Different methods of anesthesia may be used to prevent pain. A local anesthetic such as lidocaine may be injected (as a shot) into areas around the penis, or an anesthetic cream may be applied 60 to 90 minutes before the operation.

Is circumcision safe?

Circumcision is generally a safe procedure. It has a small risk of complications, most of them minor. After the initial pain and swelling go away, there are usually no problems.

The main complications are excessive bleeding, infection (usually minor), injury to the penis, problems with healing, and parents not being satisfied with the appearance of the penis. Rarely, additional surgery needed.

Some infant boys should not be circumcised right away for medical reasons: for example, if they have hypospadias (a minor birth defect involving abnormal location of the urethra, the opening where urine comes out) or possible bleeding abnormalities. If desired, circumcision can be performed after these problems are taken care of.

- Circumcision should only be done in normal, healthy newborns.

What are the advantages of having my baby circumcised?

- Boys who have been circumcised have lower rates of urinary tract infections during the first year of life. Being circumcised also reduces the risk of certain minor problems related to the foreskin in boys, such as infection or irritation.

- Circumcised males are at lower risk of developing cancer of the penis. (However, this cancer is rare even in uncircumcised men.)

- Circumcision may reduce the risk of some sexually transmitted diseases, including infection with human immunodeficiency virus (HIV), the virus that causes acquired immunodeficiency syndrome (AIDS).

What are the disadvantages of having my baby circumcised?

Circumcision has some uncommon but possible complications. Not performing the circumcision avoids the risk of these complications (listed earlier) as well as the pain of this procedure.

Should I have my baby circumcised?

This is a decision the parents must make after considering the possible benefits and risks. Talking to the doctor may help you decide.

There are a few medical situations in which it's best to have your baby circumcised and others in which it's best to avoid or delay circumcision. For many families, the decision depends on social factors:

- Having boys circumcised is traditional in some religions.

- In the past, most American boys were circumcised. Some families have their sons circumcised because that's what they're used to, or so that the boy will look "like dad."

- It may be easier to keep the penis clean if it's circumcised. However, most uncircumcised boys can easily push the foreskin back for cleaning. *Never force your son's foreskin back!* It will go back easily in time.

- Circumcision can always be performed later if needed or desired. However, the operation is simpler in newborns. If done later, general anesthesia may be have to be used.

How do I care for my baby after circumcision?

- After your baby has been circumcised, follow the surgeon's instructions for care.

- Generally, Vaseline or other ointments are applied to the circumcision area until the wound is healed and won't stick to diapers.

- Remember that the circumcision is a healing wound. At first it looks red with white areas that look like pus.

When should I call your office?

After circumcision, call the surgeon's office or our office if:

- The penis is very swollen or redness is increasing.

- You have any concerns about the appearance of the penis.

Cleft Lip and Cleft Palate

Cleft lip and cleft palate are relatively common birth defects. Your baby may have one or the other or both defects. Cleft lip is a split of the upper lip, which may extend up to the nose. Cleft palate is a split or separation in the roof of the mouth. A baby with cleft lip or palate is treated by a specialized team, including a plastic surgeon; an ear, nose and throat doctor; a speech therapist; and other professionals.

What are cleft lip and cleft palate?

Cleft lip and cleft palate are common birth defects in which a part of the lip and/or palate doesn't completely come together or close while the baby is developing in the womb, and so a split or cleft is left in that area. Sometimes they are part of a syndrome of birth defects. However, most of the time, cleft lip/cleft palate is the only abnormality.

Babies with cleft lip/cleft palate need special care to ensure proper feeding and prevent complications. Surgery is done to close the cleft lip and/or palate. Cleft lip is usually repaired by age 3 months, cleft palate by about 1 year.

Your baby may need further treatment as he or she grows, depending on the severity of the defect. Most babies with cleft lip and cleft palate are otherwise normal and do fine after surgery and other treatments.

What do they look like?

- Cleft lip and cleft palate. Clefts (splits) are visible in both the upper lip and palate (the roof of the mouth).

- Cleft lip or cleft palate may occur alone.

- The size, shape, and location of the clefts vary a great deal. Some babies have just a slight notch in the upper lip. Others have a split running all the way into the floor of the nose. Cleft palate may involve part or all of the roof of the mouth. The cleft is often in the middle of the lip or palate but also may be on either side.

- Occasionally these defects occur as part of a syndrome, with other abnormalities present.

- Many babies with cleft lip and cleft palate have trouble eating. This is because the split in their lip and/or palate interferes with their ability to suck normally. Special feeding methods are used to deal with this problem.

What causes cleft lip and cleft palate?

Usually, the exact cause is unknown. Possible causes include drugs the mother took during pregnancy, birth defect syndromes, or genetic factors.

What are some possible complications of cleft lip and cleft palate?

Immediately, babies with cleft lip and cleft palate may have feeding problems caused by their inability to suck normally. Babies with cleft palate are at risk of inhaling food (aspiration), which can lead to choking and pneumonia. Special techniques allow your baby to feed while reducing the risk of aspiration.

Later in life, cleft palate (but not cleft lip alone) may be related to other problems, including:

- Speech problems. If surgery is not completely successful, speech defects may develop. Your child's voice may sound unusual ("nasal"), or he or she may have difficulty making certain sounds.

- Ear/hearing problems. Cleft palate may result in fluid buildup behind the eardrum, leading to hearing loss.

- Dental problems may appear as your baby's teeth start to come in.

What puts your child at risk of cleft lip and cleft palate?

- The risk is higher in boys than girls.

- The risk is higher in Asian families, lower in African-American families.

- Cleft lip and cleft palate seem to run in families.

- Certain factors related to the mother during pregnancy may increase the risk of cleft palate, including:

  - Smoking.

  - Certain medications, such as drugs to lower cholesterol.

Can cleft lip and cleft palate be prevented?

Women who are pregnant or planning to have a baby can do some things to reduce the risk of cleft lip and palate:

- Taking a vitamin supplement containing folic acid (vitamin B_6) and other B complex vitamins may reduce the risk of cleft palate. This is especially important during the first 2 months of pregnancy.

- Talk to your obstetrician about any medications you are taking. For example, some medications used for epilepsy may lead to an increased risk of cleft palate.

- Don't smoke. (Using tobacco during pregnancy can harm your baby in other ways as well.)

- Some types of cleft lip/cleft palate are related to abnormal genes. Genetic counseling may help you to understand how this risk may affect future pregnancies.

How are cleft lip and cleft palate treated?

A team approach is used to treat babies and with cleft lip/cleft palate. Members of the team usually include a plastic surgeon; an ear, nose, and throat specialist (an otorhinolaryngologist); and a speech therapist. Other professionals may include a nutrition expert and a geneticist (a specialist in inherited diseases).

- *Feeding.* Feeding is a problem for many babies with cleft palate, with or without cleft lip. Until they have surgery, babies with cleft lip may also have feeding problems. These infants may have difficulty generating enough pressure to suck normally. Other babies may have problems with gagging or inhaling milk or formula.

  - Different solutions may be tried to make sure your baby gets enough food. Using a squeezable bottle with a soft nipple may be helpful. For some babies, a plastic shield called an "obturator" can be used. This device is specially shaped to cover your baby's cleft palate during feeding.

  - Many babies with cleft palate cannot breast-feed normally. Pumping breast milk and feeding it in bottles may be a way for your baby to get the health advantages of breast milk.

- *Repair/Rehabilitation.* Babies with cleft lip and palate need evaluation and treatment by a team of doctors and other health professionals. They can provide the expert services your child needs. The pediatrician is an important member of the team. Our office will continue to coordinate your child's medical care.

- A *plastic surgeon* generally plans the surgery needed to repair your child's cleft lip and palate. Surgery to repair cleft lip is usually performed when the baby is around 3 months old. Surgery to repair cleft palate is done before age 1 if possible. This operation is done to avoid problems with speech development. Additional surgeries may be needed as your child grows.

- An *ear, nose, and throat specialist* (an otorhinolaryngologist) will evaluate your child for any problems related to the ear. If ear infections are a problem, treatment is needed to prevent hearing loss.

- A *speech-language pathologist* can help in dealing with speech problems, if present.

- A *dentist or oral surgeon* can evaluate and treat any problems with your child's teeth.

- Other professionals may be involved in your child's care. These other treatments will depend on your child's individual needs.

A complete program of treatment for a child with cleft lip and palate takes many years. With expert care, most children with cleft lip and palate do fine, with no major complications.

When should I call your office?

After taking your baby home, call our office if you are having any problems with feeding, including:

- Your baby is not getting enough milk or formula.

- Choking, gagging, or milk coming out of baby's nose.

- Babies with cleft lip and palate need a lot of special care. Treatment can be pretty complicated. Call our office if you have any questions.

Clubfoot (Talipes Equinovarus)

Clubfoot is a relatively common foot deformity. Sometimes it affects the entire lower leg as well as the foot. In the most common type, clubfoot is the only birth defect present. Treatment starts with a series of casts. If this doesn't correct your child's deformity within a few months, surgery is recommended.

What is clubfoot?

Clubfoot is a congenital deformity (birth defect) in which the foot is out of position and doesn't have normal flexibility. One or both feet may be affected. The cause isn't always known, although clubfoot sometimes results from the baby's position in the womb. It is most often the only abnormality but may occur as part of a syndrome with other birth defects. Clubfoot is sometimes called by its Latin name, *talipes equinovarus*.

Clubfoot has to be treated or else your child won't be able to walk normally. Usually a series of casts are placed to stretch the foot toward the correct position; after that, a brace may be used. Surgery can be performed if needed. The treated foot isn't exactly the same as a normal foot, but your child will probably be able to walk normally.

What does it look like?

The clubfoot abnormality is obvious at birth. Sometimes it's seen on ultrasound scans before birth.

- The foot is turned inward from the normal position. Instead of facing down, the sole of the foot faces toward the inner side. The heel is higher than the ball of the foot.
- The foot is stiff; the joints can't be moved normally.
- The calf muscles may be smaller than normal.
- In about half of babies with clubfoot, both feet are affected.

What causes clubfoot?

There are three main types of clubfoot:

- *Congenital.* The most common type. The cause is unknown, but genetic (inherited) factors may play a role. Clubfoot is the only abnormality.
- *Positional.* This type of clubfoot occurs because the foot was in an abnormal position in the womb. It is the easiest to treat.
- *Teratologic.* Clubfoot accompanied by other birth defects. Clubfoot may be one sign of a general neuromuscular disorder (abnormalities of the nervous system or muscles) or part of a syndrome of birth defects. Your baby will receive a careful physical examination to look for these other abnormalities

What are some possible complications of clubfoot?

- Correction by casts or surgery may not be totally successful.
- Pain or difficulty walking. Later in life, arthritis may develop. (Most children with positional clubfoot don't have these problems.)
- Because the calf muscle may be involved, there may still be problems with use of the leg even after foot position has been corrected.

What increases your child's risk of clubfoot?

- About 1 in 1000 babies has clubfoot at birth.
- Boys are more often affected than girls.
- Genetic factors affect risk:
  - For the congenital form, if you've had one child with clubfoot, the risk in future children is about 3%.
  - If one of the parents had clubfoot, the risk in children is 20% to 30%.

Can clubfoot be prevented?

There is no way to prevent clubfoot.

How is clubfoot treated?

Treatment for clubfoot starts immediately after birth. Your baby is evaluated by an orthopedic surgeon—a specialist in treating bone and joint diseases.

- *Nonsurgical treatment.* The first choice for treatment of clubfoot is usually stretching and casting:
  - To start with, the surgeon will gently move your baby's foot toward the desired position, then apply a plaster cast to hold the foot in that position.
  - A week or two later, the cast will be removed. The surgeon will stretch the foot a little farther, then put on another cast.
  - The process is repeated until your child's foot is in the correct position. The goal is to get the foot into the correct position by the time your baby is about 3 months old.
  - After casting, your baby will receive a brace or special shoes for some period of time. Parents play a very

important role during this time. If the brace isn't worn as recommended, the clubfoot may come back.

- If your baby is born prematurely, splints or taping may be used until he or she has grown enough to begin cast treatment.

- *Surgery.* If normal foot position isn't achieved by the time your baby is about 3 months old, surgery may be recommended.

  - The operation is usually performed some time between ages 6 to 12 months. The goal is to achieve full correction by the time your child reaches normal walking age.

  - Your baby's foot is put in a cast for a while after surgery. After the cast comes off, he or she will most likely wear a brace or special shoes for a year or longer.

The orthopedic surgeon will monitor your child's condition as he or she grows. After casting or surgery, most children with clubfoot can walk, run, and play normally.

When should I call your office?

The orthopedic surgeon will plan and carry out treatment for your child's clubfoot. Our office will continue to oversee your child's general medical care.

Call your orthopedic surgeon if there are any problems with your child's cast or brace, for example, if the cast comes off. Also, call the surgeon if your child's foot seems to be turning back inward after treatment.

- During cast treatment, get medical help immediately if there is any swelling or color change of the foot.

Collar Bone Fractures in Newborns

Fracture of the collar bone is a common birth injury. It is caused by pressure on that area during birth. Although it sounds serious, collar bone fracture usually heals very quickly, often with no need for treatment.

What is collar bone fracture?

The collar bone, or clavicle, is the bone running from the breast bone to the shoulder. Fracture of the collar bone is a common birth injury. Fracture means the bone is broken; it could be a complete break or just a partial crack.

The fracture is caused by pressure on your baby's body as he or she passes through the birth canal. Collar bone fracture is more likely to occur with difficult deliveries, especially when delivering the shoulder in babies born head first. Large babies tend to have more difficult deliveries.

Your baby may be unable to move the arm on the affected side. However, many babies with a fractured collar bone have no symptoms at all. Since bone develops so rapidly in newborn babies, these fractures heal very quickly. The doctor may temporarily splint the arm on the side of the fractured collar bone. However, your baby may need no treatment.

What does it look like?

- Your baby may not be able to move one arm as much as the other. The area of the fracture may feel irregular to the doctor; it may feel "sponge-like" when pressed. The doctor may notice other abnormalities, such as a sound when moving the shoulder or lack of normal reflexes on that side.

- Your baby may be fussy, especially when the arm is moved. However, the injury often goes unnoticed.

- Other babies with collar bone fractures have mild or no symptoms. Your baby's fracture may not be recognized until you or the doctor notice a lump on the collar bone. The lump is new bone formed during healing.

What are some possible complications of collar bone fracture?

Complications are rare. Sometimes, the forces that cause collar bone fracture can also cause damage to the nerves of the arm.

What increases your baby's risk of collar bone fracture?

- Newborn's shoulder getting stuck in the birth canal during normal "head first" birth.

- Baby is larger size than usual.

- Longer than term pregnancy (beyond due date).

- Assisted delivery—for example, use of a vacuum device during birth.

Can collar bone fracture be prevented?

Most of the time, there is no way to prevent this fracture.

How is collar bone fracture treated?

- Your baby may not need treatment at all. Depending on the situation, the doctor may recommend immobilizing the arm (keeping it from moving too much). This is usually done by pinning clothing around the arm so it can't move.

- If the injury seems to be causing pain, give acetaminophen drops or other pain medication.

- The bones grow very rapidly in newborns. As a result, collar bone fractures heal very quickly. You may be able to feel strong new bone (callus) developing at the fracture area as early as 1 week.

When should I call your office?

The doctor will check your baby until the fracture has healed and he or she can move the arm normally. Call the doctor if the baby is not moving the arm normally or seems irritable after 1 to 2 weeks.

Common Newborn Rashes

Many newborn babies develop temporary skin rashes. Some common ones include *erythema toxicum*, milium, sebaceous hyperplasia, miliaria, and neonatal acne. These are harmless conditions that generally go away with no treatment. Call our office if your newborn has a rash that seems to be causing itching or discomfort.

What kinds of rashes can occur in newborns?

Newborns can develop a number of common rashes that are harmless and usually go away without treatment. However, the doctor may still want to check the rash, just to be sure that the diagnosis is correct and the condition doesn't need treatment. Any rash that seems to be bothering your baby, or a rash that is accompanied by fever, should be checked by the doctor.

What do they look like?

Erythema toxicum. Most cases begin 1 or 2 days after birth. It is rare in premature infants.

- Small, yellow/white bumps on a background of red, splotchy skin.

- Usually seen on the face and body; can occur other places as well.

- Rash may clear up in one place, only to reappear in another.

- The rash can last up to a week or so. No treatment is needed.

Neonatal acne. Sometimes called "baby acne."

- Usually begins in the first few weeks of life. The cause is unknown.

- Small, red bumps or little pustules appear on the face, particularly the cheeks. The rash doesn't bother the baby.

- Usually goes away on its own. If the rash is severe or doesn't clear up, it can be treated with acne medicine such as benzoyl peroxide (although this is rarely needed).

Infantile acne is a little different:

- Usually begins after 2 to 3 months.

- Rash looks like teenage acne: red bumps, pustules, and pimples (comedones). This rash may be related to male hormones (androgens).

- The rash usually gets better by age 12 to 16 months. If needed, treatment is similar to that for teenage acne.

Miliaria. Sometimes called "heat rash" or "prickly heat."

- Caused by plugging of the sweat glands. This rash usually appears when your baby is overheated, such as when dressed too warmly for the weather, in a humid environment, or during a fever.

- In newborns, the rash appears most often as very tiny blisters often on the back, neck, or face. The blisters break easily with mild pressure.

- More commonly in older children, the rash may look like small, red bumps or occasionally pustules. It most often appears on the neck, forehead, or areas covered by clothing.

- No treatment is needed, except to keep the baby cooler and prevent overheating.

Sebaceous hyperplasia. Caused by enlarged sweat glands.

- Rash looks like lots of small, yellow/white, smooth bumps.

- Most common on the nose, forehead, and upper lip.

- The bumps usually disappear in a few weeks; no treatment needed.

Milia. Despite their similar names, this rash is different from "miliaria" (discussed above).

- Rash looks like tiny white bumps, usually on the face, but can appear anywhere.

- The bumps are actually tiny, fluid-filled cysts. This rash looks similar to sebaceous hyperplasia, but the bumps are not yellow in color and there are not as many of them.

- This rash can occur later in infancy and childhood and usually goes away on its own.

What puts your baby at risk of these rashes?

These rashes are very common—for example, erythema toxicum occurs in about one half of babies.

Can they be prevented?

There is generally no way to prevent these harmless rashes. Miliaria may be decreased by not letting your baby get overheated.

When should I call your office?

Call our office if your baby has:

- Rash that is causing obvious itching or other discomfort.

- Rash with fever.

Congenital Diaphragmatic Hernia

Babies with congenital diaphragmatic hernia (CDH) are born with an opening in the diaphragm (a muscle that separates the lungs from the abdomen). The opening allows organs that are normally in the abdomen to enter the chest. This usually causes the lungs to develop abnormally: many babies with CDH develop breathing problems soon after birth. CDH can be a severe, life-threatening abnormality. Your baby will receive immediate evaluation and testing to find out how severe the problem is and to determine the best treatment.

What is congenital diaphragmatic hernia (CDH)?

Babies with CDH have an abnormal opening in the diaphragm. The diaphragm is a muscle, important for breathing, which separates the lungs from the abdomen. In CDH, some of the organs that should be in the abdomen go through ("herniate") the hole in the diaphragm, into the baby's chest. This can cause problems with your baby's lungs because they don't have enough room to develop normally. Other problems affecting the intestines and heart can also occur.

Some babies with CDH have a large hernia that causes serious breathing problems and other abnormalities. Others have a less severe hernia that causes fewer problems. Careful tests are needed to determine the severity and consequences of your baby's CDH. Special treatments may be needed to assist breathing for a period of time. After your baby's condition has stabilized, surgery can be done to repair the hole in the diaphragm.

What does it look like?

The medical problems of babies with CDH vary a lot, depending on the severity of the birth defect.

- Some babies with CDH develop severe breathing problems (respiratory distress) soon after birth. Less often, breathing problems develop some time after birth.

- If your infant's CDH is less severe, the symptoms may be different. Relatively mild breathing problems may occur. Vomiting or other digestive problems may result if the intestines become obstructed (blocked) in their abnormal position in the chest. In this condition, the intestines are not normally attached to the abdomen and can become twisted and obstructed (malrotation).

- Sometimes CDH is recognized before birth on a routine ultrasound scan.

- Some babies with CDH have other birth defects as well.

What causes CDH?

- CDH occurs when your baby's diaphragm develops with an abnormal opening. The opening allows some of the organs that should be in your child's abdomen to move into the chest. It is unknown what causes your child's diaphragm to develop in this way.

- Part or all of the stomach, intestine, spleen, and other organs can be found in the chest. This doesn't allow enough room for the lungs to develop normally. One lung, usually the left, is smaller than the other. The other lung may be squeezed to the side. Breathing problems occur because of the abnormally developed lungs and diaphragm.

- The lung abnormality leads to a problem called pulmonary hypertension—high blood pressure in the vessels carrying blood from the heart to the lungs. This can lead to further heart and lung problems.

What are some possible complications of CDH?

CDH is a serious birth defect. Modern treatments have greatly improved the survival rate. However, even with treatment, some infants with CDH die. The risk of death and severe complications is highest for infants with more severe CDH.

Infants who survive CDH may have medical problems related to poor lung development. Neurologic problems can also occur. The risk of these problems is higher in babies who need lifesaving extracorporeal membrane oxygenation (ECMO) treatment. Growth and nutrition problems are common as well.

Some infants with CDH need several operations or have to remain in the hospital for a long period of time for treatment and surgery.

What increases your child's risk of CDH?

- Congenital diaphragmatic hernia is a relatively common birth defect, affecting about 1 in 5000 infants. Many infants with CDH are stillborn (die in the womb).

- If anyone in your family had this birth defect, your child may be at higher risk. Otherwise, there are no known risk factors for CDH.

Can CDH be prevented?

There is no known way to prevent this birth defect.

How is CDH treated?

Infants with CDH need immediate evaluation and treatment. X-rays and other tests are performed to confirm that CDH is present and to determine how severe the abnormality is.

Treatment usually consists of two steps. Initial treatment focuses on *breathing support* to ensure that your baby is getting enough oxygen. Once his or her condition has stabilized, *surgery* is planned to move the organs into their proper position and to repair the hole in your baby's diaphragm.

- *Breathing support.* Treatments to help your baby breathe are the first priority. This often has to be done on an emergency basis in CDH babies who develop respiratory distress. Babies with CDH are treated in the intensive care unit (ICU), where they can receive constant treatment and round-the-clock monitoring.

  - Mechanical ventilation is often needed. Your baby will be connected to a machine called a ventilator to help the lungs perform the work of breathing.

  - In other infants, mechanical ventilation cannot provide enough oxygen. These infants receive a different kind of support called extracorporeal membrane oxygenation (ECMO). ECMO is a machine that takes over the functions of the lungs. It can keep your baby alive while his or her medical condition stabilizes. Your baby may need to stay on ECMO for a long time—2 weeks or even longer.

  - During either type of breathing support, your baby will receive constant medical monitoring and treatment. The goal is to allow time for your child to grow stronger before final repair of CDH is performed.

- *Surgery.* Babies with CDH eventually require surgery. More than one operation may be needed. The goals of surgery are:

  - To move the abnormally positioned organs back down to the abdomen.

  - To close the hole in your baby's diaphragm.

  - Surgery may be done as soon as 2 or 3 days after birth if your baby responds well to mechanical ventilation. If your baby requires ECMO, a delay of several weeks is more likely.

Every baby with CDH is different. Many factors affect your infant's medical condition, treatment, and chances of a good outcome.

When should I call your office?

Call our office if you have any questions about this birth defect or about your infant's treatment.

Cradle Cap (Seborrheic Dermatitis of Newborns)

Cradle cap is a common skin condition in newborns. A greasy, scaly rash develops on the baby's scalp. The rash may also occur on the face, the area behind the ears, the diaper area, and sometimes other areas. The problem generally clears up by age 1 year and responds to some simple treatments.

What is cradle cap?

Cradle cap is a usually harmless skin condition affecting infants. A rash develops on your baby's scalp and other areas, generally within the first few months. Cradle cap is also known as "seborrheic dermatitis."

The cause of cradle cap is unknown. It may be related to hormones from the mother remaining in the baby's body for a while after birth. (The hormones make the glands in the baby's skin overproduce an oily substance called sebum, thereby allowing dead skin cells to build up on the scalp.) It may take several months before cradle cap clears up completely. Simple treatments can be helpful.

What does it look like?

- A scaly, yellowish rash develops on your baby's scalp, usually in the first few months. Although often greasy, it may appear dry. The skin of his or her scalp may appear reddened at times, and the rash may become crusted.

- Scaly patches may also occur on the face, especially the forehead, behind the ears, and along the eyebrows. The underarms and diaper area may also be involved.

- The rash may or may not cause any itching or other discomfort to the baby.

How is cradle cap diagnosed?

- Cradle cap is a common condition in newborns. Usually no special tests are needed to make the diagnosis.

- When it involves the face and other areas of the body, cradle cap can look so similar to eczema that it may be difficult to tell them apart.

How is cradle cap treated?

The problem clears up over time, although it may still be present up to age 1 year. A number of different treatments may be recommended, depending on how severe the rash is.

- Massage mineral oil into your baby's scalp and leave it on for a while to loosen up scale and crusting. Then wash the scale using baby shampoo. Do this a few times a week.

- If mineral oil treatment doesn't work well enough, the doctor may recommend a weak steroid lotion. Apply this medication to the scalp a few times a week.

- Washing with dandruff shampoo can be helpful. However, be careful when using these shampoos—they can be irritating, especially to the eyes.

When should I call your office?

Call our office if the rash doesn't improve with treatment or if it gets worse.

Developmental Dysplasia of the Hip

In some babies, one of the hip joints is dislocated or can be easily dislocated at birth or shortly afterward. This is called developmental dysplasia of the hip. Early recognition and treatment are important to prevent hip-related complications later in life. Once they are recognized, congenital hip dislocations are easily treated.

What is developmental dysplasia of the hip?

Developmental dysplasia of the hip is a hip dislocation that occurs around the time of birth. Dislocation means that the end of the thigh bone (femur) is not properly fitted into the hip joint (socket). This condition used to be called "congenital hip dislocation."

The cause is unknown, but the hip is relatively unstable at birth, partly because the ligaments that hold the joint together are not very tight. That's why the doctor checks your infant's hips at every well-baby visit.

In the newborn period, there are usually no symptoms of developmental dysplasia of the hip. As your infant gets older, hip movement or leg position may appear abnormal. The earlier the dislocation is recognized, the easier it is to treat and the lower the risk of complications.

What does it look like?

- Usually, the hip dislocation is not obvious at birth. Whenever the doctor examines your infant, he or she will examine the hip to see if it dislocates or is dislocated easily. (The dislocation probably won't cause your baby any pain, because the immature hips of newborn infants are very flexible.)

- The results of the examination will tell the doctor whether your baby's hip is "unstable" (easily dislocated) or is already dislocated. Most babies with an unstable hip never develop a true dislocation.

- If there is a possible hip problem, we will probably recommend a visit to an orthopedic surgeon (a specialist in bone and joint diseases) for further evaluation and treatment.

- If developmental dysplasia is not recognized and treated, problems may develop after your child starts to walk. These may include having one leg longer than the other, limping, or waddling.

What are some possible complications of developmental dysplasia of the hip?

- If the dislocation is recognized in infancy, treatment is simple and complications are rare.

- If the dislocation is discovered later in childhood, treatment is more complicated. Surgery may be needed to put the joint back into correct position. Delayed treatment or no treatment increases the risk of arthritis and other long-term complications.

- Although uncommon, a serious complication called avascular necrosis can occur. This happens when the blood supply to the "ball" of the bone that fits into the hip joint gets cut off, causing the bone to die. Treatment is as careful and conservative as possible to prevent this complication.

What increases your child's risk of developmental dysplasia of the hip?

- Being born in breech position (bottom first).

- Genetic factors. If someone in your family had hip problems in infancy, your child may be at greater risk.

- Girls are at nine times higher risk than males.

- First-born children are at higher risk.

Can developmental dysplasia of the hip be prevented?

- There is no way to prevent this condition.

- Prompt recognition and treatment reduce the risk of complications.

How is developmental dysplasia of the hip diagnosed and treated?

Diagnosis is often made by a physical examination, although sometimes the doctor is not sure and will ask for x-rays and ultrasounds (which use sound waves to create a picture) to be sure of the diagnosis and treatment that follows.

Treatment depends on your child's age when the condition is recognized and the severity of the dislocation. If developmental dysplasia is suspected, we will recommend a visit to a bone and joint specialist (an orthopedic surgeon) for further evaluation and treatment.

- *At birth*. If an unstable hip is recognized at birth, treatment usually consists of a special harness to keep the hip in proper "turned-out" position. Keeping the hip in this position for up to a few weeks usually allows the joint to become stable.

- *From birth to about 6 months*. Use of a harness is usually enough to keep the thigh bone (femur) in its proper position in the hip joint. If not, other treatments are recommended, which may include keeping the hip in a cast for a few weeks.

- *After about 6 months*. Casting may work in some of these older infants, whereas others will need surgery.

When should I call your office?

Our office will continue to coordinate your child's medical care.

Call your orthopedic surgeon's office if you experience any problems during treatment for developmental dysplasia of the hip, such as:

- Difficulty using the harness.

- Swelling, color change, foul odor under your baby's cast, or fussiness not explained by other causes.

Diaper Rash

Diaper rash is a very common problem. It is caused by irritation in the diaper area and can be very uncomfortable for your baby. Diaper rash usually improves with simple treatments, but it sometimes can be difficult to get rid of. The irritated skin can become infected, most often with *Candida* yeast. If a yeast infection occurs, specific treatment is needed.

What is diaper rash?

Diaper rash is caused by irritation of the skin in the diaper area. It is sometimes called "diaper dermatitis."

The skin becomes red and sore. The rash can get worse if it isn't taken care of properly, and it can become quite painful for your baby. Infection can occur, including infection with the yeast *Candida*.

In most cases, diaper rash gets better if you keep the area as clean as possible, including frequent diaper changes, and apply an ointment to protect the skin. If the rash becomes large or severe, call our office.

What does it look like?

- The skin in the diaper area looks red and scaly, sometimes with scattered small bumps.

- You may notice small cracks, rubbed areas, thickening, or raw areas of the skin.

- The rash can be painful, causing fussiness and crying in your infant.

- If yeast infection occurs, the rash may become very red with well-outlined borders. Scattered bumps or pimples may appear in the skin near the borders. The rash may spread to cover the entire diaper area or beyond.

What causes diaper rash?

- Diaper rash is caused by irritation of the skin. The most important factor is the length of time the skin stays wet and in contact with urine and stool (bowel movements).

- Other irritants can also contribute to a rash in the diaper area, such as soaps and baby products.

- The rash may become infected with germs, such as *Candida* yeast. Warmth and wetness inside the diaper encourage germs to grow.

- Every baby's skin is different; some babies just get diaper rash more often than others. Changing diapers frequently can help to prevent diaper rash.

What are some possible complications of diaper rash?

- Serious complications are rare. However, diaper rash can be painful for your baby, interfering with sleep and play time.

- Yeast infection may occur. Though this causes a red and well-outlined rash, it is usually easy to treat.

- Diaper rash may become severe, with very raw sores that may take a couple weeks to heal.

- Some babies have repeated problems with diaper rash. Even with treatment, the rash seems to keep coming back.

What increases your baby's risk of diaper rash?

- Going too long between diaper changes.

- Using soaps or other products that irritate the skin.

Can diaper rash be prevented?

Frequent diaper changes, careful cleaning of the area, routinely using a protective ointment (like vaseline), and avoiding soaps or other skin irritants may help prevent these rashes.

How is diaper rash treated?

- Change your baby's diaper as soon as possible every time it's wet or dirty.

- Clean the area carefully. A clean cloth or towel with fresh water is best for cleaning; avoid using diaper wipes containing perfumes or alcohol. Be sure to clean all parts of your baby's genitals. Clean inside the deep folds in the diaper area.

- Super-absorbent disposable diapers help keep urine and stool away from the skin.

- Apply a diaper rash ointment such as petroleum jelly (Vaseline) or products containing zinc oxide (for example, Desitin). These products can help keep moisture away from the skin. Put on a light layer right after cleaning and drying the diaper area.

- If the rash takes a long time to heal or is severe, it may be a good idea to visit your doctor. He or she can check to see if the rash has become infected with yeast (*Candida*) or other germs or if some other type of skin condition is present.

- If yeast infection occurs, a prescription ointment will be recommended. Apply to the rash with each diaper change (four times per day) for a week or so.

- For a more severe rash, a weak hydrocortisone cream may be recommended. Apply a few times per day for a few days.

- Even with treatment, some babies have repeated problems with diaper rash. The same is true for diaper rash with infection, especially with *Candida*. However, diaper rash rarely causes serious problems.

- If your child is having frequent and/or severe diaper rash, call our office. The doctor may want to perform tests to see if there is some other problem that is causing the skin irritation.

When should I call your office?

Call our office if diaper rash doesn't improve with treatments.

Feeding Your Newborn: Breast Feeding and Bottle Feeding

Breast milk is the natural and recommended food for your newborn. It's not only healthful for your baby—it's also safe, convenient, and free! Some simple steps can help mothers and babies establish a good breast-feeding routine. Breast-feeding babies need vitamin drops. Most problems with breast-feeding can be solved with professional help. If you choose not to breast-feed or there are medical reasons why you can't, infant formula (bottle feeding) is an acceptable alternative.

How should I feed my baby?

Finding a comfortable and satisfying feeding pattern is an essential first step for new babies and their mothers. A good feeding routine not only provides excellent nutrition for your baby but is also a source of relaxation and emotional comfort for mother and baby alike.

For most infants, breast feeding is the preferred choice. Breast milk is the most nourishing diet for your baby and helps to reduce the risk of infections and other health problems during the first few months. Breast feeding can also be very emotionally satisfying for both mothers and babies. Unless certain health problems are present, most mothers can successfully breast-feed their infants.

Bottle feeding with infant formula is an alternative to breast feeding if necessary or desired. Modern infant formulas are good substitutes for breast milk. Your doctor and other health care professionals can provide you with information and support to establish a good feeding routine.

Breast feeding: advantages and difficulties

Advantages. Breast milk is the perfect diet for your baby. Milk is always available, at the right temperature, and totally free! It also provides antibodies that help to protect your baby against infections, especially during the early weeks when your infant's immune system is still maturing. Breast-fed babies have less diarrhea, fewer ear and other infections, and possibly fewer allergies. Many new mothers feel that breast feeding helps them establish a close emotional relationship with their new baby.

Difficulties. Although most problems can be overcome, some mothers and babies find nursing difficult. Education and support often help to deal with these problems. Breast feeding is not always convenient, especially when it's time for mothers to go back to work. However, most mothers can still breast-feed when they're at home. When the mother is at work, the babysitter can feed pumped breast milk or formula.

What if I can't breast-feed? Certain medical problems can interfere with breast feeding. For example, breast feeding is not recommended if the mother is infected with human immunodeficiency virus (HIV, the virus that causes acquired immunodeficiency syndrome [AIDS]) or if she has to take certain medications that may end up in the breast milk. Be sure to discuss these problems with your doctor. Don't worry too much if you can't breast-feed. Bottle feeding can also provide excellent nutrition and create a strong bond between mother and baby.

For some mothers, bottle feeding is more convenient than breast feeding. Some mothers may just not want to breast-feed or be unable to for various reasons. Infant formulas provide all the nutrients and vitamins needed for normal growth and development.

How do I breast-feed my baby?

Mothers will receive nursing instruction after delivery.

- Find a comfortable seat where you can support your baby's head with your arm, leaving the other hand free to hold the breast. Place the nipple and areola (the pink area around the nipple) close to your baby's mouth. Make sure that the breast doesn't block the baby's nose.

- If the baby smells milk, he or she will move his or her head in an attempt to find it. If the cheek is touched by the breast, the baby will turn his or her head to that side while opening his or her mouth. This is called the "rooting reflex."

- Putting the nipple, including the areola, into your baby's mouth will cause him or her to suck ("sucking reflex"). Once milk is in the baby's mouth, he or she will swallow ("swallowing reflex").

- When your baby is nursing at one breast, it will usually stimulate milk flow in both breasts. This is called the "let-down reflex." Feed your baby from both breasts at each feeding for the first few weeks; regular stimulation is needed to keep the milk flowing. After the milk supply is well established, you can alternate breasts between feedings.

- Nursing takes about 5 to 20 minutes per breast, but the baby gets most of the milk within the first few minutes. If the baby doesn't "unlatch" or let go of the breast within a reasonable time, gently place a finger into the corner of his or her mouth to decrease suction and release the nipple. Don't pull the baby from the breast.

- Don't let the baby use the breast for a long time as a "pacifier." This can make the nipple sore or even result in tooth decay.

- During and after feedings, the baby needs to be "burped" to let swallowed air out of the stomach. Hold your baby upright, with the head on your shoulder, while gently patting or rubbing his or her back.

- In general, it's best to avoid giving breast-fed babies extra bottles, at least until breast feeding and milk production are well established.

- All breast-fed babies need extra vitamin D. This is usually included in multivitamin drops.

- After 4 to 6 months, breast-fed babies may also need an additional source of iron. This may be given in the form of multivitamins with iron or iron-fortified formula.

- *While breast-feeding:*

  - Practice good nipple care by washing with mild soap and avoiding irritation of the breasts by clothing. Keep the nipple area as dry as possible. Wear a properly fitting bra with absorbent nipple pads or clean cloth to absorb leaking milk.

  - Mothers need to make sure they're getting good nutrition while breast feeding. Don't go on a weight-loss diet while breast feeding. There's no reason to avoid specific foods, although some mothers think certain foods "disagree" with their babies.

  - While nursing, don't smoke, drink alcohol, or take other drugs without consulting your doctor.

How do I bottle-feed my baby?

Always use a clean bottle. Washing bottles with soap and water is fine. If using powdered formula, be sure to use the correct amount of water for each scoop of formula.

- Formula is most commonly given slightly warm. However, formula can be room temperature or even cold, unless you think your baby doesn't like it. Don't microwave bottles; this can result in uneven heating, with some of the liquid being too hot. A safer way of heating is to put bottles under running warm water.

- Hold your baby comfortably and securely, just as for breast feeding. Burp him or her once or twice during feeding and afterwards.

- Always hold your baby while bottle feeding. Don't prop the bottle in your baby's mouth. Babies need physical contact. In addition, propping bottles may result in choking. Don't leave bottles in your baby's mouth; this promotes tooth decay.

- Throw out any milk that's left in the bottle; germs can grow in stored formula, even in the refrigerator.

How often? How much?

- Nursing can start immediately after birth, in the delivery room if desired, and preferably within the first hour or so. Newborns are very sleepy for the first few days of life and may not show a lot of interest in breast feeding. It's normal for newborns to lose a little weight during the first few days. Most babies "wake up" and become good nursers by the fourth or fifth day.

- Most healthy infants want to eat very frequently during the first week—every 2 to 4 hours. Breast-fed infants may need to be fed more frequently than bottle-fed infants—probably 8 times within 24 hours. Your baby should be gaining weight by the end of the second week.

- If you're breast-feeding, it can be difficult to tell how much milk your baby is getting. Generally, if your baby is satisfied after nursing, sleeps between feedings, and gains weight, he or she is getting enough milk. After the first few days, diapers should be wet every 4 hours or so.

- Solid foods are generally not recommended before 4 to 6 months. Before this age, solids are not as nutritionally important as breast milk or formula and may lead to choking.

- Juice is not needed for nutrition and can promote tooth decay. If you give your child juice, it's best to wait until he or she can drink from a cup.

When is it time to stop breast or bottle feeding?

Generally, babies gradually reduce the amount of breast milk or formula they drink as they begin to eat solid foods—around 4 to 6 months. As your baby's feedings decrease, so will the amount of breast milk produced. By age 1, most babies no longer need breast or bottle feedings, but breast feeding for a longer time is not harmful.

When should I call your office?

Especially for first-time mothers, it can be difficult to establish a good breast-feeding routine. We will probably schedule an appointment a few days after your baby goes home from the hospital to help you with this and any other problems. Call our office if:

- You are having trouble establishing milk flow or have questions or concerns about breast-feeding technique.

- Your baby is not wetting diapers every 4 hours or so (after the first few days).

- Your baby doesn't seem to be feeding properly or isn't gaining weight by age 2 weeks.

Group B Streptococcal Infection

Group B "strep" (streptococcal) bacteria can cause potentially serious infections in newborns. Early infections, usually occurring within a day after birth, are often linked to complications during labor. Later infections may develop more than 7 days after birth. Babies with group B strep infection need treatment in the hospital, including antibiotics.

What is group B streptococcal infection?

Group B streptococcal infection is a major problem for newborn babies and pregnant women. It is less common than it once was because antibiotics are given right before delivery to mothers with risk factors for group B strep infection. Infants born to mothers who have not received the proper antibiotic at the appropriate time need careful observation and sometimes treatment after birth.

In newborns, group B strep can cause various types of infection, including bacteremia (bloodstream infection), pneumonia (infection of the lungs), and meningitis (infection of the membranes lining the brain and spinal cord). Group B strep can cause serious complications and is particularly dangerous in premature infants. Infants with this infection need hospital treatment, especially with antibiotics.

What does it look like?

Group B strep infections are classified according to whether they occur early (within 1 week after birth) or late (after the first week).

- *Early infections.* These occur within the first 7 days after birth, most commonly within 24 hours. Sepsis (widespread infection) and pneumonia (lung infection) are most common.
  - *Symptoms.* Your baby may already be sick at birth; usually symptoms appear within the first day. This type of infection sometimes causes the baby to die in the womb (stillbirth).
  - Fever may or may not be present.
  - Fussiness.
  - Lack of energy.
  - Breathing problems may occur, such as grunting or apnea (not breathing), even if the infection isn't in the lungs.
  - Some infants with group B strep infection go into shock, becoming seriously ill very quickly.

- *Late infections.* These occur more than 1 week after birth.
  - Bacteremia (bloodstream infection) and meningitis are most common, although other infections may occur, for example, bone infections.
  - Symptoms are similar to those of early group B strep infection but usually less severe at first. Swollen glands and/or skin infections may appear in the jaw or neck area.
  - Group B strep infections rarely occur after the first few months of life.

What causes group B streptococcal infection?

Group B strep are common bacteria. However, they usually cause serious disease only in certain types of patients, especially pregnant women and newborn infants. (Group B strep can also cause serious disease in people whose immune systems aren't functioning properly.)

What are some possible complications of group B streptococcal infection?

- Group B strep infections are a serious disease in newborns. Although treatment is usually effective, there is a risk of death, especially in premature infants and infants with early infection.
- Complications are related to where infections occur. If infection involves the brain (meningitis), then brain damage, including hearing loss, may occur.

Can group B streptococcal infection be prevented?

- Group B strep infection most often occurs after complications of labor and delivery, such as chorioamnionitis (infection of the amniotic sac), prolonged rupture of the membranes ("bag of waters"), or early labor.
- In early group B strep infection, the bacteria are passed on from mother to baby before or during delivery. Some mothers are colonized with strep bacteria in the gastrointestinal tract or vagina. ("Colonized" means that bacteria are present in the area without causing disease.) Some babies will catch group B strep infection if the mother is infected at delivery.
- Pregnant women should undergo a screening test for group B strep late in pregnancy (between 35 and 37 weeks). If the test shows that group B strep is present, antibiotics should be given to prevent passing the infec-

tion from the mother to the baby. Antibiotics should also be given if:

- A previous baby had group B strep infection.

- Group B strep is detected in the mother's urine during pregnancy.

- No screening test was done and the mother has any of the following:

  - Fever during labor and delivery.

  - Premature birth (before 37 weeks).

  - Early rupture of the membranes (amniotic sac or bag of waters) 18 hours or longer before delivery.

- Antibiotic treatment only prevents the development of early group B strep infection. It does not affect the risk of later (after 1 week) infection.

How is group B streptococcal infection treated?

- *If your infant has group B strep infection,* immediate hospital treatment is essential. In the hospital, your baby will receive intravenous (IV) doses of antibiotics.

- Antibiotic treatment will continue for a while to make sure the infection is eliminated. Treatment lasts at least 10 days for infants with bloodstream infection, 2 to 3 weeks for those with meningitis, and up to 4 weeks for others.

- Your infant may need other types of treatment as well, depending on the nature and severity of his or her illness.

When should I call your office?

Call our office any time your newborn has signs of infection:

- Fever.

- Stops drinking fluids; starts vomiting.

- Seems irritable or very sleepy; difficult to arouse.

- Just seems "sicker."

- If your child seems to be having difficulty breathing: breathing fast, chest caving in, ribs sticking out (retractions), belly going up and down, and nostrils flaring. *This is an emergency!* Take your child to the emergency room immediately.

Human Immunodeficiency Virus and Your Newborn

Human immunodeficiency virus (HIV) is the virus that causes AIDS (acquired immunodeficiency syndrome). When a woman infected with HIV becomes pregnant, there is a risk that she will pass the virus on to her baby. Treatment for both mother and baby can reduce the baby's risk of becoming infected with HIV.

I'm HIV-positive: can I have a healthy baby?

Yes, women who are infected with HIV—the virus that causes AIDS—can become pregnant and have a healthy baby. However, there is a risk that the mother will pass the virus on to her baby during pregnancy and delivery. Mothers who are infected with HIV (HIV-positive) should not breast-feed because the virus can also be spread in breast milk. If you are HIV-positive and are pregnant or thinking about becoming pregnant, it is essential to discuss this with your doctor.

What are the facts on HIV/AIDS and pregnancy?

- Infants can catch HIV from an infected mother. Almost all children with HIV/AIDS are infected in this way. In the past, children and adults sometimes were infected with HIV through blood transfusions. However, with current testing procedures, this is now rare.

- Without treatment, 15% to 25% of pregnant HIV-positive women pass the virus on to their babies. However, with modern treatments (usually including a medication called zidovudine [or AZT] for both mother and baby), this risk can be reduced to as low as 2%.

- After birth, your baby will be closely monitored for signs of HIV infection. He or she will be tested for HIV soon after birth. However, these tests aren't accurate enough to be sure that the baby isn't infected. For this reason, your baby will be treated with specific medications for a period of time, even if he or she shows no sign of HIV infection.

- For most babies born to HIV-positive mothers, we can determine whether the baby is infected by age 4 to 6 months, with a final check at 18 months. Good medical care and follow-up give your baby the best chance of avoiding HIV infection.

What treatment will I need during pregnancy?

- As soon as you find out you are pregnant, the doctor treating your HIV will make a plan for treatment. The goal is to keep the levels of HIV in your blood ("viral load") as low as possible.

- Many factors may affect your treatment during pregnancy. The decision about which drugs to take during pregnancy is generally made after counseling and discussion with a specialist in HIV care and your obstetrician.

- Treatment with AZT reduces the chances of passing HIV on to your baby. Some HIV medicines can be harmful to the baby, so they are avoided during pregnancy. You should receive close follow-up care for your HIV disease throughout pregnancy.

- Depending on your viral load and other factors, delivering your baby by cesarean section ("c-section") may be an option. In this operation, the baby is taken out through an incision in the abdomen rather than being born through the vagina. Having a c-section can reduce the risk that the baby will come into contact with HIV in the infected mother's blood.

What treatment will my baby need after delivery?

- After birth, your baby will be tested and observed for signs of HIV. Even if the first tests don't show HIV infection, your baby will receive several weeks of treatment with AZT to prevent infection. Other treatments are needed as well: for example, antibiotics are usually given to prevent infection with bacteria called *Pneumocystis*. Although they are usually harmless, these bacteria can cause serious lung infections (pneumonia) in people infected with HIV. This treatment continues until we can be sure that the baby isn't infected with HIV.

- Your baby will receive close medical follow-up, including HIV tests after birth until about age 4 to 6 months, and again at 18 months. Of course, if HIV infection does develop, treatment will be needed.

- After birth, HIV-infected mothers should not breast-feed or feed pumped breast milk because this could pass the virus on to the baby. HIV is passed on only through contact with blood or body fluids but has not been shown to be transferred by saliva. The risk of passing HIV on to your baby after birth is very low.

- During and after pregnancy, it is important for the HIV-positive mother to take care of her own health, including proper medical care and a safe, healthy lifestyle. This is essential not only to reduce your baby's risk of getting HIV infection but also to make sure you are as healthy as possible to take care of your family.

- Your baby will most likely be cared for and followed up by an HIV specialist in addition to your regular doctor.

When should I call your office?

Call our office if you have any questions about medical care for yourself or your baby before or after pregnancy.

Where can I get more information about HIV/AIDS?

The National Women's Health Information Center. On the Internet at *www.4woman.gov/HIV*, or phone (1-800) 994-9662.

Infants of Diabetic Mothers

Diabetes during pregnancy can have harmful effects on your baby. Infants of diabetic mothers may be large in size. During the first few days after birth, they are at risk of low blood sugar (hypoglycemia) and other complications. Good prenatal care and careful monitoring and treatment of the baby after birth are essential. Keeping your diabetes under control during pregnancy also is important to your baby's health.

How does diabetes affect your baby?

Diabetes is a disease in which the body does not produce or becomes resistant to the effects of the hormone insulin, which it needs in order to use glucose (sugar) for energy. Without treatment to prevent high blood glucose levels (hyperglycemia), diabetes causes serious complications.

Pregnant women with diabetes need special care to avoid harmful effects on the developing baby. This includes women with gestational diabetes, a form that occurs during pregnancy only. Babies of diabetic mothers are often large, although some are normal-sized or smaller than expected, depending on how severe the diabetes is. These infants may have low blood sugar levels (hypoglycemia), which can cause restless or jumpy behavior among other symptoms.

Infants of diabetic mothers are at risk of other complications as well, including low calcium levels, heart problems, and certain birth defects. Treatment to keep diabetes under control during pregnancy can greatly reduce the risk of harmful effects for mother and baby alike.

What kinds of problems can occur?

Appearance.

- Infants of diabetic mothers tend to be larger than normal. They may have more than the normal amount of body fat; sometimes they look "puffy-faced."

- In some situations, the baby may be of normal size or even smaller. This is more likely if the baby is born prematurely or if the mother has diabetes-related blood vessel disease.

- Your baby may seem restless or jumpy during the first few days after birth. Trembling may occur. Other infants of diabetic mothers appear limp and inactive and show poor sucking ability. All of these may be signs of hypoglycemia (low blood sugar). Later on, similar symptoms may result from low calcium levels (hypocalcemia).

Hypoglycemia.

- Many infants of diabetic mothers are born with low blood sugar, or hypoglycemia. This can cause many different symptoms, including restlessness/jumpiness, limpness/inactivity, blue color of the skin (cyanosis), convulsions (uncontrolled muscle movements), feeding problems, and others.

- Hypoglycemia can occur with no symptoms at all. Testing and treatment for hypoglycemia are important parts of your baby's initial care.

Other complications. Diabetes can cause many harmful complications for the newborn, some of which are serious. These include:

- Premature birth.

- Breathing problems.

- Heart problems, such as enlargement of the heart (cardiomegaly).

- Low calcium levels.

- Increased hematocrit level, reflecting a higher than normal amount of blood in the body (polycythemia). This may lead to blood clots and contribute to jaundice (yellow color of the skin).

- An increased risk of birth defects, including heart, spinal cord, and kidney abnormalities.

- An increased risk of miscarriage or stillbirth. Keeping diabetes under control during pregnancy will help to reduce the risk of pregnancy loss as well as of other complications.

How can I reduce the risk of complications for my infant?

If you have diabetes and become pregnant, or if you develop diabetes during pregnancy, you'll need careful medical care. Frequent tests and follow-up examinations are needed, focusing on:

- *Keeping your diabetes under control.* Treatments are needed to keep your blood glucose level as close to normal as possible. This may include insulin shots, oral medications, diet, exercise, and education, including how to monitor your blood glucose level. With "tight" control of blood glucose levels, pregnancy outcomes in diabetic mothers are similar to those in nondiabetic mothers.

- *Monitoring your baby's development in the womb.* Ultrasound and other tests are done frequently to keep track of your baby's development and maturation.

- *Preparing for birth.* Plans will be made to ensure that specialized care is available for you and your baby at the time of delivery and after birth.

How will my baby be treated?

Specific treatments depend on your baby's situation at birth. All infants of diabetic mothers receive intensive monitoring and treatment, if needed.

- Your baby's blood glucose level will be measured frequently after birth. Hypoglycemia (low blood sugar) may be present without any symptoms. If your baby's blood sugar is too low, glucose solution may be given through a vein (intravenously).

- If your baby is healthy, frequent feedings should start as soon as possible. If there are any feeding problems, including poor sucking, your baby may receive intravenous glucose solution.

- Your baby will receive continued close follow-up examinations, as there is a risk that hypoglycemia may develop later or recur.

- *It is essential to avoid long and/or severe periods of hypoglycemia!* Serious complications may result, including brain damage resulting in reduced intelligence.

What's my baby's long-term outlook?

- Your baby should have few problems, especially if you kept your diabetes under good control during pregnancy, and there are no serious medical problems at birth. Your child will receive close medical follow-up examinations to monitor his or her physical and intellectual development, especially if there were problems with low blood sugar.

- Your child may be at increased risk of developing diabetes later in life. Infants who are large at birth also may be at greater risk of obesity.

When should I call your office?

Women with diabetes during pregnancy need regular prenatal care throughout their pregnancies. Testing for possible gestational (pregnancy-related) diabetes should be part of prenatal care for every woman.

After your baby goes home, call our office if any of the following occurs:

- Jitteriness.

- Poor feeding.

- Jaundice (yellow color of the skin).

Jaundice of the Newborn

> Jaundice in newborn babies is a very common, usually harmless condition. The color is caused by a substance called *bilirubin*. However, treatment is sometimes needed, so you should notify our office if your baby develops jaundice.

What is jaundice of the newborn?

In babies with jaundice, the skin appears yellow. Jaundice occurs in about 60% of newborns. A substance called *bilirubin* causes the yellow color. Bilirubin comes from red blood cells (RBCs) when they are destroyed as part of the body's natural process or because of certain medical conditions. The liver is the organ responsible for removing bilirubin from the blood. In newborns, the liver is often not mature enough to remove the bilirubin it needs to, and so the body becomes jaundiced. When this occurs and is not caused by a disease or condition, it is called *physiologic jaundice*. When bilirubin is abnormally high, this is called *hyperbilirubinemia. In most babies, the jaundice disappears on its own.* Very high levels of bilirubin can harm the baby's brain. When this happens, the condition is called *kernicterus*. Treatment of high bilirubin is to prevent harm to the baby's brain.

What does it look like?

- Your baby's skin appears yellow or orange. The yellow color is either present at birth or develops a few days or weeks afterward.
- After starting on the face, the yellow color may spread to your baby's belly (abdomen) and feet.

What causes jaundice?

- The most common cause is physiologic jaundice, which is a normal condition as described previously. It usually appears after the first day or so.
- Jaundice related to breast feeding occurs either because the baby is not getting enough fluid (breast milk) or because there are substances in some mothers' breast milk that increase the amount of bilirubin in the baby. The bilirubin does not usually get high enough to cause problems.
- Another common cause is blood type incompatibility. This can occur when the mother's and baby's blood types are different and can sometimes increase the baby's bilirubin.
- Less common causes include liver diseases, genetic diseases (such as deficiency of the enzyme G6PD [glucose-6-phosphate dehydrogenase]), or infections.

What puts your child at risk for jaundice?

- Your baby may be at greater risk of jaundice if he or she was born prematurely (before 8 and a half months) or if he or she feeds poorly in the first few days after birth.
- Jaundice is more likely if your baby has a brother or sister who had jaundice as a newborn.
- Newborns whose mothers have diabetes are at greater risk of jaundice.
- Jaundice is more likely to occur in babies of certain ethnic groups, including East Asian, Mediterranean, and Native American.
- Jaundice is more likely to become severe if your baby has jaundice at the time of birth or on the day afterward.

What are some possible complications of jaundice?

If your baby's bilirubin levels become very high, he or she may develop a rare but serious complication called kernicterus (bilirubin encephalopathy). Treatment to prevent bilirubin from getting too high prevents this.

How is jaundice treated?

- Most cases of jaundice are physiologic (normal). The yellow color of the skin usually goes away without treatment.
- A test may be performed to measure the amount of bilirubin in your baby's blood. The result will help to decide whether or not your baby needs treatment.
- If your baby's jaundice is too high, we may recommend treatment with phototherapy. Your baby will be placed under special lights—usually blue-colored—that help to get rid of the bilirubin in the body.
- If your baby has severe jaundice that does not improve with phototherapy, other treatments such as blood transfusions may be needed.
- If your baby's jaundice is caused by not getting enough breast milk, advice on how to improve feeding will be given. If it is caused by high levels of bilirubin in the mother's breast milk, stopping breast feeding for a day or two may eliminate the jaundice. However, because breast feeding is so beneficial for your baby, this is avoided if possible.

When should I call your office?

Call our office if:

- Your newborn develops a yellow or orange skin color after discharge from the hospital.
- Jaundice is still present 2 weeks after birth.

Meconium-Stained Amniotic Fluid

Meconium is your baby's first stool. If the baby passes this meconium stool before birth, it may lead to complications, especially breathing problems. If meconium is found in the amniotic fluid that surrounds your baby in the womb, a careful examination for possible respiratory distress (breathing difficulties) will be done, and treatment will be started if needed.

What is meconium-stained amniotic fluid?

The amniotic fluid is the liquid that supported and cushioned your baby in the womb during pregnancy. Meconium is the first stool (bowel movement), which is normally passed soon after birth.

If your baby passes the meconium before birth (while still in the womb), it stains the amniotic fluid a brownish color. This is most common in babies who suffer "stress" in the womb, often related to not getting enough oxygen or to infection.

If the baby inhales any of the meconium, it can lead to a potentially serious complication called *meconium aspiration syndrome*. This refers to the meconium getting into the lungs and causing breathing (respiratory) problems. It occurs in only about 5% of babies with meconium-stained amniotic fluid. Meconium aspiration may lead to serious complications, depending on how much meconium was in the fluid and how much of it your baby inhaled. With appropriate treatment, sometimes including mechanical ventilation to aid in breathing, most babies recover from this syndrome completely.

What does it look like?

Meconium may be seen staining the amniotic fluid at birth. Meconium stains may also be on your baby's skin. Meconium is a thick, dark green, sticky material. The amount and color of staining depend on how much meconium got into the amniotic fluid and when it occurred.

- If your baby inhaled any of the meconium, he or she may have symptoms of meconium aspiration syndrome, which include difficulty breathing:

  - Breathing very fast.
  - Working very hard to breathe. You may see your baby's chest moving up and down with each breath ("retractions") or hear grunting noises (more severe cases).

- Blue color of the skin (cyanosis—a sign of severe breathing problems).
- Severely affected babies or those who were "stressed" in the womb may be less active or limp.
- Chest x-rays often show inflammation of the lungs (pneumonia).
- Over the first few days, your infant may develop respiratory distress. If symptoms are severe, he or she may need mechanical ventilation to assist in breathing.
- Some babies develop a *pneumothorax*. This is an air leak from the lungs into the chest. It can put pressure on the lungs and can cause part of the lung to collapse, leading to more difficulty breathing.
- *Not all infants with meconium-stained amniotic fluid inhale meconium or develop breathing difficulties.* Your baby will receive close examination and follow-up to detect or prevent any problems.

What puts your child at risk of meconium-stained amniotic fluid?

- Meconium-stained amniotic fluid is fairly common; it occurs in 10% to 15% of births. Only a small percentage of these babies develop meconium aspiration syndrome or breathing problems.
- Meconium staining is most common in infants who are delivered late (past their "due date") or after a difficult labor.

Can meconium-stained amniotic fluid be prevented?

Careful monitoring during labor and delivery may help to reduce the risk of meconium aspiration. If meconium staining is present, prompt treatment may help to prevent more serious breathing problems.

How is meconium-stained amniotic fluid treated?

If your baby has meconium staining of the amniotic fluid, immediate evaluation is needed to detect and treat any complications.

- Infants who have thick meconium staining and/or difficulty breathing are checked for meconium in the throat and airway. If present, the material is suctioned (removed) using a device called a laryngoscope.

- Suctioning of the throat is done *only* if the baby is having difficulty breathing or is not as active as he or she should be. If the baby seems to be breathing normally and is normally active, trying to remove meconium by suctioning may actually increase the risk of complications.

- The doctor will carefully assess your baby's breathing. Your baby may need additional oxygen, often given through small tubes placed a short distance into the nose (nasal prongs).

- Some babies with meconium aspiration need *mechanical ventilation*. A tube is placed in the airway (trachea) and connected to a machine, which pumps oxygen into the lungs to help your baby breathe. When needed, mechanical ventilation may reduce the severity of respiratory distress. Your baby will be moved to a special newborn intensive care unit (NICU) for constant care and attention.

- Other treatments are sometimes needed:

  - Some babies with severe breathing problems receive surfactant, a substance that helps the lungs inflate more easily.

  - In very severe cases, specialized treatments may be needed to ensure your baby is getting as much oxygen as possible. *Extracoroporeal membrane oxygenation* (ECMO) is a treatment that supplies oxygen directly to your baby's blood instead of to the lungs.

- In babies with meconium aspiration syndrome, it can be difficult to tell if infection is present. Most babies are started on antibiotics until the doctor is sure there are no problems with infection (such as pneumonia).

- Your baby is monitored closely, especially to be sure he or she is getting enough oxygen. Changes in treatment may be needed over the first few days, for example, if respiratory distress or pneumonia develops.

Although meconium aspiration can be a serious problem, most babies recover completely. Breathing should begin to get better within a few days. Some babies with severe disease that resulted in not receiving enough oxygen may have some brain injury.

When should I call your office?

Call our office if you have any questions about this condition or about your infant's treatment.

Myelomeningocele

Myelomeningocele occurs when part of the spinal cord sticks out (protrudes) through your child's back. This is a serious birth defect that causes permanent neurologic abnormalities. The type and severity of your child's handicaps depend on where the myelomeningocele is located. Children with myelomeningocele need lifelong follow-up care from a team of health care specialists.

What is myelomeningocele?

Myelomeningocele is one of a group of birth defects called "neural tube defects," in which the spinal cord doesn't close normally as the fetus is developing. In babies with myelomeningocele, part of the spinal cord sticks out through the back. Most myelomeningoceles are located in the lower back, but they can occur anywhere along the spine.

Myelomeningocele usually causes some permanent damage to the spinal cord and may result in many different medical problems. Problems with bowel and bladder control are common. Surgery is done to close the spinal cord within a few days after birth; additional evaluation and treatment are provided by a team of health care professionals. Although this is a serious birth defect, most children with myelomeningocele have normal intelligence and at least some walking ability.

A "meningocele" is different from a myelomenigocele. It is an outpouching or pocket of just the membranes covering the spinal column, not the spinal cord itself. This is a much less serious condition.

What does it look like?

- Myelomeningocele is obvious at birth. Part of the spinal cord is seen sticking out of your child's spine, often covered by a thin layer of skin.

- Three fourths of myelomeningoceles are located in the lower back. However, they may be located anywhere along the spine, from the tailbone to the neck.

- Many different medical problems may be present. All children with myelomeningocele have some nervous system abnormalities caused by damage to the spinal cord. Myelomeningoceles located higher on the spinal cord (except in the neck or high upper back) cause more severe and widespread abnormalities. However, even low defects cause significant handicaps.

- Many children with myelomeningocele have some weakness and difficulties controlling the muscles in the lower body. This usually means lifelong problems related to bowel and bladder control and walking ability, depending on where the defect is and how much spinal damage is present.

- Children often may not be able to feel pain or feel being touched in the parts of the body affected.

- Many children with myelomeningocele have a problem called *hydrocephalus*, in which fluid builds up in the skull, placing abnormally high pressure on the brain. *Treatment is needed to prevent brain damage or death.*

- Other birth defects related to spinal cord damage may be present, such as clubfoot or dislocated hip.

- Most children have normal intelligence, but the risk of learning disabilities and seizure disorders (epilepsy) is increased.

- *Every child with myelomeningocele is different.* Several different factors affect the severity of your child's handicaps and medical problems. Your medical team can give you detailed information about your child's condition after a thorough medical evaluation.

What causes myelomeningocele?

The exact cause is unknown. However, many different factors probably play a role in causing myelomeningocele, including genetics. (See below.)

What puts your child at risk of myelomeningocele?

If you've had a child with myelomeningocele, future children are at increased risk of the same birth defect. Other risk factors include:

- Low levels of folic acid in the mother during pregnancy.

- Taking certain medications during pregnancy, including some drugs for epilepsy.

Can myelomeningocele be prevented?

For mothers, getting enough folic acid (vitamin B_6) during pregnancy reduces the risk of myelomeningocele and other neural tube defects. The recommended dose is at least 400 micrograms (mcg) per day. This is especially important for women who have had a child with one of these birth defects or for women taking drugs to treat epilepsy. In these cases, the recommended dose is higher.

How is myelomeningocele treated?

Myelomeningocele is a serious condition requiring a team approach to treatment. Several different doctors and other health professionals play a role in planning and carrying out your infant's treatment. Our office will continue to coordinate your baby's care.

- *Surgery* is needed to cover the exposed portion of your baby's spinal column. This operation may be performed a few days after birth if your infant's medical condition is stable.

- If *hydrocephalus* is present, surgery is usually needed to remove fluid buildup that is placing excessive pressure on the brain. A device called a shunt may be placed to drain fluid away from the skull. Excess fluid drains through a thin tube, usually emptying into the abdomen, where it is absorbed. Shunts can sometimes have problems, such as infection or malfunction.

- *Additional operations* or other treatments may be needed for other deformities that may accompany myelomeningocele, such as clubfoot or dislocated hip.

What are the long-term issues in care for myelomeningocele?

Because of spinal cord damage, children with myelomeningocele don't have normal control over the muscles of the lower body. This leads to problems with controlling bladder and bowel function and with walking ability. The severity of these problems depends on the location and severity of the spinal cord damage.

- *Bladder control.* Children with myelomeningocele may have bladder problems (neurogenic bladder). Most are unable to contain their urine (incontinence); for others, the bladder does not empty completely. Parents may have to learn to perform regular tube drainage (catheterization) of the bladder. As children get older, they can learn to do this on their own. Certain medications may also help with bladder control.

  - Surgery is usually needed only if catheterization and medications are not enough to achieve bladder control. All children need long-term medical follow-up to prevent kidney damage.

- *Bowel control.* Lack of bowel control becomes a problem after your child reaches the normal age for toilet training. When the time is right, many children can undergo bowel training, using enemas or suppositories at certain times of day.

- *Walking ability.* Assessment and treatment focus on maximizing the function of your child's legs. Nearly all children whose myelomeningocele is located in the lower spine can get around independently. Even for many of these with damage higher in the spine, walking is possible with aids such as braces or canes.

- *School and long-term function.* Most children with myelomeningocele have normal intelligence. Some have different degrees of developmental problems, such as learning disabilities. Special education services are available in every state. You are entitled to evaluation and educational services for your child. Based on the results, an Individualized Education Program (IEP) can be developed to meet your child's educational needs.

- *Long-term medical care.* Myelomeningocele is often a chronic, handicapping condition. Your child will need lifelong medical care. With good health care and support, many people born with myelomeningocele lead productive, relatively normal lives.

- *Taking care of your family.* Having a child with a serious birth defect is a traumatic event that affects your family in many ways. Doctors and other health care professionals can provide you with the information you need to understand your child's specific situation and the necessary treatments. Counseling may be helpful in helping your child and family deal with the stresses of living with a child with a chronic disease.

When should I call your office?

Call our office if you need additional information on myelomeningocele and your child's medical care.

Natal and Neonatal Teeth

Parents are sometimes surprised to find that their newborn already has teeth! In other cases, teeth appear during the first month of life. Most of the time, these natal and neonatal teeth are the only abnormality. Much less often, they occur in infants with cleft palate or other uncommon congenital syndromes. The premature teeth can be removed if they are causing pain or any other problems.

What are natal and neonatal teeth?

Natal teeth are teeth that are already present at birth. Teeth developing within the first month after birth are called neonatal teeth. Most of the time, the two lower front teeth are the only ones present. They are usually "wobbly," not firmly attached like normal "baby teeth." Sometimes they are normal teeth that have erupted (come up) early; at other times they are extra (supernumerary) teeth.

Natal and neonatal teeth are more common in babies with cleft palate and may occur in infants with certain congenital (present at birth) syndromes. The rest of the time, they are nothing to worry about. The teeth can be extracted (taken out) if needed, especially if they are causing any injury to the baby's tongue or problems with breast feeding.

What are some possible complications of natal and neonatal teeth?

- There are few or no serious complications of natal or prenatal teeth.

- The most frequent complication is injury or irritation, either of the baby's tongue or of the mother's nipple during breast feeding.

- There is some fear that a natal tooth could come loose, and the baby could aspirate (inhale) it. However, this appears to be rare.

What increases your baby's risk of natal and neonatal teeth?

- If you or any other member of your family had natal or prenatal teeth at birth, your children may be at higher risk.

- Cleft palate or any of the rare congenital syndromes linked to natal and prenatal teeth.

How are natal teeth treated?

- Your child is examined to make sure no other congenital abnormalities (birth defects) are present (for example, cleft palate or other syndromes involving abnormal development of the jaw).

- X-rays may be performed.

- Usually, no treatment is necessary. As long as no other abnormalities are present, natal and neonatal teeth are harmless and cause no serious problems.

- If necessary, the natal or prenatal teeth can simply be extracted (pulled out). This may be easily done because these teeth often aren't fixed in the jaw as firmly as normal teeth. Extraction is more likely to be recommended if the teeth are causing any injury to the baby's tongue or problems with breast-feeding or if they are very loose.

- If the teeth are left in, keep an eye on them at home. No special care is required; just wipe them with a clean cloth (the same as for regular baby teeth when they appear).

When should I call your office?

Call our office if:

- Natal or prenatal teeth seem to be causing your baby any discomfort or pain, especially if you notice a cut or other injury on the tongue.

- Natal or prenatal teeth are causing problems with breast feeding.

- The teeth become loose.

Newborn Screening

All states in the U.S. have some type of newborn screening program. Tests are done to detect certain serious diseases as soon as possible after the baby is born. For many of these diseases, early treatment can avoid serious health consequences for your baby. Screening requires only a simple blood test. In most states, screening is required by law. Call our office if you have questions about these important screening tests.

What is newborn screening?

There are many types of congenital diseases (present from birth), a large number of which are genetic (inherited). Genes contain information that determines our physical and mental characteristics. Genetic diseases may result when a baby inherits abnormal genes from one or both parents. Many families don't know about the abnormal genes until they have an infant diagnosed with a genetic disease. Many congenital and genetic diseases have serious complications (such as mental retardation) that can only be prevented if they are recognized and treated as soon as possible after birth.

For this reason, all states recommend certain screening tests for all newborn infants. The list of diseases tested for varies among states. All states test for phenylketonuria (PKU, a type of metabolic disease), and congenital hypothyroidism (a disease leading to low thyroid hormone levels). Both of these diseases can cause mental retardation, which can be prevented through proper treatment.

Most states screen for other diseases as well. The tests are done using a single blood sample obtained from a small puncture in the baby's heel. In most states, newborn screening is required by law.

What diseases will my baby be screened for?

The exact list of diseases varies by state. In addition to the required tests, your doctor may recommend other tests, depending on your family history, the baby's condition at birth, and other factors.

The number of screening tests varies widely. Some states screen for only a few diseases, whereas others screen for dozens. New automated tests have been developed in recent years, making it possible to screen for many diseases at the same time.

All states screen for:

- *Phenylketonuria* (PKU). Babies with PKU don't have a certain enzyme needed to metabolize (use) an amino acid called phenylalanine. They need a special diet to prevent mental retardation.

- *Congenital hypothyroidism*. In babies with this disease, the thyroid gland doesn't produce normal levels of thyroid hormones. These infants need treatment with thyroid hormones to prevent problems with growth, development, and mental ability.

Most states screen for:

- *Galactosemia*. Babies with galactosemia don't have a certain enzyme needed to metabolize a sugar called galactose, which is found in milk or regular infant formula. Treatment may be needed to prevent mental retardation and other complications. (Some forms of galactosemia don't cause these complications.)

- *Sickle cell disease*. An inherited blood disease that causes anemia (low levels of hemoglobin, which carries oxygen in the blood) and other medical problems. It is most common in African Americans but can occur in other racial/ethnic groups as well. Your baby may also be screened for sickle cell trait, a gene abnormality that is very common in African Americans. Although it's important to know whether or not your family has sickle cell trait, it is *not* a disease and causes no medical problems. If a child inherits this trait from both parents, he or she will have *sickle cell anemia*.

- *Hearing loss*. Most states require a hearing test for all infants. Regardless of the cause, children with hearing loss need early intervention to promote normal development.

Some states screen for other genetic and congenital diseases, such as adrenal hyperplasia, biotidinase deficiency, and cystic fibrosis.

How common are these diseases?

Fortunately, many of these diseases are rare. Of the 4 million infants who are screened each year in the United States, only about 3000 are found to have a congenital disease, excluding hearing loss. That means that only about 1 in 1300 newborns screened has any abnormal results. If your baby does have a congenital disease, then early detection and treatment provide the best chance to avoid future problems with health and development.

Does my baby have to have these tests?

In most states, newborn screening is required by law. In some states, parents can choose not to have their baby tested if it goes against their religious beliefs.

Some parents have other reasons for not wanting their baby to be tested. However, even if screening is not required by law, most pediatricians would recommend having the tests done. The screening tests are simple, are very unlikely to do any harm to the baby, and have a low but real chance of detecting a serious disease that needs immediate treatment.

Many families have concerns about privacy related to congenital and genetic diseases. Most states have laws protecting the parents' and children's confidentiality.

Are there any risks of testing?

Routine newborn screening has little or no risk for your infant. Most of the time, all tests can be performed using a single blood sample; your baby will feel a little pain from a pinprick on the heel. A simple hearing test may be performed as well.

The biggest risk is not testing! Without newborn screening, there is a small but real chance of complications occurring from unrecognized diseases.

What if there is an abnormal result?

- Every state has a system for informing the hospital, doctor, or parent about any abnormal newborn screening results. If any of the results are abnormal, further tests are performed to make sure the original result was correct.

- Depending on the disease identified, we will probably recommend a visit to a specialist (for example, a medical geneticist) for full diagnostic testing. If any genetic (inherited) diseases are suspected, the parents and possibly other family members may be tested as well.

- If a genetic disease is detected, genetic counseling will be arranged for your family. This involves education about your family's gene abnormality and the resulting disease, including the risk of disease for other children or family members. Genetic testing may be recommended for parents and other family members.

- Treatment depends on the specific disease. For example:

  - Children with PKU need a special type of formula immediately and need to follow a special diet for the rest of their lives.

  - Children with congenital hypothyroidism or congenital adrenal hyperplasia need treatment to replace the hormones that their bodies are missing.

  - Children with sickle cell disease need lifelong medical follow-up examinations. Sickle cell trait does not cause any illness, but it does mean there is a genetic abnormality that could be passed on to future children. Genetic counseling is generally recommended.

- The one thing that all of these diseases have in common is that early recognition and treatment are needed to prevent complications.

When should I call your office?

Call our office if:

- You have any questions or concerns about newborn screening.

- You have any questions about the findings of your child's screening tests, especially if there are any abnormal results.

Prematurity and Low Birth Weight

Babies born before 37 weeks of pregnancy are considered premature. Babies who weigh less than 5½ pounds are considered low birth weight. Premature infants are at increased risk of a number of problems affecting newborns: the earlier your baby is born, the higher the risk of problems. With modern medical care, even very premature infants have an excellent chance of survival.

What are prematurity and low birth weight?

- Babies born before the 37th week of pregnancy are considered premature.

- Babies who weigh less than 2500 grams (about 5½ pounds) are considered low birth weight (LBW). About 8% of babies born in the United States are LBW. Most of these babies are premature. However, other conditions can cause LBW in a baby born after a full-term pregnancy, such as smoking during pregnancy.

- Some babies with LBW are full term but underweight. Others are premature but also weight less than they should. These infants are called intrauterine growth restriction (IUGR) or small for gestational age (SGA).

- Babies who weigh less than 1500 grams (about 3⅓ pounds) are considered very low birth weight (VLBW). Nearly all of these babies are premature.

Prematurity can cause many types of health problems. The problems are related to the fact that many of your baby's organs and basic body systems aren't yet fully mature. The earlier your baby was born, the higher the risk of problems. Some problems that may occur related to prematurity, particularly in more premature infants, include breathing problems, damage to the brain and nervous system, and feeding problems. Mildly premature infants usually have few or no problems.

Treatment of premature infants has improved steadily over the years. Today, with advanced neonatal (newborn) intensive care unit (NICU) care, specialized equipment, and expert care from nurses and neonatologists (doctors specializing in the care of sick newborns), most premature infants have an excellent chance of survival. The earlier your baby was born, the higher the risk of serious medical complications.

What do they look like?

Every premature infant is different; the most important factor is how early he or she is born. Some of the things you may notice—depending on how premature your baby is—include:

- Very small size.

- Fragile skin, with veins visible underneath.

- Limp, little activity; weak cry.

- Breathing problems: baby seems unable to get enough air.

- Feeding problems; baby can't suck or swallow normally.

What causes prematurity and low birth weight?

- Several factors may lead to premature birth, including:

  - Premature rupture of the membranes (bag of water) that hold the baby and amniotic fluid in the uterus (womb).

  - Pre-eclampsia: problems with blood pressure, kidneys, and usually occurring after 20 weeks of pregnancy.

  - Chronic illnesses in the mother—for example, heart disease or sickle cell anemia.

  - Infections, such as infection of the placenta.

  - Drug abuse.

  - Problems with the placenta or uterus (womb).

  - Multiple births (twins or more).

- Reasons for intrauterine growth restriction include:

  - Infections of the fetus before delivery.

  - Chromosome or gene abnormalities (inherited diseases).

  - Problems with the placenta, not allowing enough nutrition for the fetus.

  - Poor nutrition in the mother; other problems such as chronic diseases or smoking.

What are some possible and complications of prematurity and low birth weight?

Some possible problems, particularly for the premature infant, include:

- *Respiratory problems* (related to the lungs and breathing):

  - Immaturity of the lungs can lead to newborn *respiratory distress syndrome* (sometimes called hyaline membrane disease). These babies need additional oxygen. In severe cases, they need to be connected to a machine called a ventilator to help them breathe. Some babies receive surfactant, a substance that helps the lungs to inflate and breathe.

- *Apnea*—prolonged episodes of not breathing, which result in the baby's not getting enough oxygen.

- *Nervous system problems:*

  - Bleeding into the brain ("intraventricular hemorrhage") can be a serious complication. It is more common in very premature babies.

  - Harm to various parts of the brain, causing developmental (learning) problems or problems with muscle tone or strength.

- *Infections.* Premature infants are at higher risk of infection with bacteria. The intravenous (IV) lines needed for monitoring and treatment can also increase the risk of infections.

- *Jaundice* (increased bilirubin) causes a yellow color of the skin. This problem can usually be controlled by phototherapy (special lights that lower the bilirubin level).

- *Anemia* (low blood count): often made worse because all of the blood tests needed.

- *Low blood sugar* (hypoglycemia) or low calcium level (hypocalcemia).

- *Heart problems.* A common condition is patent ductus arteriosus. This is a connection that allows blood to flow from the main artery of the right side of the heart (pulmonary artery) to the main artery of the left side of the heart (aorta) while the baby is developing in the womb. In some premature infants, this blood connection remains and can cause problems. It usually can be fixed with medications; surgery is occasionally needed.

- *Eye problems* ("retinopathy of prematurity") can occur, mainly in very premature infants.

Can prematurity and low birth weight be prevented?

- Good prenatal care is the best way to reduce your baby's risk of premature birth.

- Not smoking during pregnancy can reduce the risk of having a LBW baby.

How are premature infants treated?

Immediately after birth, your baby will have a complete examination. The focus will be on determining how premature he or she is and on looking for any related medical problems. In general, the more premature your baby is, the greater the risk of serious medical problems.

Your baby may be transferred to the neonatal intensive care unit (NICU) for special care and monitoring. This is where he or she will be treated for any of the problems or complications discussed earlier. Some general issues in NICU care include:

- *Temperature control.* Premature babies can have difficulty regulating their body temperature. Your baby will be cared for in an incubator (Isolette) or other special equipment to maintain an ideal temperature.

- *Feeding.* Feeding is one of the most important aspects of care. Less premature infants may be able to be fed by bottle or breast.

  - *Total parenteral nutrition,* or intravenous (IV) feeding, is needed for some very small or sick infants who can't be fed any other way. This is advanced care that requires very careful monitoring. There is a risk of infection and other complications.

  - *Gavage feeding.* Many babies born before the 34th week of pregnancy need to be fed through a small tube placed through the nose into the stomach (nasogastric tube) or intestine (nasojejunal tube).

  - Breast feeding often has to be delayed. However, the breast milk can usually be pumped and given to your baby in a bottle.

  - Decisions about feeding depend on your infant's particular circumstances. The goal is to provide your baby with the nutrition he or she needs to grow while limiting the risk of feeding-related complications.

- *Prevention of infection.* Premature infants are at high risk of infection. Careful attention to hand washing and other preventive measures is essential. You'll be allowed to participate in your baby's care as early and as frequently as possible.

- *Other treatments* depend on your baby's individual situation, especially on the presence of serious medical problems.

When can I take my premature or low birth weight baby home?

This decision depends on many factors, especially whether your baby has experienced any complications. As a rule, premature infants can go home when:

- They are feeding regularly from breast or bottle. Occasionally, babies are sent home while still gavage (tube) feeding, after training for the parents.

- They are gaining weight steadily.

- Their body temperature is stable.

- All medical problems are under control, and all medications are being taken orally. Babies recovering from lung disease may be sent home with oxygen.

When should I call your office?

Your premature or LBW baby will be seen regularly for follow-up visits. Between visits, call our office if you have any problems or concerns.

Respiratory Distress Syndrome in Newborns (Hyaline Membrane Disease)

Premature infants can have breathing problems because of immaturity of the lungs. The earlier your baby is born, the higher the risk of such problems. The main cause is lack of a normally produced substance called surfactant in the lungs. Depending on the severity of respiratory distress, treatment may include oxygen, surfactant, and mechanical ventilation to help your baby breathe. Most premature infants with respiratory distress syndrome do fine, but serious complications are possible.

What is newborn respiratory distress syndrome?

Respiratory distress syndrome is a disease caused by incomplete development of the lungs in premature babies. It is sometimes called "hyaline membrane disease." Other causes of respiratory distress in newborns are possible as well.

Your premature baby's lungs don't contain enough of a substance called surfactant, which helps the lungs expand with each breath. Especially if your baby is born very prematurely (before 28 to 32 weeks), breathing problems are usually apparent immediately at birth.

How is it treated?

Very small, very premature infants are at risk of various medical problems in addition to respiratory distress syndrome. These infants need a lot of special care in managing their body chemistry, temperature, blood pressure, and so forth. Careful attention to such "supportive" care may help to make respiratory distress syndrome less severe. If your baby has any other health problems related to prematurity, these need to be treated as well.

- Babies with respiratory distress syndrome often need treatment soon after birth. Your baby will be treated in the neonatal intensive care unit (NICU), where he or she can receive 24-hour care.

- If the lung problem is not too severe, additional *oxygen*, can be given through a mask that fits over the face and nose or through nasal prongs that fit in the nostrils.

- If respiratory distress syndrome is more severe, your baby may need *mechanical ventilation*. He or she will be connected to a machine to help with breathing. The type of mechanical ventilation will be selected carefully to maximize your baby's oxygen supply while minimizing the chances of damaging the lungs.

- When necessary, treatment with artificial *surfactant* can help to improve lung function. Surfactant treatment may be started at the same time as mechanical ventilation. In some babies, surfactant treatment is started immediately at birth.

- Making sure your baby has enough oxygen in the lungs is a very important part of treatment. Oxygen levels are checked frequently, especially in very premature babies.

- Most babies have an umbilical artery catheter placed to obtain blood and to check oxygen levels or to give fluids. A small catheter (thin tube) is placed in the umbilical artery; this is one of the blood vessels that connected the baby's blood supply to the placenta in the womb. A catheter may also be placed in another vessel, the umbilical vein.

- Other treatments may be needed as well. The doctors, nurses, and other specialists in the NICU have the training and expertise needed to monitor your baby's care. This team approach allows survival and full recovery of most premature infants. You will be allowed to visit and help with your baby's care as much as possible.

- Mechanical ventilation and other treatments continue until your baby's lungs have matured enough so that he or she can breathe independently. It is difficult to predict how long this will take, especially in very small premature infants.

What are some possible complications?

Respiratory distress syndrome is a serious disease, especially in very premature newborns. Treatment is needed to support your baby until his or her lungs mature enough for independent breathing. Serious complications are possible. Some are caused by the disease itself, while others are related to necessary treatments, especially mechanical ventilation.

- *Bronchopulmonary dysplasia* is injury to the lungs caused by mechanical ventilation. To help prevent or minimize this type of damage, your baby will receive only the mechanical ventilation needed to provide enough oxygen. Babies with bronchopulmonary dysplasia have more lasting breathing problems. This is a more likely complication in very premature babies who must stay on mechanical ventilation for a long time after birth.

- *Narrowing of the trachea (windpipe).* Damage may be caused by the breathing tube placed for mechanical ventilation.

- *Developmental problems.* This refers to lower intelligence and learning problems, and occurs mostly in very premature infants.

- *Blood clots.* Blood clots are related to the use of umbilical artery or vein catheters for monitoring.

Many other complications are possible in these seriously ill infants.

Can respiratory distress syndrome be prevented?

- Avoiding early labor and delivery is the best way to prevent premature birth and respiratory distress syndrome. In many cases, this is beyond the control of the mother or doctor.

- In some cases, if early delivery seems unavoidable, treating the mother with a steroid drug called betamethasone may reduce the risk and severity of respiratory distress in the infant.

When should I call your office?

Call our office if you have any questions about this condition or about your infant's treatment.

Sacral Dimple (Pilonidal Dimple)

A sacral dimple is a small indentation at the base of your child's spine (the sacrum). Sacral dimples are relatively common in newborn babies and are usually not of major concern. Less often, they are a sign of a birth defect involving the spinal cord; in most cases, the defect is a minor one. Some sacral dimples have appearances that may raise concern about a possible birth defect.

What is a sacral dimple?

A sacral dimple is a small dimple or cleft in the skin at the base of your baby's spinal cord (the small of the back, also called the "sacrum"). Especially if it is small or shallow, the dimple is harmless.

The doctor will pay attention to sacral dimples because they are sometimes a sign of birth defects involving the spinal cord or spinal bones (vertebrae). The most common of these is called "spina bifida occulta." This is a small defect of one of the vertebrae, and usually causes no problems. More serious birth defects are possible but rare.

What does it look like?

- A small dimple or pit in your child's lower back. Usually the dimple is very shallow; you can see to the bottom with no problem.
- Usually located in the crease between the buttocks.
- Certain appearances may trigger concern about accompanying birth defects, including:
  - Swelling in the area.
  - Skin tags (little pieces of "extra" skin).
  - A birthmark (nevus) in the area.
  - Sometimes a patch of hair may be present. This is often normal, especially in babies of certain racial/ethnic groups.

What causes sacral dimples?

- Most sacral dimples are minor abnormalities that occur while your baby is growing in the womb.
- Rarely, they are a sign of a deeper spinal abnormality.

What are some possible complications of sacral dimples?

- Minor, shallow sacral dimples have no complications. They are a normal variation.
- Deeper pits or sinuses can become infected, usually when the child is much older. If this happens, an abscess (infection underneath the skin) or cyst (sac of tissue under the skin) may develop. These infections may not occur until the teen years.

What increases your child's risk of sacral dimples?

- There are no known risk factors for minor sacral dimples. Some type of abnormality in the sacral region is found in about 3% of normal babies.
- Certain factors increase the risk of spinal abnormalities (for example, not enough folic acid during pregnancy or diabetes in the mother).

What tests or treatments are needed for sacral dimples?

Testing. Further testing is needed only when sacral dimples have certain characteristics previously mentioned (large, deep, unusual appearance or location).

- Shallow sacral dimples with no related abnormalities usually don't require any testing.
- When needed, ultrasound is usually the first test performed. This is a simple, painless test that can help determine if your child has any deeper abnormality associated with the spinal dimple.
- Ultrasound is usually done in the first 3 or 4 months after birth.
- If testing shows any birth defect related to sacral dimple, your child will undergo further evaluation for diagnosis and treatment.

When should I call your office?

Call our office if there is any change in the appearance of the sacral dimple, such as:

- Signs of infection (redness or tenderness).
- Fluid draining from the dimple.

Spitting Up (Gastroesophageal Reflux)

> "Spitting up" is a very common issue in infants. It involves food and acid from the stomach flowing backwards into the swallowing tube (esophagus). In most babies, spitting up is normal—it usually stops around 12 months of age. When spitting up results in harm to the baby, such as pain or not gaining weight, it is called gastroesophageal reflux disease (GERD).

What is spitting up?

Babies normally spit up breast milk or formula. Milk, along with acid made by the stomach, comes up from the stomach and out through the baby's mouth. Spitting up can happen often and the amount can be large. It's a messy problem, but it's usually normal. Nearly all babies outgrow spitting up by age 1, certainly by age 2.

Uncommonly, babies can develop a problem called gastroesophageal reflux disease (GERD), in which milk and stomach acid regularly move up from the stomach and into the esophagus, causing harm to the baby. When stomach acid is in contact with the esophagus for a long time, it can cause irritation, pain, and tissue damage.

Babies who have symptoms when spitting up, such as arching the back or refusing feedings, are more likely to have GERD. If there's a lot of reflux, it can result in your baby's not gaining enough weight or in coughing and choking. If these symptoms are present, the doctor may recommend testing for GERD.

What does it look like?

Every experienced parent knows what normal spitting up looks like.

- Milk comes out of the baby's mouth, often with burping.

- The effect is usually not too forceful; milk runs down the baby's chin.

- Spitting up is most common in the first 4 months of life. Babies usually outgrow it after age 1, almost always by age 2.

- Spitting up can be frequent and messy.

- In normal spitting up, no other symptoms are present: no pain, fussiness, choking, or coughing.

If your baby has other symptoms when spitting up, these may be an indication of problems:

- Frequent, forceful vomiting; milk goes a good distance away (projectile vomiting).

- Spitting up seems uncomfortable or painful for your baby. He or she may be fussy or cry or struggle during feeding or after spitting up.

- Hoarseness, coughing, wheezing (noisy breathing), choking, apnea (not breathing for a period of time).

What causes spitting up?

- Spitting up is related to a structure called the lower esophageal sphincter (LES), which acts like a valve separating the stomach and esophagus. Usually, the LES lets food flow from the esophagus into the stomach but not "backwards" from the stomach into the esophagus.

- Normal spitting up in babies happens because the LES hasn't started functioning normally yet. This occurs as your baby continues to grow and mature.

- In babies with GERD (as well as in older children and adults), many factors may contribute to reflux. Once the pattern of reflux has started, it can cause damage that tends to make the reflux worse.

What are some possible complications of spitting up?

- Normal spitting up has no complications, besides the mess! Almost all babies outgrow it eventually.

- Babies with GERD can have problems such as:

  - Difficulty feeding, not gaining enough weight.

  - Choking or coughing; uncommonly, *apnea* (interrupted breathing).

  - Stomach contents can be inhaled (aspirated) into the lungs, causing pneumonia.

  - GERD may also cause or contribute to breathing-related symptoms, including laryngitis (hoarseness) and wheezing.

  - GERD seems to be common in children with asthma and may even be one of the factors triggering asthma attacks.

How are reflux problems and GERD diagnosed?

- Generally, the doctor will recognize GERD by the symptoms.

- Sometimes x-rays of the esophagus and stomach (upper gastrointestinal [GI] tract) are done to make sure there is not another reason for the spitting up and vomiting. The baby drinks a dye, usually barium, that shows up on x-rays.

- In some complicated cases, a test called a pH probe is done. A small device (probe) is placed into the esophagus. This lets the doctor measure how long stomach acid stays in the esophagus.

How are reflux problems and GERD treated?

Especially before age 12 months, reflux in infants generally doesn't need any treatment if it's not causing any of the problems discussed earlier.

If problems related to GERD are present, the doctor may make a number of recommendations:

- *Position changes.* Avoid leaving the baby in the car seat when not traveling. Although babies have less reflux when placed on their stomachs, they should still generally sleep on their backs to reduce the risk of sudden infant death syndrome. When the baby is awake and being watched, he or she can be placed on the stomach.

- *Acid-reducing drugs.* Several different types of acid-reducing drugs, including cimetidine and omeprazole, may be used.

- *Thickening the formula* with cereal may help to reduce the amount of spit up. The opening in the nipple of the bottle has to made larger to let the milk flow easily. Enfamil AR ("added rice") is a special formula that thickens when it reaches the stomach. If you're using this type of formula, it's not necessary to add cereal.

If none of these treatments helps, we may recommend a visit to a doctor specializing in stomach and intestinal problems (a gastroenterologist).

When should I call your office?

Call our office if your child continues spitting up past age 1.

If your child has GERD, call our office if reflux and other symptoms continue or return, in particular:

- Frequent vomiting, especially projectile vomiting. This could be a sign of a problem other than reflux.

- Fussiness when feeding; not wanting to eat much.

- Frequent coughing, choking, or hoarseness with feeding.

- Apnea—may be related to reflux, especially if it occurs with spitting up or choking.

Swollen Scalp (Caput Succedaneum and Cephalohematoma)

Some babies are born with swelling or a large bump on the scalp. Caput succedaneum is swelling under the skin of the scalp, while cephalohematoma results from bleeding under the scalp. Both conditions are related to pressure on the baby's head during birth. They are usually harmless.

What are caput succedaneum and cephalohematoma, and what do they look like?

Caput succedaneum.

- Swelling (edema) of the scalp. The swelling is caused by pressure on the head during delivery. Sometimes there is bruising, but the swelling is not from blood in the scalp.

- There may be swelling and bruising of the face, if your baby was born face first.

- Swelling goes down after a few days. When it does, you may notice "molding," a pointed appearance of your baby's head that wasn't obvious before.

- The skull of infants is made up of pieces of bone that eventually fuse and become one. The places where the pieces meet are called "sutures."

- If high pressure is placed on the skull, the pieces of bone may overlap at the sutures. This causes the baby's head to have an unusual, often pointed, appearance. This is called "molding," and it may take several weeks to clear up.

Cephalohematoma.

- This is a collection of blood from broken blood vessels that builds up under the scalp. It is not in the brain.

- A lump or bump on one side of your infant's head. It is usually located toward the back or side of the head.

- The lump is usually caused by pressure on the skull during delivery or by the use of forceps to aid in delivery. Often, there is no bruising.

- The lump usually appears after several hours, or the day after birth. It may take several weeks or even a few months for the lump to go away.

What are some possible complications of swollen sculp?

With caput succedaneum, complications are rare.
With cephalohematoma, complications occur occasionally:

- Skull fracture may occur. These fractures usually heal without problems.

- If the collection of blood is large, it may result in anemia (low hemoglobin).

- Large cephalohematomas may result in jaundice. This is a yellow color of the skin caused by excess bilirubin, a substance produced by breakdown of blood as the cephalohematoma is resolving.

- More serious complications, such as bleeding into the brain or injury to the brain from skull fracture, occur only rarely.

- Occasionally, calcium deposits develop in the area of the cephalohematoma. This may leave a hard bump that lasts for several months.

What puts your child at risk of swollen scalp?

Caput succedaneum and cephalohematoma are common side effects of birth. A difficult labor or the use of forceps during delivery may increase the risk.

How is swollen scalp treated?

Usually, no treatment is needed.

- *Caput succedaneum* clears up in a few days.

- *Cephalohematoma.* If the doctor suspects a skull fracture, x-rays or other tests may be done. Most fractures heal with no problem. Fractures that are sunken (depressed) may need additional treatment.

- Jaundice (yellow color of the skin) is usually a minor complication. If jaundice is severe enough, light therapy may be recommended.

Many babies with caput succedaneum or cephalohematoma have "molding," resulting in a pointed or oblong appearance of the head. This is normal, although it may take several weeks to clear up. No treatment is needed.

When should I call your office?

Call our office if:

- Swelling and/or bruising of your baby's scalp do not continue to improve after your baby goes home from the hospital.

- Jaundice (yellow color of the skin) appears.

- Your baby becomes irritable or fussy for no apparent reason.

Thrush

Thrush is an infection of the mouth with the yeast *Candida*. It is common in newborn infants, resulting in white spots in the mouth. Thrush in newborns is usually a harmless problem that is easily treated. If the infection doesn't clear up within 2 weeks, contact the doctor.

What is thrush?

Thrush is a common infection of the mouth in newborns. The baby picks up the *Candida* yeast from the mother during birth. A week or so later, white spots appear in the baby's mouth. Babies can also contract thrush during breast or bottle feeding.

Thrush may cause some pain or discomfort, or it may cause no symptoms at all. In healthy infants, thrush may go away on its own, but most cases are treated. You should watch to make sure your baby's infection clears up during treatment.

What does it look like?

- White spots (plaques) appearing inside your baby's mouth: on the inner cheek, gums, or palate (roof of the mouth).

- Underneath the white spots, red tissue that may bleed easily when scraped.

- Sometimes the baby seems uncomfortable. He or she may seem fussy or may feed less because the mouth is sore. However, in most cases, the baby doesn't seem to have any pain.

- White spots usually develop 7 to 10 days after birth. Normally, they clear up gradually over the next 2 weeks. The spots sometimes come back. Thrush is unusual in children over age 1.

What causes thrush?

- Thrush is caused by infection with a yeast called *Candida*. The baby picks up the *Candida* organisms from the mother during birth.

- *Candida* is normally present in the mouth. It usually causes symptoms only in certain situations. In newborns, the immune system isn't yet mature so infection develops earlier.

- *Candida* can cause other infections as well. In newborns, *Candida* infection in the diaper area is not unusual.

- Otherwise, *Candida* usually doesn't cause serious infections in healthy people. It can be a problem in people with reduced immune function, such as those infected with human immunodeficiency virus (HIV, the virus that causes AIDS [acquired immunodeficiency syndrome]).

What increases your baby's risk of getting thrush?

Babies treated with antibiotics for other reasons (such as an ear infection) may be at increased risk of getting thrush.

How is thrush treated?

- Healthy babies with mild thrush may need no treatment. The infection often clears up on its own within 2 weeks. If it doesn't, call our office.

- Thrush and other *Candida* infections can be treated with antibiotics.

- The most common treatment is a prescription drug called nystatin suspension. It works by direct contact with the infected areas of the mouth. Apply this medication to your baby's mouth, four times per day, for about a week. Continue treatment for a day after it looks like the thrush has cleared up.

- Other treatments are available if the problem doesn't clear up with nystatin.

When should I call your office?

Call our office if:

- The white plaques in your baby's mouth haven't cleared up by 2 weeks, or after treatment.

- The thrush is severe or painful, especially if your baby is feeding less than usual.

- The thrush comes back after clearing up, or it develops after the newborn period.

- Your infant has other signs of illness, such as poor weight gain.

Umbilical Cord Care

During pregnancy, the umbilical cord is the baby's connection to the mother. After birth, the cord is cut, and the stump remains connected to the baby. This is where the navel (belly button) will be. You'll be taught some simple steps to care for the cord stump after taking your baby home. Although there are a few things to watch out for, problems with the umbilical cord stump are rare. It usually falls off within a few weeks.

What is the umbilical cord?

While your baby was in the womb, he or she was connected to you by two important organs: the placenta and the umbilical cord. The umbilical cord is the fetus's "life support system" during pregnancy; it contains blood vessels that provide oxygen and nutrition. At birth, the umbilical cord is cut, and the stump remains attached to the baby.

During the first few weeks after birth, the umbilical cord stump gradually dries and heals. It falls off on its own within a few weeks. During this time, some simple care is needed to keep the cord clean and dry. You should be alert for any signs of infection or bleeding; however, these and other complications are uncommon. If any problems occur, or if the stump hasn't fallen off within 4 weeks, call your doctor's office.

What does it look like?

- Immediately after birth, the umbilical cord is cut. A clamp is placed near the cut end to prevent bleeding. The doctor examines the umbilical cord and placenta to make sure they are normal.

- Within a few days, the stump begins to dry out and becomes darker.

- For the first few weeks, simple care is needed to keep the cord stump dry and clean. You should sponge-bathe your baby during this time rather than bathing him or her in a tub.

- The cord stump gradually becomes dry and black. It should fall off on its own around this time. The area around your baby's new belly button will be a little red at first but should soon look like normal skin.

How do you care for the umbilical cord stump?

- Keep the cord stump clean and dry until it falls off. Wash your baby with a sponge or wash cloth and warm water.

(To keep your baby warm, baths should be quick during the first few weeks anyway.)

- At every diaper change, use soap and water to clean the area around the cord stump. Pull up gently on the stump and clean around its base. A little foul odor and moisture are normal in this area.

- Some doctors may recommend cleaning the stump with rubbing alcohol. You may clean the area with a small amount of rubbing alcohol on a cotton ball or swab or use packaged alcohol wipes. Try not to use more rubbing alcohol than is necessary.

- Keep the cord stump over the diaper; it should not be inside the diaper. You may need to fold down the top edge of the diaper.

Are there any possible problems?

Problems related to the umbilical cord stump are possible but uncommon:

- *Infection.* Infection of the cord stump (called "omphalitis") is the most serious problem. Although a little moisture and foul odor can be normal, draining fluid and redness of the skin around the stump may mean infection is present. *If drainage and redness are present, see your doctor right away.* (Just fluid, without redness, is most common with granuloma—not a serious problem.)

- *Bleeding.* There should be little or no bleeding from the cord stump. Bleeding is most likely to occur if the cord is pulled off too early.

- *Granuloma.* If the skin around the cord stump is slow to heal, umbilical granuloma may be present. The granuloma looks like a small, round growth. There is usually some wetness in the belly button. Umbilical granuloma is a relatively common problem that is not serious. Simple treatment may be needed, most commonly the use of silver nitrate to speed healing.

- *Prolonged separation.* This occurs when the umbilical cord stump takes longer than 3 to 4 weeks to fall off. It is usually not a serious problem.

- *Umbilical hernia.* Part of the intestines may stick out through the belly button after the cord stump falls off. You may notice a swollen area that gets larger when your baby coughs or cries. Usually, the swelling is easily pushed back into place. Treatment is usually not needed unless the hernia is very large or doesn't go away on its own.

- *Embryologic abnormalities.* These are problems occurring when the baby was forming in the mother's womb. They may include cysts or connections between the umbilicus (belly button) and the urinary system or intestines. Surgery may be needed to repair the abnormality.

Can umbilical cord problems be prevented?

Following steps to keep the umbilical cord stump clean and dry may help to prevent infections.

When should I call your office?

Umbilical cord problems are uncommon, but it is important to watch out for signs of infection or other problems.

Call our office *immediately* if any of the following occurs:

- Redness beyond the area immediately around the base of the cord stump.

- Active bleeding—more than a drop or two of blood from the cord stump.

- Drainage or moisture—a lot of fluid coming from the cord stump, or if moisture or drainage is present for more than a few days.

- Very foul odor.

Call our office if any of the following nonemergency conditions occurs:

- The cord stump doesn't fall off on its own within 4 weeks.

- Swelling is present under the skin around the belly button area.

Section XXI ▪ Nutrition

Healthy Diet

Parents have a lot of questions about what their kids should eat. A healthy diet helps keep your child healthy now and builds good habits for the future. The goal is to provide high-quality nutrition while avoiding excess calories, which could lead to obesity. Your doctor will monitor your child's growth and nutrition at each office visit. Be sure to ask the doctor if you have any questions about this important issue.

What's a healthy diet for my child?

Children of all ages need a balanced diet, including all the different food groups: grains, vegetables, fruits, dairy products, and meats/proteins. Fats and sweets should be limited. As your child grows, the number of servings of each food will gradually increase.

No diet is perfect for every child. The best diet is one that provides a good variety of foods, with enough calories to support your child's growth and energy needs. A diet that provides too many calories, and especially too many fats and sweets, puts your child at risk of becoming overweight or obese. Providing a healthy diet in childhood will build good eating habits that will last throughout your child's life.

What foods are included in a healthy diet?

For children (and adults), a healthy diet includes a good variety of foods from the following groups:

- *Grains,* such as bread, cereals, and pasta. Whole grains are best: whole-wheat bread is better than white bread, and oatmeal is better than boxed cereals.

- *Vegetables.* Give a good mix of dark-green vegetables, like spinach or broccoli, and orange/yellow vegetables, like carrots.

- *Fruits,* such as apples, bananas, oranges, raisins. Give lots of fresh fruit, not just fruit juices. Many fruit juices have added sugar, resulting in unnecessary calories.

- *Milk.* Milk and other dairy foods (such as yogurt and cheese) provide calcium for growing bones. In children under 2, too much milk (more than 20 to 24 ounces per day) increases the risk of iron deficiency anemia.

- *Meats.* Lean meats (not too much fat) are best. This category also includes eggs, fish, beans, and tofu.

- *Fats and sweets.* Limit the amounts of these foods.

How much should my child eat?

How much your child eats depends on several factors, including age, sex, and activity level. Of course, bigger kids need to eat more. More active children and teens may also need more food because they are using extra calories through physical activity.

Although your child's diet may vary, there are some general recommendations for daily servings from each food group. The lower amounts are for boys and girls ages 2 to 3; the higher amounts are for teenage boys ages 14 to 18:

- Grains: 4 to 6 ounces per day

- Vegetables: 1 to 3 cups per day

- Fruits: 1 to 2 cups per day

- Milk: 2 to 3 cups per day

- Lean meats (or fish or beans): 2 to 6 ounces per day

For all ages, limit added fats and sweets. We tend to get enough fat and sugar in the other foods we eat, without putting a lot of butter on bread, sugar on cereal, etc.

What foods should I avoid? "Junk foods" are major contributors to overweight and obesity in American children. Cut back on snack foods like chips, cookies, candy. Avoid "fast foods" and prepackaged foods. For example, serve baked potatoes rather than French fries. For dessert, serve fresh fruit rather than sweets. For many children and teens (and parents), cutting back on or eliminating soft drinks (soda pop) can save a lot of calories.

What does a serving look like?

This is an important question; people often overestimate the amount of food that makes up one serving. Examples of appropriate serving sizes are:

- Grains: 1 slice of bread or tortilla, ½ cup of cooked oatmeal or rice

- Vegetables: 1 cup of dark green lettuce, 1½ carrots

- Fruits: 1 medium apple, orange, or banana, ½ cup of cut-up fruit

- Milk: 1 cup of milk or yogurt, 1½ ounces of cheese

- Meats/proteins: 2 ounces of meat, 1 egg, 2 tablespoons of peanut butter

What about exercise?

The latest healthy diet recommendations emphasize the importance of regular physical activity and exercise. Even the healthy diet recommended above may provide more calories per day than your child uses in energy if he or she is not physically active.

- Try to provide opportunities for your child for at least 30 minutes of physical activity every day. Build some exercise into your child's (and family's) everyday routines. For example, your child can walk to school rather than being driven.

- Exercise doesn't necessarily mean a formal exercise program or going out for team sports. For younger kids, just getting outside and playing with friends is great exercise. A daily exercise video is a good idea, and something parents can do along with kids.

- Limit your child's "screen time"—TV and video games—to 1 or at most 2 hours per day. Don't let your child have a TV in his or her bedroom.

What if my child isn't following a healthy diet?

Don't worry too much if your child's diet doesn't follow the recommendations exactly. Every child is different in food likes and dislikes, activity level, and metabolism; no diet is right for every child. Your child is probably getting adequate nutrition if he or she has enough energy for daily activities, is growing normally without being overweight, and has some variety in his or her diet. Ask the doctor if you have questions about your child's diet. If your child is not eating any foods from one of the major groups, or is on a restricted diet for some reason, vitamins or iron supplements may be recommended.

Picky eater. After the first year, toddlers are no longer growing quite so fast. Periods of lack of interest in eating are normal. Children learn by example: good eating habits by the parents are important in producing good habits in children.

When should I call your office?

The doctor will check your child's weight, growth, and nutrition at every office visit. Between visits, call our office if:

- You have questions or concerns regarding your child's diet and nutrition.

- Your child seems to be gaining (obesity/overweight) too much or too little weight.

Where can I get more information?

- The American Heart Association offers a lot of helpful information on a healthy diet and lifestyle. On the Internet at *www.americanheart.org*, or call 1-800-AHA-USA-1 (1-800-242-8721).

- The U.S. Department of Agriculture offers useful information and publications on current dietary recommendations, including recently updated "Food Pyramids" for children and adults. On the Internet at *www.mypyramid.gov*, or call 1-888-7PYRAMID (1-888-779-7264).

High Cholesterol

The high cholesterol levels that increase heart disease risk in adults may also be present in children. If high cholesterol levels are found in children over age 2 or in teenagers, diet changes may be recommended to help reduce cholesterol, along with some risk-lowering behaviors. Some uncommon genetic diseases may also cause abnormally high (or abnormally low) cholesterol levels.

What is high cholesterol and what are the health risks?

Higher than normal cholesterol levels are one of the main risk factors for heart disease in adults. Cholesterol plays a number of important roles in the body. However, when cholesterol levels rise too high, they increase the risk of atherosclerosis (narrowing or "hardening" of the arteries). Atherosclerosis that starts developing in childhood can lead to blocked arteries and heart disease in adulthood.

If your child or teenager has high cholesterol, the doctor may recommend dietary changes to reduce the amount of fat in the diet. Quite often, if the children have high cholesterol, so do the parents—your whole family may benefit from the new diet. Monitoring of cholesterol and other risk factors is especially important if your family has a history of premature heart disease.

- *It is important not to limit cholesterol in infants and toddlers less than 2 years old!* Babies need a lot of calories to support their rapid growth. Children under age 2 should rarely if ever be put on a low-cholesterol or low-calorie diet.

How is high cholesterol diagnosed?

Several types of cholesterol levels are measured. The following values are for children or adolescents at high risk:

- Total cholesterol:
  - Normal: less than 170 milligrams per deciliter (mg/dL).
  - Borderline: 170 to 199 mg/dL.
  - High: over 200 mg/dL.
- *Low-density lipoprotein (LDL) cholesterol.* Sometimes called "bad" cholesterol, high levels of LDL cholesterol lead to a higher risk of heart disease:
  - Normal: less than 110 mg/dL.
  - Borderline: 110 to 129 mg/dL.
  - High: over 130 mg/dL.
- *High-density lipoprotein (HDL) cholesterol.* Sometimes called "good" cholesterol, higher levels of HDL cholesterol lead to a lower risk of heart disease. A good balance between LDL and HDL cholesterol is healthiest for both children and adults.

What causes high cholesterol?

- In most cases, high cholesterol results from a combination of lifestyle factors (especially diet and lack of exercise) and genetic (inherited) factors.
- Less commonly, high cholesterol in children results from specific inherited diseases.
- Like adults, children and teens with high cholesterol may have additional risk factors for heart disease:
  - Obesity.
  - Lack of exercise.
  - Diabetes.
  - High blood pressure.
  - Smoking.

Can high cholesterol be prevented?

Encouraging a healthy lifestyle—including proper diet, regular exercise, and avoiding obesity—may reduce your child's risk of high cholesterol. This is especially important if you or others in your family have had high cholesterol or premature heart disease.

How is high cholesterol treated?

The doctor's recommendations will depend on your child's situation, including:

- Your child's total, LDL, and HDL cholesterol levels.
- Your family's history of cardiovascular disease.
- Lifestyle factors, especially obesity and lack of exercise.
- Other risk factors, such as diabetes and high blood pressure.

Diet is the first step in managing your child's high cholesterol. Dietary changes are generally recommended for children, teens, and adults with LDL ("bad") cholesterol levels over 110 mg/dL.

- The "Step I" diet is a low-fat diet (no more than 30% of calories from fat). It also limits the amount of cholesterol, which comes from animal fats, in the diet. In some situations, the doctor may recommend a diet that is even lower in fat.
  - The doctor may recommend a visit with a dietitian, who can help develop a diet plan. It's usually best to introduce the new diet gradually.

- In most cases, we recommend that all family members over age 2 follow the Step I diet; when the children have high cholesterol, the parents often do too.

- *Infants and toddlers under age 2 should not be put on a low-fat or low-calorie diet.*

- The doctor will check your child to see if the new diet is lowering your child's cholesterol levels. If target levels aren't reached, the doctor may recommend another diet ("Step II").

- Don't get discouraged if your child doesn't reach the target levels; it can be hard to make major reductions in cholesterol through diet alone. Even if your child doesn't reach the ideal cholesterol level, the dietary changes will help to reduce his or her long-term risk of cardiovascular disease.

Other risk factors may need attention too, including obesity and lack of exercise. Losing weight and increasing physical activity will not only help to reduce your child's cholesterol levels but also make him or her feel and look better. Teens (and adults) who smoke may need help in quitting. It is also important to treat any related health problems, such as high blood pressure or diabetes.

Drugs may be recommended for some children over 10 years old whose cholesterol levels remain high despite changes in diet. We will probably recommend visits to a specialist with expertise in this area.

Other causes of high cholesterol, including specific inherited disorders, also require specialist treatment.

When should I call your office?

Call our office if you have any questions about treatment for your child's high cholesterol, including planning a healthy diet for your family.

Where can I get more information?

The American Heart Association offers a lot of helpful information on a healthy diet and lifestyle. On the Internet at *www.americanheart.org*, or call 1-800-AHA-USA-1 (1-800-242-8721).

Obesity

Obesity is an increasingly common problem in American children. Being obese can have lifelong harmful effects on your child's health as well as in other areas of his or her life. A diet that reduces calories and fat, along with increased exercise, is the recommended treatment. Although losing weight can be difficult, the doctor can help your family make important changes for a healthier lifestyle.

What is obesity?

Children are considered obese when their body mass index (BMI) is higher than that of 95% of children their age. The BMI is a calculated number based on the person's height and weight—the higher the BMI, the heavier the person is for his or her height. If the doctor says your child is "above the 95th percentile," that means his or her BMI is higher than that of 95 out of 100 children of the same age.

In the United States, obesity rates are rising fast in children (and adults). Some of the many health problems related to obesity, including diabetes and high blood pressure, are also becoming more common in children.

Although genetic factors play a role, obesity nearly always results from a combination of too much food (especially high-fat foods) and not enough exercise. In many cases, childhood obesity is a sign that the whole family needs to make changes toward a healthier lifestyle. Losing weight can be difficult. However, a healthy diet and regular exercise can help to reduce your child's risk of serious health problems, now and later in life.

How is obesity diagnosed?

- Obesity in children is defined as a BMI (body mass index) above the 95th percentile for children of the same age.

- Children who are between the 85th and 95th percentiles are considered "overweight." Children in this group are at high risk of continued weight gain.

- In older teens (and adults), obesity may be defined as a BMI of 30 or higher. (Occasionally, athletic teens will have a high BMI because they are very muscular, not obese or overweight.)

What are the causes and risk factors for obesity?

- Some children and teens are obese because of specific medical conditions, for example, hypothyroidism (low activity of the thyroid gland) or specific genetic abnormalities.

- *However, in the vast majority of cases, obesity results from too many calories and not enough exercise.* The main risk factors are lifestyle, including a diet that provides too many calories and not enough physical activity (exercise). Genetic (inherited) factors also play a role.

- Psychological issues can contribute to obesity; other times they are caused by obesity.

- There is a direct link between obesity and time spent watching television and playing video/computer games. The more time your child spends in front of a video screen, the higher his or her risk of obesity.

- Having obese parents—especially the mother—increases the chances of being obese as an adult. Overweight children or teens are more likely to be obese as adults.

- Breast-fed babies are at lower risk than bottle-fed babies.

- The risk is higher for African Americans (especially girls) and Hispanics.

What are the health risks of obesity?

Because it leads to so many other diseases, obesity shortens your child's life expectancy. Some of the many health problems related to obesity are:

- Type 2 diabetes.
- High cholesterol and triglycerides.
- High blood pressure.
- Cardiovascular (heart and blood vessels) diseases, including heart attacks and strokes.
- Obstructive sleep apnea (breathing problems during sleep).
- Bone and joint problems.
- Psychological problems (like depression and anxiety).

Can obesity be prevented?

Prevention is extremely important, because treatment of obesity is so difficult. Your family should build healthy eating and exercise habits while your children are young. Children learn from their parents—including eating behaviors.

How is obesity evaluated and treated?

Treatment of obesity starts with a complete physical examination, including measurement of blood pressure. Although uncommon, if a medical problem causing obesity (like hypothyroidism) is suspected, certain tests or visits to specialists will be recommended.

Depending on your child's age and the presence of risk factors for diabetes and cardiovascular disease (especially if parents or grandparents have diabetes or if anyone in your family has had a heart attack or stroke before age 55), certain blood tests may be recommended:

- Cholesterol and triglyceride levels—indicators of heart disease risk.

- Tests to determine whether your child has or is at risk for diabetes, such as fasting blood sugar level.

Diet and exercise are the main treatments for obesity:

- *Diet.* Your doctor will recommend a diet that is lower in calories and fat and higher in fiber. In most cases, we recommend that all family members over age 2 follow the new diet; when the children are obese, the parents may have weight problems as well.

  - Infants and toddlers under age 2 should not be put on a low-fat or low-calorie diet, but should follow a healthy diet.

  - Your doctor may recommend a visit with a dietitian, who can help develop a diet plan. It's usually best to introduce the new diet gradually.

  - Recommendations may vary, but for most families "counting calories" is not the best approach. Usually, the results are best when the whole family makes changes in eating and exercise behaviors:

    - Serve a good variety of foods from all food groups: grains, vegetables, fruits, milk and other dairy foods, and meats and beans. Limit the amount of fats and sweets. The doctor or dietitian may recommend specific numbers of servings from each food group per day, including advice on proper serving sizes.

    - Cut back on snack foods like chips, cookies, candy. Avoid "fast foods" and prepackaged foods. For example, serve baked potatoes rather than French fries. For dessert, serve fresh fruit rather than sweets. For many children and teens (and parents), cutting back on or eliminating soft drinks (soda pop) can save a lot of calories.

  - Children should be praised and rewarded for healthier behaviors (of course, the reward shouldn't be food!). Praise for healthy changes works better than criticizing or nagging for unhealthy behaviors.

  - Diets should never be restricted so much so as not to supply necessary nutrients and vitamins.

- *Exercise/physical activity.* Calories provide energy—your child needs exercise to use up some of that energy. Being more active will not only help your child lose weight, but it will improve his or her general health.

  - Try to provide opportunities for at least 30 minutes of physical activity every day. Build some exercise into your child's (and family's) everyday routines. For example, your child can walk to school rather than being driven.

  - Exercise doesn't necessarily mean a formal exercise program or going out for team sports. For younger kids, just getting outside and playing with friends is great exercise. A daily exercise video is a good idea, and something parents can do along with kids.

  - Limit your child's "screen time"—TV and video games—to 1 or at most 2 hours per day. Don't let your child have a TV in his or her bedroom.

- Things to avoid:

  - In general, avoid "low-carb" and other fad diets. The goal is to build healthy eating habits for a lifetime, not just a temporary weight-reducing diet. Medications, "diet pills," and other products are generally not recommended.

  - In special cases, such as extreme obesity or obesity causing medical problems that don't improve with diet and exercise, prescription medications may be recommended. We may recommend a visit to an expert in treating obesity, often an endocrinologist (a specialist in hormone problems).

  - Don't smoke! Some teens (and adults) use smoking as a diet aid, believing that it will help them lose weight. This is not necessarily effective, and smoking leads to even more health problems.

- *Medical follow-up.* Regular weight checks are appropriate to see how well your child is doing.

  - Don't get discouraged if weight loss isn't immediate or dramatic. For many children, just staying at the same weight for a time is a reasonable goal. For older children and teens, the recommended amount of weight loss depends on age, how overweight the child is, and whether complications like high blood pressure are present.

Weight loss should be gradual. Remember, your child needs enough calories and a good variety of foods to ensure proper nutrition. Sustained changes in diet and exercise habits are needed to control weight.

When should I call your office?

Call our office if you have any questions about treatment for your child's weight problem, including planning a healthy diet for your family.

Where can I get more information?

The American Heart Association offers a lot of helpful information on a healthy diet and lifestyle. On the Internet at *www.americanheart.org*, or call 1-800-AHA-USA-1 (1-800-242-8721).

Section XXII ▪ Respiratory

Cystic Fibrosis

Cystic fibrosis (CF) is an inherited disease that mainly causes problems with the lungs and gastrointestinal system. The genetic defect causes the mucus to become thick, leading to blockage of the airways and respiratory infections. Children with CF also have problems with digesting and absorbing enough nutrients to grow properly. There is no cure, but medical advances have greatly improved the length and quality of life for patients with CF.

What is cystic fibrosis (CF)?

CF is the most common cause of severe, chronic (ongoing) lung disease in children. Children with CF have an abnormal gene that affects the cells producing mucus and other fluids in various parts of the body, especially the lungs and pancreas. The mucus of children with CF is very thick, sticky, and difficult to clear; this causes problems with plugging and blockage of the airway and lungs. Lung infections are a frequent and long-term problem for most children with CF and are the most common cause of death.

CF also causes abnormalities of the digestive organs, especially the pancreas—an organ in the abdomen that makes enzymes that help with digestion. Children with CF don't make enough of these enzymes to digest and absorb certain foods and minerals (called "malabsorption"). CF can also affect the liver and other organs.

In the past, patients with CF usually died in childhood. Today, with good medical care, children with CF can live well into adulthood. The results are best when families work in close partnership with doctors, nurses, and other health professionals.

What does it look like?

The symptoms of CF vary, depending on the gene causing the disease and other factors. Symptoms can begin at different ages—sometimes in the first few months of life, sometimes later. Some children have severe lung disease and digestive problems, others have fewer symptoms.

- *Respiratory symptoms* (breathing-related) include:
  - Cough. Coughing occurs as the body tries to eliminate thick, sticky mucus. Cough may be worse in the morning or after your child has been active.
  - Repeated respiratory infections, including pneumonia (lung infection), bronchitis (infection of the airways), and sinusitis (infection of the sinuses). Children with CF may need many hospital stays to treat these infections.

- Wheezing (noisy breathing) and asthma-like symptoms may develop.
- As the lung disease of CF gets worse, your child may have low energy and shortness of breath.
- With time, the chest can become "barrel-shaped." The fingertips may appear swollen—this is called "clubbing."

- *Digestive symptoms*:
  - Some CF babies are born with intestinal obstruction (blockage), so stools can't pass out of the body. The blockage occurs when the baby's first stool, called meconium, doesn't pass. Other symptoms include bloating of the abdomen and nausea.
  - Abnormal function of the pancreas leads to poor digestion, with poor growth and weight gain. Your child may have frequent, foul-smelling BMs. The stools may float because they contain large amounts of fat.

- *Other symptoms*:
  - Children with CF lose too much salt in their sweat; their skin may even "taste" salty. This can lead to problems with low sodium levels (hyponatremia), especially during times of warm weather or illness.
  - Other problems may develop later in childhood, including diabetes and delayed sexual development.
  - Many other medical problems are possible, including cirrhosis (scarring and damage) of the liver.

How is cystic fibrosis diagnosed?

The doctor may first suspect CF because of typical symptoms or a family history of CF. In some states, all newborns are tested for CF as part of newborn screening for many diseases.

Several tests may be done to confirm that CF is present:

- *Sweat testing.* This is the best test to make the diagnosis. A machine is used to produce and collect a sample of sweat (usually from the arm) and measures the level of chloride. The sweat of children with CF contains increased levels of chloride.

- *Genetic tests* can be done to look for the defective gene causing CF. These tests detect 90% of patients with the disease. They are usually done if the child is too little (such as newborns) to obtain enough sweat for sweat testing, or to identify carriers, that is, people who have the abnormal CF gene but don't have the disease.

What causes cystic fibrosis?

One of many different gene abnormalities (mutations) occurs. Which specific mutation your child inherits has a major impact on the severity of CF.

Your child has CF because he or she inherited a copy of the mutated gene from *both parents*. People who have just one copy of a mutated gene do not develop CF; they are *carriers* of the CF gene.

Genetic testing is done to identify the gene mutation causing your child's CF. Parents and other family members need to be tested as well. Genetic counseling can help you to understand the risk of passing CF on to future children.

What are some possible complications of cystic fibrosis?

- CF progresses gradually over time. Most people with CF eventually die of complications related to the lungs and heart.

- Respiratory complications include pneumothorax (air leaking out of the lungs into the chest) and bleeding into the lungs and airways.

- Digestive problems and malabsorption can lead to vitamin deficiencies.

- Diabetes mellitus may occur if the pancreas does not make enough insulin. Some patients with CF develop diabetes as they get older.

- Fertility problems may occur, especially in males.

- Other complications are possible as well. Prevention, early identification, and treatment of complications are major goals of treatment for CF.

What increases your child's risk of cystic fibrosis?

Inheriting a gene mutation from both parents is the only cause of CF. These genes are most common in families of central or northern European origin. In the United States, CF is much more common in whites (1 in 3500 infants) than in African Americans (1 in 17,000).

If your family has a history of CF, genetic testing and counseling may help you understand your risk of passing the abnormal gene on to your children.

How is cystic fibrosis treated?

Your child will most likely be referred to a pulmonologist, an expert in lung diseases. Your child may see other specialists as well, including a gastroenterologist, an expert in diseases of the digestive system, and a nutritionist or dietitian.

A comprehensive plan will be developed to manage your child's CF. He or she will receive regular medical follow-up. The goal is to keep your child in stable condition for as long a time as possible.

Treatment of respiratory/lung problems includes:

- *Percussion and postural drainage.* Your child's body needs help to clear thick, sticky mucus more effectively. Postural drainage means positioning your child's body to help secretions drain. Chest percussion means tapping on the chest to help loosen secretions. These steps help your child get the secretions out of the body by coughing. They are among the most important things you can do to keep your child's lungs working as well as possible.

- *Aerosolized saline solution.* Using a device called a nebulizer, your child breathes in a fine mist of salt water. This helps to thin the mucus so that it can be better removed by coughing.

- *Antibiotics* are used to control infections. Sometimes they are given through a vein (intravenously, or IV), sometimes orally, sometimes inhaled.

- *Human recombinant DNAse (Pulmozyme).* This is an enzyme that helps thin and clear mucus from the airway. It is inhaled using an inhaler or nebulizer.

- *Bronchodilators.* Commonly used for asthma, drugs called "bronchodilators" can help to reduce airway blockage for some children with CF. They are especially useful for patients with asthma-like symptoms such as wheezing, which may be called "reactive airway disease." These drugs, such as albuterol, are given through an inhaler or nebulizer.

- *Steroids.* Oral steroids may be used for some severe lung problems. Inhaled steroids are often used for patients with asthma-like symptoms.

Other treatments may include:

- Macrolide antibiotics: a type of antibiotic that also helps reduce inflammation.

- Ibuprofen is commonly used, also because of its effect on inflammation.

- Oxygen may be needed, especially during sleep.

- Lung transplantation is an option for CF patients with very severe lung disease.

- *Nutritional therapy.* Without treatment, most CF patients have severe problems digesting fats, proteins, vitamins, and minerals. Treatment may include:

  - Pancreatic enzymes to replace those not produced normally.

  - Special diets to increase calories. A nutritionist or dietitian can help in planning a diet.

  - Other methods may be tried to get more food and calories into the child. These may include placing a feeding tube into the stomach or through the nose (nasogastric tube) or through the skin of the abdomen. Your child may receive hyperalimentation, that is, food in the form of proteins, fats, and sugars, along with vitamins and minerals, given through a vein (IV).

  - Treatments may be needed for other digestive problems, including obstruction of the intestines and liver disease.

- *Mental health care* and support are also important. Having a child with such a serious disease can be overwhelming for parents. Several national and local organizations are available to provide information and support for children with CF and their families.

When should I call your office?

Your child with CF will receive specialized team care, with frequent health visits and monitoring. Regular medical follow-up is essential to keep your child in the best possible health and avoid complications. Between appointments, contact your treatment team or doctor immediately if any problems occur.

Where can I get more information about cystic fibrosis?

The Cystic Fibrosis Foundation is on the Internet at *www.cff.org* or call 1-800-FIGHT CF (1-800-344-4823).

Laryngomalacia

Laryngomalacia is a relatively common problem that can cause difficulty breathing in infants. A part of the airway, the larynx (voice box) collapses easily. This can lead to noisy and sometimes difficult breathing. Feeding problems may be present as well. Laryngomalacia usually clears up on its own. If not, or in severe cases, treatments are available.

What is laryngomalacia?

Laryngomalacia is a relatively common problem involving the larynx ("voice box"). The exact cause is unclear, but the cartilage and other tissues supporting the larynx seem "too soft" in babies with laryngomalacia. The larynx is sometimes described as "floppy." It may partially collapse and become narrow easily, interfering with the flow of air. In some infants, laryngomalacia is related to neurologic problems, such as cerebral palsy.

Laryngomalacia causes episodes of noisy breathing, usually when your baby inhales. Feeding problems may occur. Laryngomalacia can be diagnosed with certainty by an office procedure called laryngoscopy, usually done by an ear, nose, and throat (ENT) specialist. This involves looking through a tube placed into the larynx through the mouth.

Fortunately, the typical child with laryngomalacia usually gets better over several months. Your child will need close follow-up to make sure this occurs. Surgery may be needed in severe cases, but this is rare.

What does it look like?

The main symptom of laryngomalacia is noisy breathing. This may be called *stridor*—a sharp, high-pitched sound caused by the upper part of the airway closing up when your child breathes in. Stridor is the same sound made by babies with croup.

- Noisy breathing typically starts within the first 2 weeks after birth

- This is most noticeable when your child is breathing in.

- It usually gets better with time; most cases clear up by 18 months to 2 years.

- Episodes of noisy, difficult breathing are more frequent when your child is very active or excited, for example, such as when crying or feeding.

- In more severe cases, other symptoms can occur:

  - Feeding problems. These may lead to slow growth.

  - "Spitting up" milk/formula from the stomach.

What are some possible complications of laryngomalacia?

Complications are possible, especially if laryngomalacia is severe:

- Episodes of interrupted breathing (apnea).

- Reflux, with stomach acid causing damage to the larynx and airway. If your child inhales the stomach contents, a form of pneumonia called "aspiration pneumonia" can occur.

- Feeding problems, leading to slow growth.

What increases your child's risk of laryngomalacia?

Laryngomalacia is more common in boys than girls.

Can laryngomalacia be prevented?

There is no known way to prevent this condition.

How is laryngomalacia diagnosed?

- If your baby is having episodes of stridor within the first 2 weeks after birth, your doctor will consider the possibility of laryngomalacia. Next to infections, it is the most common cause of stridor in infants.

- To make sure of the cause, we may recommend a visit to a specialist: either an ENT doctor (an otorhinolaryngologist) or a specialist in lung and breathing problems (a pulmonologist).

- This specialist may perform an office procedure called *laryngoscopy,* using a long, flexible instrument like a telescope to examine your child's upper airway and larynx. It is often done to make sure there is not another cause of stridor. Your baby will receive anesthesia for the laryngoscopy procedure.

- In more severe cases, other tests may be recommended:

  - Chest x-rays to check the lungs.

  - Other x-ray tests to assess the esophagus (swallowing tube) and stomach.

How is laryngomalacia treated?

- Usually, no treatment is needed. The problem eventually clears up, as the cartilage in the larynx becomes firmer and better developed.

- In most infants, symptoms begin to decrease by age 6 months.

- The condition usually clears up by age 18 months to 2 years.

- During this time, your child will need regular medical visits to ensure that problems with laryngomalacia are resolving.

- If laryngomalacia is severe or persistent, the ENT doctor or pulmonologist may continue to care for your child. Rarely, if laryngomalacia is very severe, surgery is needed to restore normal airway and swallowing function.

When should I call your office?

Call our office (or the specialist who is caring for your child) if you have any questions about your child's treatment, or when you expect that the problem should have cleared up and it has not.

Call the doctor if breathing problems get worse, or if problems with feeding or swallowing occur (choking or gagging).

- If your child is having severe difficulty breathing, call 911 or go to the emergency room.

Obstructive Sleep Apnea

Apnea is interruption of breathing for a certain amount of time, or when accompanied by a change in skin color. Obstructive sleep apnea (OSA) is an increasingly recognized problem in children. Symptoms include snoring at night and feeling sleepy during the day. Diagnosis and treatment are available.

What is obstructive sleep apnea?

Obstructive sleep apnea is an interruption in breathing for longer than the normal time because air (oxygen) is blocked (obstructed) from getting into the airway. Sometimes the obstruction is partial, allowing less air than normal to get in.

Obstructive sleep apnea (OSA) occurs most commonly in adults but is being recognized more often in children and teens. For various reasons, the upper airway temporarily gets blocked and doesn't stay as open as it should while your child is sleeping. This can cause noisy breathing and snoring. The episodes of apnea may or may not wake your child up. Sometimes the airway is just partially blocked, so it's not "true" apnea. However, this can still result in less air getting to the lungs (called "hypoventilation").

What does it look like?

The main symptoms of OSA are:

- *Snoring*. Especially in severe OSA, snoring is the most noticeable symptom. (*However, not all kids who snore have OSA!*)

  - A period of loud snoring may be followed by a few moments of silence. You may hear a snort as your child starts breathing again; then snoring may start again. Some children may appear to be struggling to breathe. In others, you may hear very loud snoring through most of the night.

  - Snoring is often quieter and less noticeable in children than in adults. This may make it more difficult to recognize OSA.

- *Restless sleep*—your child may wake up frequently during the night.

  - Sleeping in odd positions, for example, with the neck stretched out.

- *Daytime sleepiness*—your child may lack energy for the usual activities. Sleepiness at school may lead to poor grades and other problems. Some children with OSA have symptoms similar to those of attention deficit–hyperactivity disorder (ADHD): inattentiveness, hyperactivity, behavior problems.

- *Mouth breathing* may be a symptom, although most children with OSA breathe normally when they are awake. Children with more severe OSA may breathe noisily during the day as well.

What causes obstructive sleep apnea?

- The most common cause of OSA in children is enlarged tonsils and adenoids. The tonsils and adenoids are lymph tissue that are part of the immune system. The tonsils are located in back of the throat and can be seen when the mouth is open wide. The adenoids are farther down and cannot be seen. The main cause of enlarged tonsils and adenoids is repeated respiratory infections (such as sore throats). In children, OSA is most frequent between ages 2 and 5, when the tonsils and adenoids are relatively large compared with the airway.

- Congestion in the nose, such as caused by allergies, can occasionally cause OSA. These children usually also have enlarged tonsils and adenoids.

- Some physical abnormalities can also increase the risk of OSA. These include having a large tongue and small jaw, which may occur in children with certain genetic conditions. Obesity also increases the risk of OSA, but children with OSA are not necessarily obese; in fact, most are not. Children with certain neurologic conditions, such as cerebral palsy, are also at increased risk.

What are some possible complications of apnea?

- If it is severe and frequent, OSA can lead to complications affecting the heart, lungs, and brain, related to lack of oxygen. Most cases of severe childhood OSA are detected and treated before these problems occur.

- Poor growth and weight gain (failure to thrive).

- Complications related to intellectual functioning and behavior. Daytime sleepiness can interfere with your child's school work and other daily activities.

Can obstructive sleep apnea be prevented?

- Most cases of OSA in children are probably not preventable.

- In obese children and teens with OSA, the problem is more likely to continue into adulthood. Weight management should be a long-term goal.

How is obstructive sleep apnea diagnosed?

- The doctor will often recognize OSA from the child's symptoms. In these cases, the problem is often enlarged tonsils and/or adenoids.

- If there is a lot of swelling and congestion in the nose, usually from allergies, the doctor may recommend treatment with allergy medications to see if that improves the OSA symptoms.

- *Polysomnography* (sleep study). If the doctor isn't sure whether there is a sleep-related breathing problem or how severe it is, he or she may recommend a sleep study called polysomnography (PSG). This is an overnight test, done at the hospital in a special sleep laboratory.

    - Your child will be hooked up to various machines that measure how he or she is breathing while asleep, how much oxygen is in the blood, how frequently episodes of interrupted breathing (apnea) occur and how long they last, and how difficult it is for your child to breathe during sleep.

    - The test is not painful, although it could be scary for a younger child. A parent is usually allowed to stay overnight with the child.

    - The information gathered by PSG answers a lot of important questions about the presence and severity of OSA. This helps determine the most effective treatment.

How is obstructive sleep apnea treated?

Treatments for OSA depend on your child's situation. Other doctors may be involved in your child's treatment, depending on the cause of the problem. We may recommend a visit to a doctor specializing in ear, nose, and throat problems (an otorhinolaryngologist or ENT) or to a specialist in lung and breathing problems (a pulmonologist).

- *Surgery.* For most children with OSA, the problem is caused by enlarged tonsils and adenoids. Treatment involves removing the tonsils and adenoids to create more room in the throat for your child to breathe. This operation is called adenotonsillectomy—"taking the tonsils (adenoids) out."

- For children who are otherwise healthy, this operation has a very high success rate. Problems with OSA usually clear up quickly. If your child is underweight or has been growing slowly, he or she may have "catch-up growth" after surgery.

- If problems other than enlarged tonsils and adenoids are present—such as obesity, cerebral palsy, or genetic diseases—there is an increased risk that sleep apnea will still be present or will return after surgery, if done. Your child will need continued medical follow-up.

- *Treatment for allergies.* If your child has problems with allergies, these may be treated first to see if the OSA symptoms improve. Oral antihistamines and decongestants may be used. Often, steroids sprayed into the nose (nasal steroids) are more effective.

- *Continuous positive airway pressure (CPAP).* If the doctor feels that surgery would not be helpful, or if surgery did not solve the problem, he or she may recommend a treatment called CPAP.

    - The CPAP machine produces mild air pressure to keep the airway open while your child is sleeping. The machine delivers air through smell tubes that fit in your child's nose and mouth. Although it takes a little getting used to, CPAP is highly effective in reducing episodes of apnea. Most patients requiring CPAP are cared for by a specialist.

- *Other operations* may be recommended in certain situations. For example, in children with facial deformities, reconstructive surgery may improve the problem with sleep apnea.

When should I call your office?

Call our office (or your ENT doctor or pulmonologist) if your child continues to have symptoms of OSA after treatment:

- Snoring, noisy breathing.

- Waking up at night for no obvious reason, especially with snoring.

- Daytime sleepiness.

Peritonsillar and Retropharyngeal Abscesses

A peritonsillar abscess is a localized infection (pus) involving the tonsils. Retropharyngeal abscesses occur in the back of the throat. Although these two infections have some differing symptoms, both usually cause fever, sore throat, and difficulty eating. Treatment in the hospital is usually needed, including intravenous (IV) antibiotics and sometimes surgery.

What are peritonsillar and retropharyngeal abscesses?

An abscess is a localized area of infection with pus, usually caused by bacteria. Abscesses can develop in lymph nodes behind the throat ("retropharyngeal") or in the area of the tonsils ("peritonsillar"). The tonsils are lymph tissue located at the back of the mouth; they can easily be seen when enlarged. Like the lymph nodes, the tonsils contain cells that play a role in the immune system.

The bacteria causing peritonsillar abscesses include "strep" (group A streptococci) and other bacteria from the mouth. Retropharyngeal abscesses are caused by the same bacteria as well as by "staph" (*Staphylococcus*) bacteria. Peritonsillar abscesses usually start from a throat infection, like strep throat. Retropharyngeal abscesses may begin from throat infections or sometimes from dental infections or trauma (such as a laceration or cut in the throat).

What do they look like?

Peritonsillar abscess is more common in older children and teens. Symptoms include:

- Sore throat.
- Fever.
- Difficulty eating.
- Difficulty opening the mouth very wide because of pain.
- The doctor may see that one tonsil is much larger than the other.
- Enlarged glands in the neck.
- Muffled voice.

Retropharyngeal abscess is more common in younger children, usually less than 3 or 4 years old. Symptoms include:

- Many of the same symptoms as peritonsillar abscess (fever, sore throat, difficulty eating).
- Drooling—child refuses to move the neck.
- Sometimes swelling in the back of the throat causes difficulty breathing. Call our office!

What are some possible complications of peritonsillar and retropharyngeal abscess?

- The main complication of both infections, especially retropharyngeal abscess, is blockage of the airway, causing difficulty breathing.
- There is also a risk that the infection will spread to other areas nearby.

How are peritonsillar and retropharyngeal abscess diagnosed and treated?

Diagnosis.

- The doctor will examine your child's throat to see if there are any obvious areas of swelling or redness. The diagnosis is suspected from the symptoms and medical examination. Especially for retropharyngeal abscess, a special kind of x-ray test called a CT scan is often needed to be sure of the diagnosis.

Treatment.

- *Antibiotics* will be given to kill the bacteria causing the infection. Your child usually needs to go to the hospital so that antibiotics can be given through a vein (intravenous, IV).
  - Antibiotic treatment will continue for at least several days, until your child is feeling better. After the IV antibiotics are stopped, your child will receive oral antibiotics.
- *Incision and drainage* may be needed to drain infected material. This is a relatively simple operation in which a small cut (incision) is made in the abscess to allow removal of the pus and other infected material (drainage). This is done if your child is experiencing difficulty breathing or is not getting better with antibiotics.
  - A sample of the infected material will be tested (cultured) to identify the exact bacteria present. This is important to make sure your child is receiving effective antibiotic treatment.

- For peritonsillar abscesses, a simpler procedure called needle aspiration may be performed. A needle is used to remove as much fluid as possible from the abscess.

- Needle aspiration can often be done using local anesthesia only. General anesthesia may be needed in younger children.

- If the infection doesn't improve after needle aspiration, incision and drainage may still be needed. In some cases, surgery to remove the tonsils (tonsillectomy) may be needed.

Follow-up.

- Make sure your child finishes his or her antibiotic prescription completely! This is very important in order to eliminate the bacteria causing the infection. Don't stop giving antibiotics just because your child is feeling better.

- Your child will receive follow-up care to make sure the infection doesn't return.

When should I call your office?

Call our office if symptoms return (fever, sore throat, etc.) soon after treatment.

Sudden Infant Death Syndrome

Sudden infant death syndrome (SIDS) occurs when an apparently healthy infant (under age 1) dies suddenly in his or her sleep, and no other cause of death is identified. It is sometimes called crib death. Although it's not always possible to prevent SIDS, certain steps can reduce the risk. The most important is placing babies on their backs to sleep, not on their stomachs or sides.

What is SIDS?

SIDS isn't a specific disease. Instead, it is defined as the sudden death of an infant for which no explanation can be found, despite a thorough medical history, investigation of the death scene, and autopsy. Most SIDS deaths occur in babies less than 6 months old.

The cause of SIDS is unknown. Some babies have apparent life-threatening events such as apnea (interrupted breathing) or cyanosis (turning blue) but don't die. These infants may be targeted for close monitoring.

What causes SIDS?

- The cause of SIDS is unknown—a combination of genetic and environmental factors seems to be involved.

- There is also evidence of subtle, mild abnormalities of the brain that affect breathing and heart rate. Autopsies of babies who died of SIDS often show signs that the infant was not getting enough oxygen for weeks or months before death.

What increases your infant's risk of SIDS?

Many risk factors for SIDS have been identified:

- Smoking increases the risk of SIDS. This includes smoking by the mother during pregnancy and smoking around the baby after birth.

- Babies who sleep on their stomachs are at higher risk.

- Risk is increased for premature babies, and for infants whose mothers didn't get adequate medical care during pregnancy.

- Other factors related to the baby's sleep environment increase the risk of SIDS, including sleeping on a soft mattress or pad or a sheepskin; and sleeping with pillows or heavy blankets.

- Babies who are overheated or overbundled may be at higher risk.

- Sleeping with parents may increase the risk of SIDS. In particular, bed sharing has been linked to increased risk if the mother smokes, if other children or adults other than the parents are in the bed, if the baby and parent are sleeping on a sofa, and if the parents are using alcohol and other drugs.

- There may be a small increase in risk if a previous child died of SIDS.

- Babies who have had an apparent life-threatening event (such as apnea or cyanosis) may be at increased risk.

- Risk is higher for African-American babies than white babies and lower for Hispanic and Asian babies.

- The SIDS rate is higher for boys.

Can SIDS be prevented?

Although SIDS cannot always be prevented, there are several things you can do to reduce your baby's risk:

- *Place babies on their backs to sleep!* This is an important step toward reducing your infant's risk of SIDS. Since the American Academy of Pediatrics started its national "Back to Sleep" campaign, the SIDS rate has decreased by about half.

  - Each day give your baby some "tummy time" while he or she is awake. Spending time on their stomachs is normal and natural for babies. It also helps to avoid a problem called "positional plagiocephaly," in which the baby's head develops a flattened shape from spending too much time in one position.

- *Don't* place the baby on soft surfaces like waterbeds or sofas. Don't put pillows, loose blankets, or stuffed toys near the baby.

- *Avoid tobacco smoke!* Don't smoke during pregnancy. After birth, don't allow anyone to smoke around the baby. Not smoking reduces many other child health risks as well.

- Giving your baby a pacifier at sleep time may help to reduce the risk of SIDS, but should not be started until breast feeding is well established.

- If bed sharing, parents shouldn't smoke or use alcohol or other drugs that could change the way they sleep.

- Avoid letting the baby get too hot in the crib—use pajamas appropriate for the room temperature. Don't overbundle the infant.

- Avoid products marketed as SIDS-prevention devices (for example, designed to keep the baby in a certain position or monitoring devices). None of these products has been proven effective in preventing SIDS.

- Home monitors (apnea/cardiac monitors) have not been shown to prevent SIDS, except in certain circumstances.

When should I call your office?

Call our office if you have any questions about SIDS risk factors or about strategies to reduce your child's risk of SIDS.

Where can I get more information?

The National Institute of Child Health and Human Development offers more information on SIDS and the "Back to Sleep" campaign on the Internet at *www.nichd.nih.gov/sids/sids.cfm*, or call 1-800-370-2943.

Vocal Cord Nodules (Screamer's Nodes)

Vocal cord nodules are the most common cause of prolonged hoarseness in children. Caused by repeatedly overusing or misusing the voice, they are sometimes called "screamer's nodes" or "singer's nodes." The nodules usually go away, and the voice returns to normal after the patient stops abusing his or her voice. Speech therapy (voice therapy) can be helpful.

What are vocal cord nodules and what do they look like?

Vocal cord nodules are swollen or hardened areas that develop on the edges of the vocal cords. They are caused by excessive yelling, screaming, or other forms of overusing the voice. For example, vocal cord nodules may result from excessive crying in infants, in toddlers from tantrums or screaming fits, and in teenagers from cheerleading or singing in a rock band. One episode of screening can irritate the vocal cords. However, for nodules to develop, the abuse must be repeated over a long time.

The nodules cause the voice to become hoarse or rough. It may be hard for your child to speak in a normal voice. Usually the damaged area will heal if the voice is allowed to rest and the misuse is stopped. Other treatments may be recommended, but surgery is rarely needed.

What are some possible complications of vocal cord nodules?

- Usually none. In infants and toddlers, the problem generally resolves as the child grows and the bad voice habits go away.

- However, if your child continues abusing his or her voice, the problem is likely to continue. In some cases, vocal cord damage requires special treatment.

- There is a risk that the nodules will come back after treatment, especially if the harmful voice habits are not corrected.

What increases your child's risk of vocal cord nodules?

Besides overusing the voice, other factors may increase the risk of vocal cord nodules:

- Smoking, or exposure to second-hand smoke.

- Gastroesophageal reflux disease (GERD): damage to the vocal cords caused by stomach acid.

How are vocal cord nodules diagnosed?

- Any child (or adult) with hoarseness lasting longer than 2 weeks should be examined by a doctor. There are other possible causes of hoarseness.

- The doctor usually makes the diagnosis by asking about overuse of the voice. If there's any doubt, or if treatment doesn't solve the problem, we may recommend a visit to a doctor specializing in ear, nose, and throat problems (an otorhinolaryngologist, or ENT).

  - The ENT doctor can examine the vocal cords using an instrument called a laryngoscope. If vocal cord nodules are present, the doctor can see how severe they are and recommend proper treatment.

How are vocal cord nodules treated?

- If vocal cord nodules are present, the first step is *resting the voice!* Your child will need to stop whatever habits are irritating the vocal cords, especially yelling and screaming. In many cases, your child's voice will improve after a few weeks' rest.

- For younger children, behavioral therapy may be needed. This involves rewarding and praising your child for not carrying out the behaviors that are irritating the vocal cords, like screaming and shouting. Younger children usually outgrow the behavior causing vocal cord nodules. Talk to your doctor if you need help handling temper tantrums.

- For children who are old enough to cooperate, voice therapy is helpful. This is usually done by a speech therapist, who can teach your child proper techniques of speaking to correct the harmful habits that led to vocal cord nodules. This type of therapy is especially helpful for singers, actors, or others who use their voices a lot.

- If any contributing factors are present (such as GERD), treatment may help to improve the voice problem as well.

- Rarely, surgery may be needed to remove the nodules that are causing voice changes. This is sometimes done with the use of lasers. After the operation, your child will need voice therapy.

When should I call your office?

Call our office if your child's hoarseness doesn't get better after a few weeks of resting the voice, or if the hoarseness returns.

Section XXIII • Skin and Nails

■ Acne ■

Acne is a very common skin condition, affecting 80% of teenagers. Topical (placed on the skin) medications, such as benzoyl peroxide or tretinoin (Retin-A), can treat and control acne in most patients. Other medications, such as oral antibiotics, certain birth control pills for girls, or oral isotretinoin (Acutane), may be used for more severe cases.

What is acne?

Acne refers to various types of pimples or blemishes. They occur because of blockage of the *sebaceous glands*. These glands produce an oil-like substance called sebum, which comes to the skin surface through hair follicles (pores). This blockage causes different types of pimples, depending on how much inflammation occurs. Certain bacteria that are normally found at the sebaceous glands are also involved in producing inflammation.

All kinds of acne start with a very small (cannot be seen) *comedone*—a blocked pore without inflammation. Acne generally occurs around puberty because the increase in sex hormones affects the sebaceous glands in a way that promotes blockage. There are a few types of acne, depending on where in the pore the blockage occurs and how much inflammation occurs. Medications used to treat acne are meant to unblock or prevent blockage of these pores and to control the inflammation.

Even when mild, acne can be very embarrassing for children and teens. Basic treatments can help them feel and look better. Treatment can also reduce the chances of scarring.

What does it look like?

There are a few kinds of pimples:

- Open or closed comedones ("blackheads" or "whiteheads")—very small bumps without redness or inflammation. As the names suggest, they have "whiteheads" (closed comedones) or "blackheads," with black specks in the center (open comedones).
- Reddened bumps (papules).
- Pimples filled with pus (pustules).
- Deeper nodules or cysts, which may occur if inflammation occurs deeper in the skin. This is the most severe type of acne and the most likely to cause scarring.

Pimples most commonly appear on the central part of the face, but they may also occur on the chest, upper back, or shoulder area.

Boys are more likely to have acne on the chest, where hair is developing.

As pimples heal, they may leave some redness and increased skin color, which take some months to go away. In more severe acne, scarring may occur.

What puts you at risk for acne?

- Around 80% of young people develop some amount of acne during puberty or the teen years.
- Anything that blocks the pores can make acne worse. This includes greasy ointments or creams, as well as hair products.
- Blockage of the pores causing pimples can occur under sweat bands worn during sports or exercise.
- Trying to "pop" pimples is likely to cause increased inflammation.
- Acne is not caused or made worse by eating particular foods.
- Emotional stress and fatigue may make acne worse.
- Acne may be less severe during the summer months (because of exposure to sunlight and subsequent peeling) and more severe in the winter.
- Acne may also be caused by certain medications, such as topical steroids, and by certain hormonal conditions.

What are some possible complications of acne?

- Scarring may occur in severe acne.
- Even if relatively mild, acne can have a significant emotional impact on teens.

How is acne treated?

There are a number of different medications to treat acne, and the doctor will decide which is best for you. If acne is severe or doesn't respond to treatment, we may recommend a visit to a dermatologist (a doctor specializing in skin diseases).

Basic treatments can keep acne under control until it goes away on its own:

- Cleaning with mild soap and water helps the skin look less oily but won't prevent pimples. Avoid repetitive cleaning, because it may cause the skin to become irritated and chapped.
- Products that contain alcohol or other substances that kill surface bacteria won't help prevent new acne pimples. In fact, they may make the skin more irritated.

Topical medications, or medications applied to the skin, can control most cases of acne that are not too severe. Often, more than one type of medication is used to get

459

the best results. Typically, it takes 4 to 8 weeks to see any improvement. Many of these medications can make the skin dry or irritated. If this is a problem, a "non-comedogenic" moisturizer can be used.

- Benzoyl peroxide is a commonly used and effective medication that is available over the counter (in products such as Clearasil). It comes in different strengths and is used once a day. Benzoyl peroxide is often used along with other drugs, such as Retin-A. However, it can be irritating to the skin, especially if too much is used. The water-based gel products are best.

- Tretinoin (Retin-A) is a form of vitamin A. It is very effective in preventing and treating blockage of the pores, which is how all acne starts. Tretinoin comes in different strengths and is used once a day. It can be very irritating to the skin, so it's best to start slow—for example, use every other day at first. This medication may also make your skin more sensitive to sunlight. For best results, apply 30 minutes after washing.

- Topical antibiotics can help control bacteria involved in causing acne and are often used in combination with other medications. They include topical erythromycin and clindamycin. These drugs are also available in combination with benzoyl peroxide in one product, such as Benzamycin or BenzaClin.

- Other topical medications are available, including azelaic acid (Azelex) and salicylic acid.

Oral antibiotics are often used if topical medications don't work or if acne is more severe. They are frequently used along with topical medications. Commonly used antibiotics include tetracycline, doxycycline, minocycline, and trimethoprim-sulfamethoxazole (Bactrim). These drugs have various side effects. Reactions to sunlight are especially common with doxycycline and tetracycline.

- Oral isotretinoin (Acutane) is used for nodular or cystic acne, or for severe acne that doesn't respond to other treatments. It is very effective, and its positive effects last for a long time—in about 30% of patients, the problem never comes back. Isotretinoin has many side effects. Most important, it is a "teratogen"—that means it will cause birth defects if taken during pregnancy. That is why all girls who are taking this drug are required to be on effective birth control, Other side effects include cracked lips, very dry skin, and increased levels of cholesterol and triglycerides in the blood. If needed, this medication is usually prescribed by a dermatologist.

- Birth control pills can be helpful for girls whose acne is difficult to control. They work by decreasing the amount of certain sex hormones.

- Some newer treatments are now available—for example, laser treatment for patients who have trouble taking the medications listed earlier or for whom they are not working well.

After you start treatment, your doctor may have you come back every few months to check on your acne. You may need a change in medications because of side effects or if your treatment is not working well.

When should I call your office?

Call our office if:

- Acne becomes a noticeable or socially embarrassing problem.

- Acne doesn't get better with recommended treatment.

Athlete's Foot (Tinea Pedis)

> Athlete's foot is an infection of the foot with certain types of fungi called dermatophytes. The infection causes itching, tenderness, and foot odor. Medications can be used to kill the fungus, though treatment may need to be continued for several weeks.

What is athlete's foot?

Athlete's foot is a common foot infection caused by infection with certain types of fungi, called dermatophytes—these are the same fungi that cause ringworm and jock itch. Dermatophytes grow best in moist, damp places, which is why infection commonly spreads in the shower areas of gyms and swimming pools.

Active people who wear tight, thick socks and heavy shoes are at increased risk of getting this infection, especially in hot weather. Athlete's foot is more common in teens than in younger children.

What does it look like?

- The feet become itchy and tender, especially in the spaces between the toes. One or both feet may be affected.

- Peeling and cracking of the skin occur between and under the toes and on soles of the feet. Unpleasant foot odor may occur.

- Sometimes, especially in younger children, blisters and pustules (pimples) develop.

- If the infection is present for a long time, the bottom of the foot may become thickened and scaly.

What are some possible complications of athlete's foot?

- Even with treatment, the infection may be difficult to eliminate completely or may come back frequently.

- The infection may spread to other areas, especially the toenails.

Can athlete's foot be prevented?

It's a good idea to wear shower shoes or sandals in public showers and locker rooms, rather than going barefoot.

How is athlete's foot diagnosed?

The doctor may recognize athlete's foot from the appearance of the infection. Other conditions, such as eczema or irritation from some type of material in the shoes (contact dermatitis), may look like athlete's foot.

To be sure of the diagnosis, the doctor may collect a sample by scraping the infected area. He or she can then look at the sample under the microscope to see if fungus is present or may send it for culture. If culture is performed, it may take a week or longer to get the results.

How is athlete's foot treated?

- It is important to keep the feet clean and dry.

- For mild cases, a topical (placed on the skin) antifungal power or cream may be effective—for example, Desenex or Tinactin. Your doctor may recommend a prescription antifungal cream. Apply the medication to the foot for at least a few weeks.

- The infection can return quickly and can be hard to control with just topical medications. Some patients may need to take oral antifungal medications plus a longer period of treatment with topical medications.

- Athlete's foot sometimes becomes a chronic or frequent problem. Treatment may need to be repeated.

When should I call your office?

Call our office if the infection doesn't clear up or if it returns after treatment.

Eczema

There are many causes of eczema (atopic dermatitis), a skin rash that may cause severe itching. Children with eczema often have allergies. Some children "outgrow" eczema, while for others it is a lasting problem. Children with atopic dermatitis have high rates of other allergic diseases, including asthma and hay fever (allergic rhinitis).

What is eczema?

Eczema is a chronic skin disorder—a rash that comes and goes and can cause severe itching. Atopic dermatitis is the most common cause of eczema in children. It is often seen in children with allergies or whose families have lots of allergies.

Eczema is very common, affecting more than 10% of children in the United States. Especially when it appears in babies and young children, eczema may be the first sign that your child has allergies.

What does it look like?

- An itchy skin rash. The itching may be severe, making it difficult for your child to sleep.

- The rash may look red and scaly or crusting. Small blisters may occur, especially in African-American children.

- The skin is often dry, including the hair and scalp. The skin may also become thickened.

- The rash can appear in many different parts of the body. In babies, it often occurs on the cheeks and forehead, then spreads to the trunk, arms, and legs. As children grow, the rash may spread to other areas and become quite large. In older children, the rash commonly occurs in the elbow crease and behind the knees, wrists, and ankles. In teens and adults, eczema may appear on the face, neck, and back.

- The skin where the rash is located may become darkened. This discoloration may take some time to clear up.

- The rash may get worse in areas where your child scratches. The skin may become infected.

What causes eczema?

Atopic dermatitis may be caused by anything your child is allergic to, including:

- Foods, such as peanuts and eggs.

- Pollen—eczema may occur at the same time or before symptoms of asthma or hay fever.

- House dust mites.

Other causes may lead to eczema or make the skin rash worse. Some examples are:

- Anything that irritates the skin, such as wool clothing, skin lotions or ointments, or household cleaners or chemicals.

- Weather extremes—especially high heat and humidity, causing increased sweating.

- Sometimes no specific cause of eczema is found.

What are some possible complications of eczema?

- Occasionally, areas of eczema may become infected with bacteria. If so, the skin may become redder and more crusty and start oozing.

- Skin problems related to scratching, including scarring.

- Children with eczema have high rates of other allergic diseases, including potentially severe allergic reactions.

What puts your child at risk of eczema?

- Allergies, including food allergies, asthma, or hay fever (allergic rhinitis).

- Having parents or other family members with allergies.

- Certain types of clothing: wool may irritate the skin, while nylon or other synthetic fabrics trap sweat.

- Extremes of weather, especially high heat and humidity.

- Girls are affected about twice as often as boys.

Can eczema be prevented?

- There is no known way to prevent eczema.

- If the cause is allergies, avoiding exposure to whatever your child is allergic to may help to reduce eczema outbreaks.

- You can learn to take care of your child's skin and to avoid anything that has triggered or worsened eczema outbreaks in the past:

  - Avoid any products that irritate your child's skin, such as wool, harsh soaps, and perfumes.

  - Use mild, unscented soaps. Right after bathing, put a nonperfumed moisturizer on the skin.

  - Wash new clothes before your child wears them.

  - Have your child wear loose, cotton clothing to absorb sweat.

- Sports involving intense sweating or heavy uniforms or equipment may make eczema worse. Rinse off skin after swimming.
- To reduce damage caused by scratching, keep your child's fingernails short. Wearing soft gloves at night may be helpful.

How is eczema treated?

- If your child's eczema is caused by a food allergy, avoid that food. Some common food allergens can be difficult to avoid (for example, peanuts or soy).
- If the cause is allergy to house dust mite, special pillow and mattress covers may be helpful. Keep household dust under control.
- *Simple treatments* can help to keep your child's eczema under control:
  - Use moisturizers. Use unscented moisturizers, because perfumes may irritate the skin.
  - For more severe eczema, have your child soak in lukewarm water for 20 minutes, then apply a moisture-retaining skin ointment (such as Vaseline, Aquaphor, or Eucerin).
- *Steroid creams or ointments* are an important part of treatment.
  - To avoid side effects, these medications should be used carefully, as directed by your doctor.
  - Avoid using strong steroids on the face or diaper area, unless recommended by your doctor.

- Steroid creams or ointments usually don't interfere with your child's growth, unless used at high doses for a long time.
- Other topical treatments may be helpful:
  - Products containing coal tar can help to keep your child's eczema under control. They can also help to reduce the amount of steroid cream needed.
  - Protopic cream (generic name: tacrolimus) and Elidel cream (generic name: pimecrolimus) are helpful and are not steroids.
  - Treatment with special ultraviolet light (phototherapy) is sometimes recommended.
  - Antihistamines such as Benadryl (generic name: diphenhydramine) may be used to control itching. Because these drugs cause drowsiness, they may be particularly useful at night.
- If your child has severe eczema, a visit to a dermatologist (a specialist in treating skin conditions) may be helpful.

When should I call your office?

Call our office if:

- Your child's rash does not improve with treatment, or if there are signs of infection (redness, crusting, oozing).
- Your child develops fever or uncontrolled itching during a flare-up of eczema.

■ Fungal Infections of the Nails (Onychomycosis, Tinea Unguium) ■

Infections of the nails with fungi are uncommon in children, but they do occur. These infections are caused by dermatophytes—the same fungi that cause ringworm and athlete's foot. The nails slowly become discolored, thickened, and brittle. Oral antifungal drugs are effective, but may require treatment for up to 3 months.

What are fungal infections of the nails?

Although not as often as adults, children and teens may get fungal infections of the nails. These infections are usually caused by dermatophytes—the same fungi that cause ringworm and athlete's foot. In fact, when a nail does become infected, it is usually a toenail and occurs with athlete's foot. These infections are also called "onychomycosis" or "tinea unguium."

Candida, a type of yeast, can also cause nail infection, usually on the hand. These infections are less common.

What do they look like?

- The infection usually starts at the end of the nail and develops very slowly.

- The nail becomes whitish in color; over time, it becomes yellow or brown.

- The nail becomes thicker, with a collection of dead skin underneath.

- If the infection is present for a long time, the nail can become loose.

Nail infections caused by *Candida* are different. They usually occur on the hand, and there is inflammation (redness, swelling) of the skin around the nail.

Bacterial infections only involve the skin around the nail. These infections produce redness, swelling, and pain (like an ingrown toenail).

What increases your child's risk of fungal infections of the nails?

- Because the fungi that cause nail infections like warm, moist areas, they are most likely to spread in hot, humid weather or when your child wears heavy shoes during long periods of exercise or activity.

- Athlete's foot (fungal infection of the foot) may be present as well.

How are fungal infections of the nails diagnosed?

Dermatophyte infections of the nails can look like a number of different conditions—for example, psoriasis or trauma. Because treatment involves taking oral antifungal drugs, the doctor may perform some tests to be sure of the diagnosis.

The doctor may obtain a sample of the nail and examine it under the microscope to see if fungus is present. The doctor may also send a sample for fungal culture. It may take a week or longer to get the culture results.

How are fungal infections of the nails treated?

- Several different antifungal medications can be used to treat dermatophyte infections of the nails. Some commonly used drugs are terbinafine (Lamisil) and itraconzole (Sporonox). Your child will have to continue taking these drugs for a fairly long time—up to 3 months, depending on the drug and whether the infection is in the toenail or on the fingernail.

- The antifungal medications used to treat nail infections can cause side effects, especially liver problems. Close follow-up is needed, including tests of liver function.

- After treatment, there is a significant risk that the infection will return. Even if treatment is successful, it takes several months for the nail to grow back completely.

When should I call your office?

Call our office if your child has a fungal nail infection that does not improve with treatment or comes back after treatment.

During treatment with oral antifungal medications, call our office if your child develops abdominal pain, especially on the right side.

Head Lice (Pediculosis Capitis)

Head lice is the presence of a bug called a "louse" living on the scalp. It can cause itching of the scalp, which is sometimes severe. Outbreaks of head lice may occur at day-care centers and schools. The eggs of the louse, called "nits," are often visible on the hair. Special shampoos are needed to kill the lice and nits. Using a fine-toothed comb can help remove them from your child's hair. Washing and cleaning items like clothes and hairbrushes may be needed to eliminate lice from your home.

What are head lice?

Lice are tiny bugs that live on the human body, where they feed on blood. Although there are different types of lice (body lice, pubic lice), head lice are the main problem in children. This condition is also called *pediculosis capitis.*

Head lice are spread from person to person, or from contact with items used by a person with lice (such as brushes, combs, or towels). The lice can live for a few days on objects without being on a person. The lice themselves are hard to see, but you can see their eggs (called nits) stuck to your child's hair.

What do they look like?

- Itching of the scalp is the most common symptom. However, many parents find out about the infestation when a note is sent home from school or day care.

- Nits (the eggs of the lice) can be seen. They are tiny white specks, stuck to the side of a hair. The nits are difficult to remove from the hair—they won't just come off easily, like dandruff. The lice are harder to see—they are very small, gray-white bugs.

- Itching may lead to scratch marks on the scalp and neck.

- Inflammation may lead to enlarged lymph nodes (glands) in the neck and back of the head.

- Occasionally, infection with bacteria (usually "staph") may be caused by scratching. This results in crusted, oozing sores (soreness, tenderness) of the scalp, often with visible pus.

What are some possible complications of head lice?

Although not very common, the main complication is bacterial infection, caused by scratching.

What increases your child's risk of head lice?

- Contact with other children who have head lice, or with their personal items, is the main risk factor. Head lice are a common problem, especially in places like schools and day-care centers. Having head lice doesn't mean your child isn't clean—the lice spread easily from person to person.

- Lice infestations are most common in warm climates and during the summer months.

Can head lice be prevented?

Most of the time, there is no practical way to avoid head lice. The personal items of children with head lice, such as combs and hats, need to be cleaned. If there are cases of head lice in the school or community, children should not share personal items.

How are head lice diagnosed?

The diagnosis should be confirmed by finding a louse or live nits on the scalp.

- To find lice, the hair is repeatedly combed with a fine-toothed comb, looking for the bugs.

- If nits are seen within one-quarter inch of the scalp, they are probably alive. Nits seen farther up on the hair are not alive. If the diagnosis is in doubt, the doctor may look at the nit under a microscope.

- Sometimes, especially in outbreaks, nits and lice are found before any symptoms occur.

How are head lice treated?

The goal of treatment is to eliminate the lice from your child's hair and from the home environment. Careful attention may be needed to achieve this.

Medications—Several products can be used to help eliminate head lice. Many are available at drug stores, without a prescription. These are pesticides and should be used as directed.

- One percent permethrin (Nix) is usually effective in killing lice and nits and is often recommended. Apply this product to your child's hair and leave it there for 10 minutes before rinsing. Another application is often recommended after a week or so.

- Your doctor may recommend another product. Other over-the-counter products include RID, A200, and Kwell, which also contain pesticides. These medications should be used as directed and not overused.

- Some patients are hard to cure and need prescription medications. Malathion (Ovide) is a lotion that is also a pesticide and is sometimes used for difficult cases. Some oral medications are sometimes used, such as trimethoprim-sulfamethoxazole (Bactrim), an antibiotic, or ivermectin (Stromectol).

- Talk to your doctor before using lice-killing products on newborns and young infants!

- Other over-the-counter products are available, but less is known about their effectiveness.

Combing—A fine-toothed comb can help in removing all nits from the hair. This can be difficult to do, because the nits produce a substance that makes them stick very closely. An equal mix of vinegar and water may help eliminate the nits, or your doctor may be able to recommend a product. Combing must be done carefully, as it is easy to overlook the tiny nits.

- Removing nits is usually done for appearance—after treatment, any remaining nits are usually dead.

Other family members should be checked for lice and live nits. Family members who sleep with a child who has head lice should probably be treated.

Careful cleaning of your home is probably a good idea to eliminate lice and nits:

- Vacuum all areas of your home carefully, including floors and furniture.

- Wash in hot water all items your child might have come into contact with, including clothes, sheets, and blankets. Hats, jackets, and other articles need to be washed or dry-cleaned as well. Items that cannot be cleaned can be placed in a sealed plastic bag for 2 weeks.

- Brushes and combs can be treated with lice-killing products and cleaned in boiling water, but it may be easier just to throw them away.

When can my child go back to school? It is reasonable to let children return to school or day care after the scalp and hair have been treated with one of the products listed earlier. However, your school board may have a different policy.

When should I call your office?

Call our office if:

- Your child has symptoms of infection (crusty, scaling rash on the scalp) or a rash on the neck, ears, or elsewhere on the body.

- You have difficulty eliminating lice or nits or if the infestation returns after treatment.

Heat Rash (Miliaria Rubra)

Heat rash is a common skin rash that occurs when there is increased sweating under warm, humid conditions. It is caused by blockage of the sweat glands. It most commonly appears as small red bumps, sometimes looking like little blisters, within the skin. The skin may feel prickly when touched. The rash most commonly develops on the neck, upper chest, and back and in skin folds. Heat rash usually clears by keeping the affected area cooler.

What is heat rash?

There are a few types of heat rash, but the most common is called miliaria rubra, or "prickly heat." It occurs when there is a lot of sweating and blockage of the sweat glands. This most often occurs during hot weather. However, it can also result from being overdressed, especially in babies, or from fevers. Miliaria rubra is a harmless rash that clears up quickly.

What does it look like?

- Little red bumps appear on the skin, sometimes looking like small blisters or pimples. The skin often feels prickly when touched.

- The rash may be a little itchy—but otherwise, there are no other symptoms.

- The rash most commonly occurs in body creases or places where clothes rub up against the skin. Common sites include the neck, diaper area, armpit, upper back, and chest.

- Another form of heat rash, called "miliaria crystallina," occurs most often in newborns. This rash looks like tiny, clear blisters (not red) that break easily.

- Heat rash goes away within a few days, especially after keeping the area cooler.

What increases your child's risk of heat rash?

- Excessive exposure to high temperatures and humidity.

- Wearing too many heavy clothes for the weather (even on cold days).

How is heat rash treated?

- Usually, cooling your child down is all the treatment needed. On hot days, get your child out of the heat and into an air-conditioned room, if possible. Remove any excess clothing. A cool compress (a washcloth soaked in cool water) can be helpful.

- No need to put anything on the skin—for example, lotions or creams. These may actually make the rash worse by contributing to blockage of the sweat glands.

- The rash should clear up within a few days. If not, call our office.

When should I call your office?

Call our office if:

- Heat rash doesn't clear up within a few days.

- Your child has repeated episodes of heat rash.

Other conditions can cause a rash similar to heat rash. Call our office if your child has other symptoms, including fever, or just "acts sick."

Ingrown Toenails

Ingrown toenails are a common and painful problem occurring when the edge of a toenail grows into the skin. Keeping the nails properly trimmed is the best way to prevent ingrown toenails. If severe, simple surgery involving removal of part of the nail can be done to correct the problem.

What are ingrown toenails?

An ingrown toenail happens when the edge of a nail, often on the big toe, grows into the skin at the side of the nail. This can cause redness, swelling, and pain. There may also be infection in the area. Simple prevention and treatment steps are effective.

What do they look like?

- Ingrown toenails cause soreness and redness along the edge of the nail, in the little fold of skin next to the nail. Depending on severity, the area may be quite painful.
- The inside edge of the nail of the big toe is affected most often.
- In some cases, a sore may develop in the skin alongside the nail. If this happens, there is a risk that the area may become infected.
- Pus may be seen draining from the area.
- Redness and tenderness from infection can extend beyond the skin bordering the nail (cellulitis).

What causes ingrown toenails?

- Improper cutting or trimming of nails can cause an ingrown toenail. Toenails should be cut straight across—not in a curve—so that the nail edges grow past the fold of skin alongside the nail.
- Tight-fitting shoes that put pressure on the toes can increase the risk of ingrown nails.

What are some possible complications of ingrown toenails?

- Infection may occur in the inflamed skin around the ingrown toenail.
- Ingrown toenails are a commonly recurrent problem.

Can ingrown toenails be prevented?

To prevent ingrown toenails or to keep them from coming back:

- Wear properly fitted shoes; avoid shoes with high heels or pointed toes.
- Keep nails properly trimmed—cut straight across, not in a curve. Don't tear or pick at the nails, especially at the corners.

How are ingrown toenails treated?

If the problem is not too severe, you may be able to treat it at home:

- Soak the foot in warm water a few times a day to soften the skin.
- Place a small piece of cotton under the edge of the nail.
- Leave the cotton in place until the nail grows out over the skin fold.
- Once the nail has grown out, keep the nails properly trimmed to prevent the problem from coming back.
- If infection is suspected, antibiotics will be prescribed.

If home treatment doesn't work or if pain and tenderness are getting worse, the doctor may recommend a minor operation to correct the problem:

- The area is numbed with a local anesthetic during the procedure, and the surgeon removes the part of the nail that is growing into the skin.
- In some situations, the entire nail is removed.
- Follow the surgeon's instructions for care of the area after surgery.

When should I call your office?

Call our office if:

- Pain and swelling of ingrown toenail continue or get worse despite home treatment or if the problem recurs after treatment.
- Signs of infection develop (increasing redness and tenderness, sometimes with an oozing or crusting wound).

Jock Itch (Tinea Cruris)

Jock itch is infection of the groin area with certain types of fungi called dermatophytes. The infection causes a rash in the groin, with itching that is sometimes severe. The infection usually clears up after treatment with antifungal medications and by avoiding moisture and irritation in the groin area.

What is jock itch?

Jock itch is a common infection of the groin (crotch) area caused by infection with certain types of fungi, called dermatophytes, the same fungi that cause ringworm and athlete's foot. Jock itch is also called "tinea cruris."

Jock itch most often occurs when the groin area is moist and irritated—for example, in teenaged boys wearing a tight-fitting athletic supporter ("jock strap"). However, this infection can also occur in females.

What does it look like?

- It usually starts as a small, scaly, red patch in the groin area, especially in areas around skin creases.

- Over a few days, the rash spreads over the inner thighs, although usually not the scrotum (the sac containing the testicles). Distinct areas of scaly rash may occur.

- The rash can be very itchy, especially at first. It may spread to other areas of the body.

What increases your child's risk of jock itch?

Jock itch occurs more often when the groin area gets moist and irritated, as on hot, sweaty days. Active people who wear tight-fitting clothes and underwear are at increased risk. Jock itch is also more common in people who are overweight or obese.

How is jock itch diagnosed?

- The doctor may recognize jock itch from the appearance of the rash. Other conditions, such as yeast infections or irritation from clothing or products used in the area (contact dermatitis), may look like jock itch.

- To be sure of the diagnosis, the doctor may collect a sample by scraping the rash. He or she can then look at the sample under the microscope to see if fungus is present or may send it for culture. If culture is performed, it may take a week or longer to get the results.

How is jock itch treated?

- Keep the groin area clean and as dry as possible. Wear loose-fitting cotton underwear.

- Use topical (placed on the skin) antifungal medications. Over-the-counter products like Tinactin may be effective, or your doctor may recommend a prescription medication. The rash usually clears up after a few weeks of treatment.

When should I call your office?

Call our office if the rash doesn't clear up or if it returns after treatment.

Minor Burns

Burns are a common and potentially serious cause of injuries in children. Burns that extend to the deeper layers of the skin (second- and third-degree burns) and cover a large part of the body surface (10% or more) require hospital treatment. Hospital treatment is also needed for burns involving large portions of the hands, feet, or genitals. Especially with young children, it is very important to take steps to prevent burns.

What are burn injuries in children?

Children are at high risk of burns. Burns are the second most common cause of accidental death in children and teens (after motor vehicle crashes). Scald injuries (caused by hot water) are especially common in children under age 4. Most burns are thermal, caused by flame or heat. Other types of burns include electrical and chemical burns.

Small burns of the skin surface can be safely managed at home. However, larger or deeper burns require medical attention. Burns that are very large or involve a large proportion of the hands, feet, or genitals often require hospital care. Fortunately, most burns in children are not that severe.

Especially with young children, it is very important to take steps to prevent fires and burn injuries. These steps include wearing flame-retardant clothing, having working smoke detectors, paying attention to water-heater settings, and not smoking.

What do they look like?

In assessing burn injuries, there are three main things the doctor needs to know: how deep the burn is, how large the burn is, and whether there are any other injuries.

- *How deep is the burn?* Burns are classified as first-degree, second-degree, or third-degree:

  - First-degree: Mild surface burns. The skin is red, painful, and sometimes swollen, like a mild sunburn. There are no blisters, although skin peeling may occur. Pain usually goes away in 2 or 3 days.

  - Second-degree: Burns that destroy the top layer of the skin (epidermis) and cause damage to parts of the deeper layer (dermis). You may see blisters on the injured skin. Some second-degree burns are extremely painful. There is a risk of infection, which can delay healing. Milder second-degree burns heal within a week or two, but more severe burns take longer to heal and may require skin grafting (surgery to cover the area damaged by the burn).

  - Third-degree: Burns that destroy both the epidermis and dermis. Because the skin in the area is completely

destroyed, it cannot heal without surgery or scarring. These are serious injuries with many possible complications.

What are some possible complications of burns?

- Infection is one of the most important complications of burns. The skin plays an important role in protecting against germs. If it is damaged or destroyed, the risk of infection is much higher. Even for relatively minor second-degree burns, infection can lead to longer healing time.

- Scarring may occur after more severe burns. The more skin damage that has occurred, the less the skin will be able to heal normally.

What increases your child's risk of burns?

- Children under age 4 are at high risk of scald injuries—for example, from being put in a bath that is much too hot or pulling a pot full of hot liquid off the stove.

- Playing with matches is a major source of fires and burns in young children.

Can burns be prevented?

- Make sure your home has working smoke detectors! This is the most important step in preventing fatal house fires. Check smoke detector batteries regularly.

- Don't set the hot water heater thermostat too high. A setting of 120°F (49°C) is recommended.

- Be careful with matches, lighters, and smoking materials. Keep them out of the reach of young children.

- Choose flame-retardant pajamas and other clothing for infants and toddlers.

How are burns treated?

Seek medical attention for large burns, burns that cause visible skin damage (worse than a minor sunburn), or burns that are causing a lot of pain.

- For first-degree burns (no blisters, just redness and sometimes swelling):

  - Use a cool compress (washcloth soaked in cool water) and pain medications such as ibuprofen.

  - Pain clears up in 2 to 3 days; peeling may occur.

- For mild second-degree burns (with blisters), the main goals are to prevent infection and speed healing. Unless the burn is very small, see the doctor for second-degree burns.

- Leave blisters alone. Cover the burned area with an antiseptic cream, such as bacitracin or another ointment recommended by the doctor, and a bandage.

- Each day, remove the bandage, wash the area with lukewarm water, and apply antiseptic cream and a fresh bandage. Give pain medication, if needed, 1 hour before dressing changes.

- For some burns, the doctor may want your child to return to the office every few days to remove dead skin (*debridement*) and check on the healing process.

- The burn should heal within 10 to 20 days. If not, call our office—it may be that the burn was deeper than originally thought. It can be particularly difficult to judge the depth of scald burns.

(!) More severe burns require medical attention! See below.

When should I call your office?

After home or doctor's office treatment for burns, call our office if your child has any of the following:

- Signs of infection: increased pain, redness or swelling of the burned area, fluid or pus draining from the wound.

- Severe pain or pain that is not controlled by medications.

Get immediate medical attention for:

- Burns producing blisters, unless very small.

- Burns on the hands, feet, or genitals.

- All electrical burns.

Pityriasis Rosea

Pityriasis rosea is a common rash in children and young adults. It usually looks like round or oval scaly pink/brown patches and occurs mainly on the chest and back, although the rash may appear at other places as well. Itching occurs sometimes. Pityriasis rosea usually goes away without any specific treatment, but it may take several weeks to clear up completely.

What is pityriasis rosea?

Pityriasis rosea is a common rash in teens and young adults, although it may occur in younger children. The cause is unknown—infection with a virus may be involved. The rash usually begins gradually, with a single "herald patch," followed by a more widespread rash on the back, chest, and abdomen. Other patterns are possible.

What does it look like?

- Before the rash develops, your child may have symptoms of a cold or "flu," such as fever, aches, and swollen glands.

- The rash often begins with a herald patch—a single pink or brown circle or oval up to a few inches in size. The spot is scaly with raised edges.

- Five to ten days later, smaller round or oval spots develop, usually on the trunk, shoulders, and upper thighs. Less often, the rash may spread to the face and scalp and further down the arms and legs or may appear only in those areas. New spots come out over a few days.

- These new spots are also pink/brown with scaly, raised edges, like the herald spot. Less often, the spots may just be bumps.

- The spots tend to follow certain lines of the skin, which can result in a typical pattern on the back or chest. This pattern is often described as like a "Christmas tree."

- Itching may or may not be present.

- The rash clears up on its own, but that may take a while, from a few weeks to a few months.

What are some possible complications of pityriasis rosea?

- Usually, there are no complications.

- After the rash clears up, the skin may be slightly darker or lighter where the spots were. This goes away eventually, after several weeks or months.

How is pityriasis rosea diagnosed and treated?

Diagnosis and testing. The doctor usually recognizes pityriasis rosea from the appearance of the rash. It can be confused with other skin conditions, such as eczema. The herald patch can sometimes be mistaken for ringworm (tinea corporis). In some cases, tests will be performed to exclude other possible causes.

Treatment. Usually, no treatment is needed. The rash goes away on its own. It may take a few weeks to a few months to clear up completely.

- Moisturizing lotion, or a weak steroid cream or ointment, may help relieve scaling and itching of the skin.

When should I call your office?

Call our office if the rash of pityriasis rosea hasn't started to clear up within a few weeks or if it goes away but comes back.

Poison Ivy

Poison ivy is a plant that causes a very itchy, red rash. The rash is an allergic response to a chemical in the plant's resin (sap). The resin can remain on skin, clothing, pets, and other surfaces, so it can cause a rash even if your child doesn't come into direct contact with the poison ivy plant. Other plants, including poison oak and poison sumac, can cause similar reactions.

What is poison ivy?

Poison ivy is a plant that causes an intense, sometimes severe skin rash with itching. The rash develops after the skin comes into contact with a chemical found in the plant's resin. It is a type of allergic reaction called "contact dermatitis."

In addition to direct contact with the plant, the resin can be spread over other parts of the body by scratching or rubbing, or from contact with clothing or animal fur. If one has had poison ivy before ("sensitized"), the rash usually develops within a few days after coming into contact with the resin. If not, it may take longer—up to a few weeks.

Poison ivy is found in most parts of the United States and can grow as either a shrub or vine. The leaves are notched and grow in threes on a stem. *Poison oak* and *poison sumac* are less widespread plants that cause similar allergic contact dermatitis reactions. Poison oak is a shrubby plant with three leaves that look like oak leaves. Poison sumac is a woody plant with paired leaves on either side of a long stem.

What does it look like?

A red, itchy rash develops in areas of the skin that have come into contact with the poison ivy resin.

- Red bumps appear, often with blisters of different sizes.

- The skin may become crusted, scabbed, and oozing.

- The rash can appear in streaks where the skin brushed up against the plant. However, other patterns are possible, depending on how the resin got into contact with the skin. For example, if a dog has been in poison ivy and your child then pets or hugs it, the rash will appear in those areas that touched the pet.

- The rash may be mild or severe, depending on whether you've had poison ivy before and how your particular skin reacts to it.

- If the rash is severe, especially when it's on the face, lots of swelling may occur.

- The rash and itching often get worse for a few days before they start to get better. It may take a few weeks for the rash to go away completely.

What are some possible complications of poison ivy?

- Once you've had one reaction to poison ivy, future reactions are likely to appear more rapidly and be more severe.

- Especially with scratching, bacterial infections of the skin (such as impetigo) may occur.

Can poison ivy be prevented?

- The best prevention is to recognize poison ivy and stay away from it!

- Another good preventive step is to wear long sleeves and pants while walking in wooded areas. (This also lowers the risk of tick bites.) However, the resin can still get on your clothes if you come into contact with poison ivy. Wash your clothes as soon as possible.

- If you come into contact with poison ivy, wash the skin as soon as possible—preferably within 30 minutes. Wash thoroughly, including under the fingernails.

- If trying to eliminate the poison ivy plant, don't burn it because smoke can carry the resin onto the skin, particularly the face.

How is poison ivy treated?

Once the rash of poison ivy has appeared, treatments can help control itching and inflammation.

- Mild cases are treated with lotions that reduce itching, such as calamine lotion, or a weak steroid cream, such as 1% hydrocortisone. Both can be bought over the counter.

- A cool compress (washcloth soaked in cool water) can be helpful, especially if the rash is crusting or oozy.

- For more severe cases, the doctor may prescribe a stronger topical (placed on the skin) steroid cream. These medications help reduce inflammation and itching.

- The doctor may also recommend oral antihistamines to help control itching.

- For severe cases—including swelling of the face or genitals—the doctor may prescribe an oral steroid for a week or longer.

Removing poison ivy—If you have the poison ivy plant on your property, it can be difficult to eliminate. Herbicides may work but can kill other plants as well. You can eliminate the plant by pulling it up by hand, but make sure to wear appropriate gloves and other protective clothing. *Never burn poison ivy!* (For more removal tips, see the Internet resource listed at the end of this topic.)

When should I call your office?

Call our office if any of the following occurs:

- Medications aren't helping after a few days.

- The rash becomes more severe or starts to involve the face or genital area.

- Signs of bacterial infection develop, especially pus oozing from skin blisters.

Where can I get more information?

The U.S. Food and Drug Administration has a useful article on "Outsmarting Poison Ivy and Its Cousins," including more tips for prevention, treatment, and removal. Go online at *http://www.fda.gov/fdac/features/796_ivy.html.*

■ Psoriasis ■

Psoriasis is a common, chronic skin disease that often develops in childhood or adolescence. It causes outbreaks of a scaly rash—most commonly raised, red patches covered with scale, which is often silvery. The rash may develop anywhere on the body but is especially common on the scalp, knees, and elbows. The nails may be involved, and some patients may have arthritis. There is no cure for psoriasis, but treatments can help relieve symptoms.

What is psoriasis?

Psoriasis is a skin disease consisting of outbreaks of skin rash (exacerbations), alternating with episodes of clearing (remissions). It's difficult to predict how often the outbreaks will occur. The disease can affect many different areas of the body; involvement of the nails is fairly common. One form of psoriasis, called "guttate psoriasis," usually follows infections like a sore throat. Some patients develop arthritis.

One third of people with psoriasis develop the disease by age 20. Psoriasis often runs in families, although the exact cause is unknown. Current research suggests that psoriasis is caused by an abnormal immune system reaction. Psoriasis is a chronic (long-lasting) disease with no known cure. However, effective treatments can help keep psoriasis outbreaks under control.

What does it look like?

- The skin rash consists of red, raised patches, which are often itchy.

- The patches develop a scaly, silvery, or yellow-white appearance. These patches are often called "plaques."

- If the scale is removed (for example, scratched off), areas of pinpoint bleeding may occur.

- The rash may occur anywhere, but common sites include the scalp, knees, elbows, stomach, buttocks, and genital area. Abnormalities of the fingernails and toenails are fairly common. The nails may develop pits and become discolored. The skin underneath the nails may become thickened, or the nails may become loose.

- Outbreaks are followed by periods of clearing. As the psoriasis rash heals, it may leave areas of lighter than normal skin color. This is most noticeable in patients with dark skin. Sometimes psoriasis causes severe outbreaks that are bad enough to require hospital treatment.

- Guttate psoriasis, seen more often in children, consists of small, round or oval patches. The rash occurs most often on the chest, abdomen, back, and upper arms and legs. It

often follows a case of strep throat or other infections with streptococcal bacteria.

- Other patterns are possible, but uncommon. These include having many pustules ("pustular psoriasis") or when involved skin areas become very red ("psoriatic erythroderma").

What causes psoriasis?

- The exact cause is unknown. Psoriasis seems to be an "immune-mediated" disease—the person's own immune system is causing the problem in the skin. Psoriasis is not contagious.

- Genetic factors seem to play a role, especially when psoriasis develops in children.

- Many factors may increase the risk of psoriasis outbreaks, including minor injuries, dryness of the skin, changes in the weather, or even stress.

What are some possible complications of psoriasis?

- Arthritis develops in some patients ("psoriatic arthritis"). The arthritis is generally mild but can be severe. Psoriatic arthritis is less common in children.

- Skin infections may occur. This complication is most common in plaques that have become cracked or injured due to scratching.

- Psoriasis is a chronic disease (lasting a long time) that can be embarrassing for children and adults. Psychological difficulties can occur.

What increases your child's risk of psoriasis?

Girls are affected more often than boys. Whites are affected more often than other racial/ethnic groups.

How is psoriasis treated?

Unfortunately, there is no cure for psoriasis. However, treatments are available to relieve symptoms, and some practical steps can help keep psoriasis outbreaks under control. Many patients with psoriasis are treated by a *dermatologist* (a doctor specializing in skin diseases), especially if outbreaks are severe or frequent. Treatment options depend on your child's age, the type of psoriasis, and the location and severity of the rash.

General skin care—Use moisturizers and other types of skin creams to help reduce dryness and irritation of the skin. Moisturizers also help reduce itching and scratching, which can lead to further skin damage. These products work best if applied right after a shower or bath.

Medications. Various medications are used, including the following:

- Topical (applied to the skin) steroid creams or lotions.

- Tar preparations—These topical medications are used less frequently now. They are available as shampoos (for example, T-Gel) or as products to be placed in bathwater or applied directly to the skin.

- Calcipotriene (Dovonex)—A topical medication related to vitamin D.

- Topical retinoids—Drugs related to vitamin A, including tazarotene (Tazorac).

- Calcineurin inhibitors—For example, tacrolimus (Protopic) or pimecrolimus (Elidel). These drugs help by affecting the immune system in the skin.

Very severe outbreaks of psoriasis can be serious and may require immediate evaluation, sometimes followed by hospital treatment. Get medical help immediately if your child has a psoriasis outbreak covering all or most of the body surface, especially if the rash is very red.

Psychological issues—Living with psoriasis can be difficult, causing embarrassment and self-esteem issues. If psoriasis is having a major impact on your child's emotions or self-esteem, talking to a psychologist or other mental health professional may be helpful.

When should I call your office?

Call your dermatologist or our office if:

- Your child is having severe or frequent outbreaks of psoriasis.

- The skin shows any signs of infection (redness, oozing, or crusting).

- Medication side effects occur.

If your child has a very severe psoriasis outbreak covering all or most of the body surface, get medical help immediately.

Where can I get more information?

The National Psoriasis Foundation: go online at *www.psoriasis.org* or call 800-723-9166.

Ringworm (Tinea Corporis)

Ringworm is infection of the skin with types of fungi called dermatophytes. The name comes from the distinct, circle-shaped rash produced by this infection. The infection is spread by contact with infected people or animals or with objects that have infected scales on them. Treatment with topical (placed on the skin) antifungal medications is usually effective.

What is ringworm and how is it spread?

Ringworm is a common infection caused by various dermatophytes, a type of fungus. Ringworm is also called "tinea corporis." Ringworm is most common in young children, but it can occur in any age group. The fungus spreads from person to person or from animals (pets)—if from a pet, the animal may have patches of fur loss ("mange"). The infection may also be spread by objects containing infected scales, such as clothing.

Dermatophytes can also cause infections of the feet (athlete's foot) or groin (jock itch). These infections are different, because of the unique characteristics of the skin in the infected areas. Ringworm can also appear on the scalp, where it is called "tinea capitis."

What does it look like?

- Ringworm usually starts as a small, scaly, red patch on the skin almost anywhere on the body.

- The rash spreads outward over a few days. The edges of the rash are often raised, with little bumps. As the rash spreads, the middle of the round area clears, causing the typical circle or ring shape.

- Sometimes there are blisters, pimples, or lots of red bumps instead of scales, but they still usually occur in a circular pattern. Sometimes there is no central clearing, so the ring-shaped pattern doesn't occur.

- The rash can look similar to several different skin conditions. Sometimes it looks like eczema—with dry, scaly patches of skin. Children with immune problems may have a larger, more severe rash.

What are some possible complications of ringworm?

Serious complications are very rare.

What increases your child's risk of ringworm?

Ringworm is most common in young children but may occur at any age. The fungus may be passed to several people by one infected person (or pet).

How is ringworm diagnosed?

The doctor may recognize ringworm from the appearance of the rash. Because ringworm can look like other conditions, a sample of the scale may be collected by scraping the rash. The doctor can look at the sample under the microscope to see if fungus is present or may send it for culture. If culture is performed, it may take a week or longer to get the results.

How is ringworm treated?

- Ringworm is usually treated with a topical (placed on the skin) antifungal cream or ointment.

- The doctor may recommend an over-the-counter antifungal medication, such as Monistat or Lotrimin, or may recommend a prescription medication. Apply the topical medication on the rash daily for about 3 weeks, depending on how severe it is.

- If the infection is severe or does not improve with topical treatments, your doctor may recommend an oral antifungal medication.

- The rash usually clears up after a few weeks of treatment. Follow your doctor's instructions.

When should I call your office?

Call our office if the rash isn't eliminated after treatment or if it returns.

Ringworm of the Scalp (Tinea Capitis)

Ringworm is infection with certain types of fungi called dermatophytes. The name comes from the distinct, circle-shaped rash formed when the infection involves the skin. When ringworm infects the scalp and hair, it can look several different ways. The scalp can look scaly (like dandruff) and have bald spots or sores. Treatment with antifungal medications is effective. If bald patches are present, the hair will usually grow back once the infection is eliminated.

What is ringworm of the scalp?

Ringworm of the scalp is a common infection caused by certain fungi called dermatophytes. Ringworm of the scalp is also called "tinea capitis." Dermatophytes also cause infections of the feet (athlete's foot) or groin (jock itch). Ringworm of the scalp is most common in young children, especially African Americans but can occur in any age group.

The fungus most commonly spreads from person to person. It can also spread from objects on which there are infected hair or skin cells—for example, pillows, combs, hats, or barber's tools (if not cleaned properly). In some cases, the fungi causing ringworm can be spread by animals, like dogs and cats.

What does it look like?

Typically, ringworm starts as a patchy rash on the scalp. However, the infection may appear in several different ways:

- The scalp may have scales that look like dandruff. There may be scaly patches throughout the scalp, with or without hair loss.

- A typical round, ringlike scaly patch may be present.

- There may be sores with crusting or pustules (pimples).

- Bald spots with little black dots may appear. The black dots are hairs broken off at the follicle (root).

- In more severe cases, red, tender, swollen areas that look like an abscess (*kerion*) may appear.

What are some possible complications of ringworm of the scalp?

Serious complications are rare. With severe infection, permanent hair loss is possible.

Can ringworm of the scalp be prevented?

There are some things you can do to help prevent ringworm of the scalp. However, the infection is difficult to prevent because it is easily passed from person to person—for example, children playing together. (See under "How is ringworm of the scalp treated?")

Family members and other people with whom your child has been in contact should be checked for infection. Other family members, including adults, can carry the infection without having any symptoms. They can be treated with medicated shampoo, as described later.

How is ringworm of the scalp diagnosed?

- The doctor often suspects the diagnosis from the appearance of the rash on the scalp. However, it may be confused with other conditions, such as dandruff.

- Tests can be done to make the diagnosis for sure—usually by culture of the fungus. The doctor will obtain a sample of the scale and hair from your child's scalp. This procedure is not painful—a toothbrush is often used. It takes a few weeks to get the results.

- Sometimes the doctor will look at a sample of scale and hair under the microscope to see if fungus is present. However, the fungus is not found as often this way.

How is ringworm of the scalp treated?

It is important to check for infection in family members and other people your child has been in contact with, especially other children. If infected, these contacts will also need to be treated.

Oral antifungal medication can be used to kill the fungus causing the infection. The most commonly used medication is griseofulvin.

- Treatment usually lasts for 6 to 8 weeks. Give this medication with milk or with a meal containing some fats.

- Griseofulvin is generally a very safe drug. Newer oral antifungal medications are available but are not yet used widely. When more is known about their safety and effectiveness, they may be used more often because they can shorten treatment time.

- The doctor may want to check your child's scalp to be sure the infection is gone before stopping oral antifungal medications.

Antifungal shampoos are used along with oral medications. These shampoos can help remove scale from the scalp and may help prevent spreading the infection to others. However, they are not as important as the oral medications and are not very effective treatment on their own.

- Some of these products contain selenium sulfide (for example, Selsun Blue) or zinc pyrithione (for example, Head & Shoulders).

- Most experts recommend antifungal shampoos for family members of an infected patient. This is because family members may be "carriers"—they have the fungus on their scalps, but no symptoms of the infection. Treatment with shampoos can kill the fungus and possibly reduce or prevent the spread of infection.

When should I call your office?

Call our office if:

- Your child's scalp rash isn't eliminated after treatment.

- Scaling and other problems return.

- Other children who may have ringworm of the scalp, or who have some type of rash or other symptoms—on the scalp or elsewhere on the body—should be seen by the doctor.

Scabies

Scabies is caused by a certain type of mite living on the skin. It causes a very itchy rash. The rash looks like little red bumps, most commonly between the fingers and toes, on the wrists and ankles, under the arms, and around the waist. In infants, the rash may be located elsewhere and may look a little different. Medication can eliminate the scabies mites, but the rash may take a while to clear up completely.

What is scabies?

Scabies is a skin reaction caused by the scabies mite (scientific name *Sarcoptes scabiei*), a tiny bug that lives only on humans. Mites usually spread from person to person, but generally only after close contact. Much less often, they can spread from clothing and other personal items. The mites dig into the skin, where they lay their eggs. The rash is caused by the burrowing into the skin and by the body's reaction to the mites and some substances they produce.

There is a form of scabies that comes from animals. However, because these mites don't live on people, the rash goes away fairly quickly on its own. The animal often has hair loss ("mange").

What does it look like?

- The first sign of scabies is usually itching over most of the body. The itching can be severe and is worse at night.

- A red, bumpy rash appears. If the area is not scratched, a little tunnel or burrow may be seen where the mite dug into the skin.

- The rash can also look like pustules (pimples with "whiteheads") and blisters, especially in infants. If the rash is present for a while, areas of skin can become thick and scaly, looking like eczema.

- Streaks of scratch marks may be seen.

- In infants, the rash may appear on the palms and soles, or on the face and scalp. Sometimes, especially in infants, firm red-brown spots that feel like a lump under the skin (nodules) may develop.

- If infection with bacteria occurs, crusted, oozy areas may appear or sores may become red and tender.

What are some possible complications of scabies?

The main complication is bacterial infection of the skin, including impetigo or boils (abscesses).

What increases your child's risk of scabies?

The scabies mite generally spreads from person to person, which requires close contact. Scabies can spread fairly easily in day care or in families, especially among young children.

Can scabies be prevented?

Most of the time, there is no practical way to avoid scabies. Children should not have close contact with an infected child or family member, until about 24 hours after treatment. Children should avoid using other people's personal items (such as clothing).

How is scabies diagnosed?

Often, the doctor recognizes scabies from the typical appearance of the rash. However, scabies can be confused with other diseases, such as eczema or insect bites, or sometimes even chickenpox, if blisters are present.

If unsure, the doctor may collect a sample of the sores by scraping and then looking under the microscope for mites and eggs. In some cases, we may recommend a visit to a dermatologist (specialist in skin diseases) to make the diagnosis.

How is scabies treated?

Treatment is usually recommended for the entire family and other close contacts of the person with scabies.

- *Medications*

  - Five percent permithrin (Elimite) is a topical (placed on the skin) medication that is very effective. It is usually the treatment of choice, except for very young infants. This drug is applied from the neck down, left on the body for 8 to 12 hours, and then washed off. In infants, the scalp and face may be included. The doctor may recommend repeating the treatment after 1 week.

  - Lindane (Kwell) is another topical medication. It is usually not the first choice for treatment because of possible toxic effects on the nervous system, especially if overused.

  - Sulfa ointment is often used for infants younger than 2 months old or when other medications are avoided because of possible toxic effects.

  - Oral ivermectin (Stromectol) is occasionally used for patients with severe scabies.

- *Treatments to control itching*—The doctor may recommend a steroid cream to help with itching. Oral antihistamines and moisturizing creams may also be helpful.

- *After treatment*—By about 24 hours after treatment, your child will no longer be able to spread the scabies mite to others. He or she can return to school or day care at this time. Itching may continue for a few days, but it may take up to several weeks for the rash to clear up completely.

- *Other treatment issues*
  - Family members and other people your child has come into close contact with should be treated as well (for example, day-care providers). It may take up to 4 weeks after the initial infestation before symptoms of scabies develop.
  - Wash all clothing, sheets, and blankets in hot water and then dry at a high temperature. Items that can't be washed should be dry-cleaned or placed in a sealed plastic bag for about 1 week.

When should I call your office?

After treatment for scabies, call our office if itching and rash are still present after 2 weeks or if they come back. It's possible the mites have not been eliminated or that they have returned.

Sunburn

Sunburn is a common problem in children. In addition to causing painful burns, excessive sun exposure increases the risk of skin cancer, skin aging, and other skin conditions. Especially during the summer months, it's important to take steps to prevent excessive sun exposure, such as wearing sunscreen.

What is sunburn?

Sunburn is redness, pain, and sometimes other symptoms caused by ultraviolet (UV) rays from the sun. Sunburn occurs within 6 to 12 hours after skin exposure. In addition to redness and pain, it can cause tenderness of the skin, swelling, and blisters. Severe sunburn can also cause nausea, chills, and just "feeling sick." The burned area remains red and painful for a few days. Later, peeling may occur as the skin heals.

What causes sunburn?

- Excessive exposure to sunlight on unprotected skin.
- Exposure to artificial light sources, such as sun lamps and especially tanning beds.

What are the long-term risks of sunburn and excessive sun exposure?

Excessive exposure to sunlight in childhood greatly increases the risk of skin cancer later in life. It can also cause premature aging and wrinkling of the skin, actinic keratoses (rough spots and skin growths caused by sun damage), and other problems.

- Severe sunburns causing blistering when young greatly increase the risk of an especially serious type of skin cancer called *malignant melanoma.*
- Although sunburn results from a type of ultraviolet radiation called UV-B rays, the same long-term damaging effects—including skin cancer—are also caused by UV-A rays. Tanning booths, which use UV-A light, are not healthy and not recommended.

What increases your child's risk of sunburn?

- People with fair skin are at highest risk. Sunburns occur most easily and fastest in people with very light skin, especially those with freckles or red hair and those who do not tan.
- Sunburn can also occur in people whose skin does tan and in those with darker skin, including African Americans. Getting a suntan *does not* protect against sunburn. There is no such thing as a "healthy tan"—if skin is tanned, that means it has been sun-damaged.
- Sunburn is most likely to occur if your child is out in the sun during the middle of the day, when the sun is strongest: about 10:00 a.m to 2:00 p.m. However, your child can still get enough sunlight to cause a burn at other times of day and even on hazy or partly cloudy days.
- Younger children have higher rates of sunburn, partly because they spend more time outdoors, especially in the summer. It is estimated that most people receive one half of their total lifetime dose of sunlight exposure by age 20.
- Infants and young children can quickly develop serious sunburns.

Can sunburn be prevented?

Yes. Especially if your child has fair skin and does not tan, take protective steps every time he or she is out in the sun. On sunny summer days, sunburns can occur very rapidly: after as little as 15 to 30 minutes in the sunlight!

Put on sunscreen. Make sure the sunscreen has a "sun protection factor" (SPF) of *at least* 15. (This means you can stay out in the sun 15 times longer before sunburn occurs, compared to without sunscreen.)

- Apply sunscreen a half-hour before your child goes out in the sun. Apply again every 2 to 3 hours and after swimming or sweating.
- There is not enough information on the use of sunscreen in infants younger than 6 months old, so it is generally not recommended. Keep babies covered and out of the sun. *However,* if this is not possible, it might be best to use sunscreen.
- Wear protective clothing, especially a hat and a shirt that covers the shoulders. (Also, wear sunglasses—exposure of the eyes to UV rays increases the long-term risk of cataracts.)
- Be especially careful to provide sun protection when your child is out in the middle of the day. As much as possible, try to limit outdoor activities during the midday hours. If children are out playing or exercising on hot, sunny days, make sure they take frequent breaks for rest (out of the sun) and water. (This will also help prevent heatstroke and heat exhaustion.)

How is sunburn treated?

When sunburn occurs, your child should stay out of the sun until the burn is completely healed. Make sure he or she has on sunscreen and other sun protection before going out again.

- Apply cool washcloths to help relieve pain.

- Give anti-inflammatory pain medications, such as ibuprofen, to reduce pain and tenderness.

- Sprays and other products containing local anesthetics (such as benzocaine or lidocaine) that numb the skin may help some, but they may also cause skin rashes or irritation.

- Especially after the skin has begun to heal, apply moisturizing lotion. Products containing aloe vera may help soothe the skin.

Tinea Versicolor

Tinea veriscolor is a common, harmless fungal infection of the skin. It produces reddish-brown or light-colored oval spots, covered with a very fine scale. The spots may join together to cover a larger area of the skin. The rash is most often found on the chest, back, and upper arms. Effective medications are available, but tinea versicolor may return after treatment.

What is tinea versicolor?

Tinea versicolor is a fungal infection of the very top layer of skin cells. The yeast form of the fungus that causes tinea versicolor is normally found on the skin. The rash occurs when there is increased growth of the fungus—this most commonly occurs in hot, humid conditions or on areas of the body where there is excessive sweating. The infection is harmless. It usually improves with treatment, but the problem may return.

What does it look like?

The rash of tinea versicolor can look several different ways.

- There may be flat, oval spots covered with a very fine scale. The spots vary in color. In light-skinned people, they are usually reddish-brown. In dark-skinned people, the spots may be either light or dark.

- The rash occurs most commonly on the upper arms, chest, and back. It may also appear on the face, arms and hands, and groin.

- Over time, the spots may grow and join together into large patches of rash. The area under the rash does not tan.

- There is usually little to no itching.

What increases your child's risk of tinea versicolor?

- Most often, it occurs in hot, humid weather. The rash may go away if the weather gets cool.

- It is most common in teens and young adults and usually doesn't occur in younger children (but can occur at any age, especially in warm climates).

How is tinea versicolor diagnosed?

- The doctor often recognizes tinea versicolor from the appearance of the rash. If unsure, the doctor may collect a sample of scale by scraping the rash. He or she can look at the sample under the microscope to see if fungus is present.

- The doctor may shine a special light, called a Wood's lamp, on the rash. This produces a certain color (fluorescence) if fungus is present.

How is tinea versicolor treated?

- Tinea versicolor can be treated with a topical (placed on the skin) lotion, cream, or ointment. These may include selenium sulfide (Selsun) or antifungal creams like clotrimazole (Lotrimin). When using antifungal creams, they should be placed on the rash twice a day for 2 to 4 weeks.

- The doctor may recommend an oral antifungal drug, such as fluconazole (Diflucan) or ketoconazole (Nizoral). These drugs are given in a single dose, and the dose may be repeated in a week.

There is a risk the rash may return after treatment. If this happens, call our office because repeat treatment is usually effective.

When should I call your office?

Call our office if the rash isn't eliminated after treatment or if it returns.

■ Warts ■

Warts occur most frequently in children and teens. They are caused by infection with a certain family of viruses. Warts may vary in appearance, partly depending on where they occur on the body. The hand is a common location for warts. Another is the sole of the foot, where they are called "plantar warts." Warts can be unsightly and sometimes painful. Several different treatments are available, and treatment may have to be repeated several times to eliminate warts completely.

What are warts?

Warts are caused by infection with a family of viruses called "human papillomavirus" (HPV). The virus is usually spread by direct contact with an infected person, but it can also be spread from objects or from one part of the body to another. Little breaks or cuts in the skin allow the virus to enter. Because the hands, feet, and elbows often have some breaks in the skin, they are common sites for warts. It may take 1 month or longer after HPV infection occurs before warts appear.

Warts usually look like small bumps or lumps of rough, hardened skin. Their appearance varies depending on several factors, including the type of HPV, the part of the body where the infection occurs, and the person's health. People with warts in noticeable locations, such as the face or hands, are concerned about their appearance. Warts can cause pain in some locations, such as the feet (plantar warts).

What do they look like?

- Most often, warts appear as small, hard bumps on the skin. The surface of the wart is usually rough and "horny" looking.

- Warts may appear practically anywhere on the body. Common sites include the following:

  - On the fingers, including around the nails, or on the back of the hand.

  - On the face.

  - On the knees or elbows.

  - On the soles of the feet (plantar warts).

- The rough skin on the surface of the wart can usually be scraped away without causing pain. Underneath, black dots may be visible. People sometimes think these dots are the "roots" of the wart, but they're really just clots at the ends of tiny blood vessels.

- Pain and tenderness may result from warts in certain areas, including around the fingernails and on the feet.

- The appearance of warts may vary, depending on the cause and location.

  - Plantar warts are flattened because of pressure from the body's weight on the soles of the feet. There may be a ring of calloused skin—sometimes making it difficult to identify the growth as a wart—around a hollowed-out middle.

  - Warts may fuse together, causing a larger area of hardened skin ("mosaic warts").

  - "Flat warts" are most common on the face and neck. They appear as small, slightly elevated pink or brown spots and are smoother than the usual wart.

- Other appearances are possible.

What are some possible complications of warts?

- Warts can be difficult to get rid of. They may spread to other parts of the body or may come back after treatment.

- Although warts can be an unsightly and embarrassing problem, they do not usually case serious complications.

- The exception to this is *genital warts*. When warts occur on the genitals, they are usually a sign of a sexually transmitted disease; however, warts in the genital area are not always caused by sexual contact. In women and girls, HPV infection of the cervix (the opening of the uterus) may increase the long-term risk of cervical cancer. Pregnant women with genital warts may spread HPV infection to their baby at birth.

- Always get medical attention for warts in the genital area.

How are warts treated?

There are several treatments for warts. Many warts eventually go away on their own. However, because of problems with appearance or pain or to avoid the risk of spreading to other sites, warts are usually treated. Your doctor can recommend the most appropriate treatment, based on the type of wart, where it is located, and whether it is causing pain or other problems.

Wart removers—Especially if warts are small and located in easy-to-reach places like the hands, they can be treated at home using prescription or nonprescription wart-removal products (for example, Compound W). These products contain mild acids that slowly and painlessly destroy the warts. They can be effective but may take a long time to eliminate warts.

- Before applying wart-removal products, soak the area in warm water and use a pumice stone or emery board (nail file) to remove excess skin. This will help speed treatment. Cover the area with a bandage after applying wart remover.

Tape method—Another approach is to cover the wart with tape (usually duct tape). Leave the tape on continuously for a week or longer. Reapply tape each week until the wart is gone—this may take several months or longer. The tape method is especially useful for warts around the nails, which can be difficult to treat.

Other treatments—The doctor may recommend other treatments or recommend a visit to a dermatologist (doctor specializing in skin diseases). With all of these options, repeated treatment may be needed to eliminate warts completely.

- *Liquid nitrogen* is a common method of treatment in which a very cold substance called liquid nitrogen is used to freeze the wart (cryotherapy). Blistering can occur, and treatment can be painful. However, the pain usually goes away after an hour or so.

- Topical (placed on the skin) medications are available in several forms:

  - *Cantharidin (Cantharone)*: causes blistering.

  - *Imiquimod (Aldara)*: stimulates part of the immune system.

- *Acids*.

- *Oral cimetidine*: most often used to control stomach acid for heartburn and ulcers, but is sometimes used for warts.

- *Laser treatments* are sometimes used.

Treatment for plantar warts—Warts on the soles of the feet are often treated by freezing with liquid nitrogen. Another option is the use of 40% salicylic acid plasters, which are placed over the wart and changed every few days. Soak the area and remove dead skin when changing plasters. There are a number of different ways to treat these kinds of warts.

When should I call your office?

Call our office if:

- Warts come back after treatment.

- Increased redness, tenderness, or pus develops in the skin around the wart.

- Call our office about treatment of warts in the genital area.

Index of Topics

Our book is organized by body system/specialty for easy browsing. To help in finding specific handouts, the following list presents all topics in alphabetical order. Topics are cross-referenced under both medical and lay terms (e.g., conjunctivitis and pinkeye).

A

Abscesses, skin, 306
Abrasions. *See* Skin wounds
Acne, 459–460
Acute otitis media. *See* Middle ear infection
Adjustment disorder, 43–44
Adoption, 3–4
ADHD. *See* Attention-deficit hyperactivity disorder
AIDS. *See* HIV/AIDS
Alcohol, use and abuse, 59–60
Allergic dermatitis. *See* Eczema
Allergic rhinitis. *See* Hay fever.
Allergic shock. *See* Anaphylaxis.
Allergies, food, 35–36
Ambiguous genitalia, 383–384
Anal fissure, 183–184
Anaphylaxis, 29–30
Angioedema. *See* Hives.
Anorexia nervosa. *See* Eating disorders.
Antibiotics, preventive, for children with heart disease, 94–95
Anxiety, 45–46
Apnea of the newborn, 385–386
Appendicitis, acute, 121–122
Arrhythmias, 241–242
Asthma, 31–32
Athlete's foot, 461
Attention-deficit hyperactivity disorder, 47–48
Autism, 101–102

B

Baby's first weeks, 387–388
Bacterial vaginosis, 255
Bed-wetting, 327–328
Bee stings and other insect stings, 33–34
Bell's palsy, 367
Below normal height. *See* Short stature.
Bipolar disorder, 49–50
Bites, animal and human, 123–124
Blocked tear duct, 171
Blood clots, 77–78
Blood pressure, high. *See* High blood pressure.
Bottle feeding. *See* Feeding your newborn.
Bowlegs, 345
Breast enlargement in boys, 153–154
Breast enlargement in infants, 155–156
Breast-feeding. *See* Feeding your newborn.
Bronchiolitis, 256–257
Bulimia nervosa. *See* Eating disorders.
Bullying, 51–52
Burns, minor, 470–471

C

Candida vaginitis. *See* Yeast infections.
Caput succadaneum. *See* Swollen scalp.
Carbon monoxide poisoning, 125–126
Cat-scratch disease, 258–259
CDH. *See* Congenital diaphragmatic hernia.
Celiac disease, 185–186
Cellulitis. *See* Skin infection.
Cephalohematoma. *See* Swollen scalp.
Cerebral palsy, 368–369
CF. *See* Cystic fibrosis.
Chickenpox, 260–261
Child passenger safety, 5–6
Childproofing your home, 7–8
Cholesterol, high. *See* High cholesterol.
Chronic diarrhea, 262–263
Circumcision, 389–390
Cleft lip, 391–392
Cleft palate, 391–392
Clubfoot, 393–394
Cold sores, 264–265
Colds, 266–267
Colic, 187–188
Collarbone fractures, in newborns, 395
Concussion. *See* Head trauma, minor.
Conduct disorder, 53–54
Congenital diaphragmatic hernia, 397–398
Conjunctivitis, 172
Constipation, 189–190
Corneal abrasions, 173–174
Cradle cap, 399
Croup, 268–269
Cystic fibrosis, 443–445

D

Day-care guide, 9–10
Dehydration, 127–128
Dental trauma, 93
Depression, 55–56
Developmental dysplasia of the hip, 400–401
Diabetes mellitus, type 1, 157–159
Diabetes mellitus, type 2, 160–161
Diaper rash, 402–403
Diarrhea, acute, 253–254
Diarrhea, chronic, 262–263
Diet, healthy, 435–436
Discipline—the basics, 11–12
Divorce, 57–58
Down syndrome, 211–212
Drugs, use and abuse, 59–60

E

Earwax problems, 111
Eating disorders, 61–62
Eczema, 462–463
Epididymitis, 225–226
Enlarged lymph nodes, 79
Eye injuries. *See* Corneal abrasions.

F

Fainting, 129–130
Febrile seizures, 131–132
Feeding your newborn, 404–405
Fetal alcohol syndrome, 103–104
Fever management, 13
Fifth disease, 270–271
Flatfoot, 346
Food poisoning, 272–273
Foreign bodies, 133–134
Foreskin problems, 227–228
Fractures, 347–348
Fragile X syndrome, 213–214
Frostbite, 135–136
Fungal infections of the nails, 464

G

Ganglion cyst, 349
Gastroenteritis. *See* Diarrhea, acute.
Gastroesophageal reflux, newborn. *See* Spitting up.
Gastroesophageal reflux disease, 191–192
Genetic counseling, 215–216
GERD. *See* Gastroesophageal reflux disease.
German measles, 274
Glaucoma, 175–176
Glomerulonephritis, 329–330
Group B streptococcal infection, 406–407
Growing pains, 350
Guillain-Barré syndrome, 370–371
Gynecomastia. *See* Breast enlargement in boys.

H

Habits, 14–15
Hand-foot-and-mouth disease, 275–276
Hay fever, 37–38
Head lice, 465–466
Head trauma, minor, 137–138
Headaches, 372–373
Healthy diet, 435–436
Heart disease, preventive antibiotics for children with, 94–95
Heart murmurs, 243
Heat rash, 467
Heat-related illness, 139–140
Height, below normal. *See* Short stature.
Hemolytic-uremic syndrome, 331–332
Henoch-Schönlein purpura, 333–334
Hepatitis, A, B, or C, 277–278
Herpes simplex. *See* Cold sores.
Herpes zoster. *See* Shingles.
High blood pressure, 244–245
High cholesterol, 437–438
Hirschsprung's disease, 193–194
HIV/AIDS, 279–280
HIV and your newborn, 408–409

Pomeranz, 978-1-4160-0296-3

Hives, 39–40
Hodgkin's disease, 87–88
Hordeolum. *See* Stye.
Hyaline membrane disease. *See* Respiratory distress syndrome in newborns.
Hydrocele, 229–230
Hydrocephalus, 374–375
Hypertension. *See* High blood pressure.
Hyperthyroidism. *See* Thyroid disorders.
Hypospadias, 231–232
Hypothyroidism. *See* Thyroid disorders.

I

IBD. *See* Inflammatory bowel disease.
Immunizations, 16–17
Impetigo, 281
Infants of diabetic mothers, 410–411
Infection of the vagina. *See* Vulvovaginitis.
Infectious mononucleosis. *See* Mononucleosis.
Inflammatory bowel disease, 195–196
Influenza, 282–283
Ingrown toenails, 468
Inguinal hernia, 197–198
Innocent murmurs. *See* Heart murmurs.
Insect stings. *See* Bee stings.
Interrupted breathing in newborns. *See* Apnea of the newborn.
Intersex conditions, 383–384
Intestinal obstruction, 199–200
Iron-deficiency anemia, 80–81
Irritable bowel syndrome, 201–202

J

Jaundice of the newborn, 412
Jock itch, 469

K

Kawasaki disease, 246–247
Kidney stones, 335–336
Klinefelter's syndrome, 217–218
Knock-knees, 345

L

Lacerations. *See* Skin wounds.
Laryngitis, 284
Laryngomalacia, 446–447
Lead poisoning, 141–142
Learning disabilities, 105–106
Legg-Calvé-Perthes disease, 351–352
Leukemia, 89–90
Lockjaw, 313–314
Low birth weight, 420–421
Lyme disease, 285–286
Lymph nodes, enlarged, 79

M

Marfan's syndrome, 219–220
Measles, 287–288
Meconium-stained amniotic fluid, 413–414
Meningitis, viral and bacterial, 289–290
Middle ear infection, 112–113
Migraine. *See* Headaches.
Mononucleosis, 291–292
Mumps, 293
Muscular dystrophy, 376–377
Myelomeningocele, 415–416

N

Nail-biting. *See* Habits.
Nails, fungal infections of, 464
Natal teeth, 417
Neonatal teeth, 417
Newborn care. *See* Baby's first weeks.
Newborn screening, 418–419
Nightmares and night terrors, 63–64
Nocturnal enuresis. *See* Bed-wetting.
Nonfebrile seizures. *See* Seizures, without fever.
Nosebleeds, 143–144
Nursemaid's elbow, 353

O

Obesity, 439–440
Obsessive-compulsive disorder, 65–66
Obstructive sleep apnea, 448–449
Onychomycosis. *See* Fungal infections of the nails.
Osgood-Schlatter disease, 354
Otitis media with effusion, 114–115
Otitis media, acute. *See* Middle ear infection.
Outer ear infection, 116–117

P

Palpitations, 241–242
Pancreatitis, 203–204
Panic attacks and panic disorder, 67–68
Patellofemoral pain syndrome, 355
Pediculosis capitis. *See* Head lice.
Peptic ulcer disease, 205–206
Peritonsillar abscess, 450–451
Pertussis, 294–295
Pes planus. *See* Flatfoot.
Phobias, 69–70
Pinkeye. *See* Conjunctivitis.
Pinworm infection, 296
Pityriasis rosea, 472
Plantar warts. *See* Warts.
Pneumonia, 297–298
Poison ivy, 473–474
Poisoning, 145–146
Posterior urethral valves, 337–338
Premature thelarche. *See* Breast enlargement in infants.
Prematurity, 420–421
Preventive antibiotics for children with heart disease, 94–95
Psoriasis, 475–476
Puberty, 162–163
Pulled elbow. *See* Nursemaid's elbow.
Punctures. *See* Skin wounds.
Pyloric stenosis, 207–208

R

Rabies, 299–300
Rashes, common newborn, 396
Respiratory distress syndrome in newborns, 422–423
Retropharyngeal abscess, 450–451
Rheumatic fever, 248–249
Rheumatic heart disease, 248–249
Ringworm, 477
Ringworm of the scalp, 478–479
Rubella. *See* German measles.
Rubeola. *See* Measles.

S

Sacral dimple, 424
Scabies, 480–481
Scarlet fever, 311–312
SCFE. *See* Slipped capital femoral epiphysis.
Scoliosis, 356–357
Screamer's nodes. *See* Vocal cord nodules.
Screening, newborn. *See* Newborn screening.
Seborrheic dermatitis, of newborns. *See* Cradle cap.
Seizures, with fever. *See* Febrile seizures.
Seizures, without fever, 147–148
Sex, talking to teens about, 22–24
Sexually transmitted diseases, 301–302
Shingles, 303
Short stature, 164–165
Sickle cell disease and sickle cell trait, 82–83
SIDS. *See* Sudden infant death syndrome.
Sinusitis, 304–305
Skin abcesses, 306
Skin infection, 307–308
Skin wounds, 149–150
Sleep problems and bedtime issues, 18–19
Slipped capital femoral epiphysis, 358–359
Smoking: risks and how to quit, 20–21
Sore throat, 309–310
Spitting up, 425–426
Sprains, 360–361
Sprue. *See* Celiac disease.
STDs. *See* Sexually transmitted diseases.
Strabismus, 177–178
Strains, 360–361
Strep throat, 311–312
Streptococcal infection, group B. *See* Group B streptococcal infection.
Stuttering, 107–108
Stye, 179
Sudden infant death syndrome, 452–453
Suicide, 71–72
Sunburn, 482–483
Swallowed objects. *See* Foreign bodies.
Swimmer's ear. *See* Outer ear infection.
Swollen scalp, newborn, 427–428
Syncope. *See* Fainting.

T

Talipes equinovarus. *See* Clubfoot.
Talking to your teens about sex, 22–24
Tear duct, blocked, 171
Temper tantrums, 73–74
Tendinitis, 362
Tennis elbow, 362
Tension headaches. *See* Headaches.
Testicles, undescended, 235–236
Testicular torsion, 233–234
Tetanus, 313–314
Thrombotic disorders. *See* Blood clots.
Thrush, 429
Thumb sucking. *See* Habits.
Thyroid disorders, 166–167
Tics, 378–379
Tinea capitis. *See* Ringworm of the scalp.
Tinea corporis. *See* Ringworm.
Tinea cruris. *See* Jock itch.

Tinea pedis. *See* Athlete's foot.
Tinea unguium. *See* Fungal infections of the nails.
Tinea versicolor, 484
Toilet training, 25–26
Tooth decay, 96–97
Torticollis, 363–364
Tourette's syndrome, 378–379
Transient synovitis of the hip, 315
Trisomy 21. *See* Down syndrome.
Tuberculosis, 316–317
Turner's syndrome, 221–222

U
Umbilical cord care, 430–431
Undescended testicles, 235–236
Urinary tract infections, 339–340
Urolithiasis. *See* Kidney stones.
Urticaria. *See* Hives.

V
Vaccinations. *See* Immunizations.
Vagina, infection of. *See* Vulvovaginitis.
Varicella. *See* Chickenpox.
Varicocele, 237–238

Vesicoureteral reflux, 341–342
Vocal cord nodules, 454–455
Vulvovaginitis, 318–319

W
Warts, 485–486
West Nile virus infection, 320–321
Whooping cough. *See* Pertussis.

Y
Yeast infections, 322–323

Pomeranz, 978-1-4160-0296-3